A COMPREHENSIVE GUIDE TO CHINESE HERBAL MEDICINE

A Comprehensive Guide to
Chinese
Herbal Medicine

Ze-lin Chen, M.D. and Mei-fang Chen, M.D.

CASTLE BOOKS

This edition published by Castle Books,
a division of Book Sales, Inc.
114 Northfield Avenue
Edison, NJ 08837
1999
Published by arrangement with and permission of
Keats Publishing, Inc.
27 Pine Street
New Canaan, CT 06840

ISBN 0-7858-1076-5
Printed in the United States of America

*This book
is dedicated to the memory of*
**Dr. Hong-yen Hsu
(1917-1991)**,
*who sought to bridge Eastern and Western under-
standings of health and healing through
his research and writings.*

*His many decades of work
in herbal science and other forms of
oriental medicine continue to serve as an inspiration
to students, scholars, academicians and
practitioners alike.*

Contents

Editor's Note

The authors have adopted *Standard Acupuncture Nomenclature*, published by the World Health Organization's Regional Office for the Western Pacific in Manila, as their guide for assigning names to the acupuncture points presented in this book.

Source books are footnoted in the text and cited in the references for each of the formulas. For the most part, the English and *pinyin* names, ingredients and doses are the same as those given in *Commonly Used Chinese Herb Formulas with Illustrations* by Drs. Hong-yen Hsu and Chau-shin Hsu, while literal translations of the *pinyin* terms are those given in *Chinese Herbal Medicine Formulas and Strategies*, compiled and translated by Dan Bensky and Randall Barolet. A few minor changes, such as the italicizing of *pinyin* terms, have been made in Bensky and Barolet's transliterations in order that they might more closely conform with the style of this text.

Ancient texts, many of which are no longer being published, have been omitted from the references. The authors have seen fit to only include more recent authoritative texts.

In this text, dosages of individual herbs are given in *qian*. Though China converted to the metric system in 1979, many herbalists, especially in Taiwan and the United States, still employ the *qian* and *liang* system. The situation is further complicated by the fact that herbal formulas are now available in a variety of forms--decoctions, powders, pills, capsules and granules--each having its own appropriate dose, depending on the concentration of the constituent herbs. It is important to note that, though the units may change, the ratios between the ingredients remain constant. For instance, in Magnolia and Ginger Formula, presented below, the 1:1 ratio which exists between licorice and ginger will be maintained whether the units are *qian*, grams, pounds or metric tons. Further note that, in order to convert *qian* to grams, simply multiply the dosages by 3, e.g., 1 *qian* = 3 grams.

Magnolia and Ginger Formula (*Ping Wei San*)

Ingredients		Daily Dosage for Decoctions		Powders, Pills or Granules	
Common Name	*Pinyin*	*Qian*	Grams	Ratio (parts/ total parts)	Percent of Total
Atractylodes	*Cang zhu*	4	12	4/14	28.57
Magnolia bark	*Hou pu*	3	9	3/14	21.43
Citrus peel	*Chen pi*	3	9	3/14	21.43
Licorice	*Gan cao*	1	3	1/14	7.14
Jujube	*Da zao*	2	6	2/14	14.29
Ginger, dried	*Gan jiang*	1	3	1/14	7.14

For most powders and pills, the standard dosage is 3 *qian* of the formula given once daily, though a few are given two or three times daily in 1-*qian* doses. Concentrated granules are usually taken two or three times daily in 2- or 3-gram doses.

Foreword

Never before have I seen a book like this among the publications on traditional Chinese medicine in the United States--one that so thoroughly combines clinical experience with systematic presentation of the differentiation and treatment of diseases and conformations. Internal medicine, surgery, gynecology and pediatrics are covered as to the etiology, symptomatology, pulse and tongue diagnosis, herbal treatment and effective acupuncture points for diseases associated with these branches of medicine. Perhaps the most outstanding feature of this book, however, is found in the chapter on differentiation and treatment in terms of visceral conformations and their etiology--something which is rarely seen among publications either in this country or abroad.

The authors, Professors Ze-lin Chen and Mei-fang Chen, both graduated from Zhejiang Medical University, after which they undertook systematic training in traditional Chinese medicine at China's Academy of TCM in Beijing. For the next three decades, they collected prescriptions from multifarious sources and skillfully treated many obstinate and peculiar diseases with traditional Chinese medicine and Chinese medicine in combination with Western therapies. Due to their remarkable therapeutic techniques, they have garnered the praise and respect of their colleagues, as well as that of countless patients over their many years of practice.

Since moving to the United States, they have worked and lectured at the Oriental Healing Arts Institute, Santa Barbara College of Oriental Medicine, South Baylo University and the University of California, Los Angeles. As TCM professors and scholars, the authors were approached by acupuncturists, academicians and students who urged them to write a comprehensive text which would systematically explain disease conformations and provide instructions as to how herbal therapy could be combined with acupuncture to treat these diseases.

Taking time from their busy schedules, Drs. Ze-lin Chen and Mei-fang Chen wrote this text. I salute their work as a truly noteworthy achievement. It is my unqualified belief that this book will gain great notoriety among practitioners and students alike.

Hong-yen Hsu, Ph. D.

President

Oriental Healing Arts Institute

May 1990

Preface

While in the United States in 1988, we taught at two oriental medical universities in California. During that time, we met with many acupuncturists and practitioners of traditional Chinese medicine who told us they urgently needed a practical textbook of Chinese therapeutics. Encouraged and supported by Drs. Hong-yen Hsu, Chau-shin Hsu and Daniel Hsu, we wrote this book as a useful reference for American acupuncturists.

Included within these pages is information essential to acupuncturists and TCM doctors who base their practices on the principle of diagnosis and treatment through an analysis of signs and symptoms. Through 35 years of clinical experience in China, we have gained much insight into the nature of conformations, tongue and pulse diagnosis, treatment principles and the enhancing effect of herbal formulas on the healing process, particularly when formulas are combined with acupuncture and moxibustion. All of this we have attempted to share with our readers in this book.

The majority of the formulas discussed in the following chapters can be purchased in the United States. For a more detailed discussion of herbal formulas, their efficacy and their contraindications, please refer to Drs. Hong-yen and Chau-shin Hsu's *Commonly Used Chinese Herb Formulas With Illustrations*, also published by the Oriental Healing Arts Institute.

It would be impossible in a brief preface to express appreciation to all who have helped in preparing this work. We would, however, like to single out a few of our colleagues for special recognition.

We would like to express our gratitude for the constant support and encouragement of Dr. Chau-shin Hsu and Dr. Daniel Hsu. Our thanks as well to Mr. Wei-din Chen for his assistance in translating this work into English; our editor, Heidi Ziolkowski, for her care and polishing of our manuscript; acupuncturist Oda S. Halverson for her valuable input and Mrs. Yeen-wun Chu for her long hours of typesetting.

Ze-lin Chen, M.D., O.M.D.

Mei-fang Chen, M.D., O.M.D.

November 1991

Chapter 1

Causal Differentiation of Conformations and Their Treatment

Traditional Chinese medicine (TCM) holds that a relatively stable, dynamic equilibrium exists between *zang* and *fu* (the solid and the hollow organs) and the rest of the human body. Disruption of these functions causes an imbalance in *yin* and *yang*. If equilibrium is not promptly restored through self-regulation, the body will contract diseases.

The conditions which upset this balance are the six excesses (also known as the six climatic factors), the seven emotions, the retention of phlegm, and stagnant blood. What follows is a discussion of all but the seven emotions, which are dealt with in Chapter 3.

Section 1
The Six Excesses

Wind, cold, summer heat, dampness, dryness and fire are the six climatic variations in nature, also known as the six *qi*. If, due to a decline in vital resistance prompted by abrupt climatic changes, the body cannot adjust to its environment, the six *qi* will become pathogenic conditions, attacking the body and causing diseases. Under such circumstances, the six *qi* are called the six excesses, the six evils or the six evil *qi*. Diseases caused by the six excesses have the following characteristics:

1. They are generally related to the seasons, the climate, one's dwelling place or other factors in one's immediate environment. For example, wind-evil diseases prevail in the spring, while cold-evil diseases are most common in the winter, and heat evil is generally a problem in the summer. In late summer or early autumn, or in damp, moist environments, some persons are susceptible to dampness diseases, whereas dryness diseases are common in late autumn.

2. The six excesses can attack the human body either singly or in combinations of two or three to cause diseases such as the wind-cold type of common cold or jaundice due to heat-dampness evil or even wind-cold-dampness arthralgia.

3. At the onset of the illness, the six excesses can be subdued, but if cold evil is not controlled, it will transform into heat after having penetrated the body's interior, where it will impair body fluids and induce dryness.

4. During drastic temperature changes and seasonal transitions, climatic influences invade the body from the outside through the mouth, nose or skin, or through all these surfaces at once. The consequent diseases are known as diseases of the external pathogens, though diseases which are not caused by external pathogenic factors may also have symptoms similar to those caused by wind, cold, dampness, dryness or heat. To distinguish them from the six external pathogenic factors, they are named interior wind, interior cold, interior dampness, interior dryness and fire.

Wind

Since wind is the principal *qi* of spring, diseases caused by the wind usually occur at this time. Cold, dampness and heat may invade the body along with wind, resulting in wind-cold, wind-dampness and wind-heat combinations. In "Bone Cavities," a section in *Su Wen* (Plain Questions), it is stated: "Wind is the initial pathogenic factor of many diseases."

Wind is a *yang* evil characterized by an upward and outward movement which attacks the upper body, especially the head and face. Such an assault on the body can cause excess perspiration and/or an aversion to drafts.

Wind is characterized by constant movement and rapid changes. Wind diseases begin abruptly and their symptoms migrate to different parts of the body. For instance, *feng bi* or *xing bi* (arthralgia due to wind) is characterized by migratory pains, while skin diseases such as urticaria are characterized by constantly changing lesions which erupt one after another.

Due to its active nature, many clinical symptoms, such as dizziness, tremors, convulsions of the limbs, rigidity of the neck, opisthotonos and the upward turning of the eyes, are associated with wind. Thus in *Su Wen* it is stated: "When wind evil dominates, abnormal movements arise in the human body." And: "Violent spasms and rigidity of the muscles are due to wind."

Symptoms caused by interior wind are generally related to abnormalities of the muscles and eyes. The liver stores blood, is related to the tendons and has the eyes as its opening. Therefore, disturbances in liver functions are the main cause of wind arising inside the body.

Pathological changes originating from the abnormal movement of wind evil are seen in symptoms of diseases caused by external pathogenic factors and internal injuries. For example, the dizziness and apoplexy of some forms of hypertension and the epileptiform convulsions appearing during the course of some acute infectious diseases, most notably epidemic cerebrospinal meningitis and encephalitis B, are all pathological changes resulting from the movement of wind evil inside the human body.

External-wind Conformations

1. Wind-cold

Wind-cold is characterized by fever, an aversion to wind and cold, headache, body aches, a cough, thin sputum, a floating and tense pulse, and a tongue with a thin, white coating. The patient should be treated with warm, pungent diaphoretics to relieve exterior symptoms, ventilate and soothe the lungs and dispel cold. Schizonepeta and Siler Formula (*jing fang bai du san*) can be used.

Schizonepeta and Siler Formula[1]
Jing Fang Bai Du San
(Schizonepeta and Ledebouriella Powder to
Overcome Pathogenic Influences)[2]

Schizonepeta	*Schizonepetae herba*	*Jing jie*	1.5
Siler	*Ledebouriellae radix*	*Fang feng*	1.5
Chiang-huo	*Notopterygii rhizoma*	*Qiang huo*	1.5
Forsythia	*Forsythiae fructus*	*Lian qiao*	3.0
Tu-huo	*Angelicae tuhuo radix*	*Du huo*	1.5
Cnidium	*Cnidii rhizoma*	*Chuan xiong**	1.5
Bupleurum	*Bupleuri radix*	*Chai hu*	1.5
Peucedanum	*Peucedani radix*	*Qian hu*	1.5
Chih-ko	*Citri fructus*	*Zhi ke*	1.5
Platycodon	*Platycodi radix*	*Jie geng*	1.5
Licorice	*Glycyrrhizae radix*	*Gan cao*	1.0
Mentha	*Menthae herba*	*Bo he*	1.0
Lonicera	*Lonicerae flos*	*Jin yin hua*	3.0
Ginger, dried	*Zingiberis siccatum rhizoma*	*Gan jiang*	1.0

**Ligustici rhizoma*, also known as *chuan xiong*, may be substituted.

Herbs commonly used for expelling wind-cold are:

siler (*fang feng*)	cinnamon twig (*gui zhi*)
schizonepeta (*jing jie*)	ma-huang (*ma huang*)
perilla leaf (*zi su ye*)	chiang-hou (*qiang hou*)
fresh ginger (*sheng jiang*)	

All are diaphoretics with warm, pungent properties for dispelling wind-cold. Siler and cinnamon twig are used for those patients who have an aversion to drafts, while schizonepeta and *ma-huang* are for those with an aversion to cold. Patients who experience congestion should be given perilla leaf, and those who complain of muscular pain or arthralgia should be given *chiang-hou* or siler. If pain is accompanied by nausea and vomiting, fresh ginger is recommended.

2. Wind-heat

Wind-heat is characterized by a high fever; a slight aversion to cold; headache; a cough with yellow sputum; a swollen sore throat; a floating, rapid pulse; a pale red tongue tip; and a white- or yellow-tinged tongue coating.

The patient should be treated with cool, pungent diaphoretics to relieve exterior symptoms, ventilate and soothe the lungs, and clear heat. Either Morus and Chrysanthemum Combination (*sang ju yin*) or Lonicera and Forsythia Formula (*yin qiao san*) can be used.

Morus and Chrysanthemum Combination[1]
Sang Ju Yin
(Mulberry Leaf and Chrysanthemum Decoction)[2]

Morus leaf*	*Mori folium*	*Sang ye*	4.0
Chrysanthemum	*Chrysanthemi flos*	*Ju hua*	3.0
Mentha	*Menthae herba*	*Bo he*	1.5
Apricot seed	*Armeniacae semen*	*Xing ren*	3.0
Platycodon	*Platycodi radix*	*Jie geng*	1.0
Forsythia	*Forsythiae fructus*	*Lian qiao*	4.0
Phragmites	*Phragmitis rhizoma*	*Lu gen*	18.0
Licorice	*Glycyrrhizae radix*	*Gan cao*	6.0

* also known as mulberry leaf

Lonicera and Forsythia Formula[1]

Yin Qiao San

(Honeysuckle and Forsythia Powder)[2]

Lonicera*	*Lonicerae flos*	*Jin yin hua*	4.0
Forsythia	*Forsythiae fructus*	*Lian qiao*	4.0
Arctium	*Arctii fructus*	*Niu bang zi*	3.0
Mentha	*Menthae herba*	*Bo he*	1.0
Schizonepeta	*Schizonepetae herba*	*Jing jie*	2.0
Soja	*Sojae semen praeparatum*	*Dan dou chi*	3.0
Platycodon	*Platycodi radix*	*Jie geng*	2.0
Bamboo leaf	*Bambusae folium*	*Zhu ye*	3.0
Phragmites	*Phragmitis rhizoma*	*Lu gen*	5.0
Licorice	*Glycyrrhizae radix*	*Gan cao*	1.5

*also known as honeysuckle

Cool, pungent diaphoretics are used to dispel wind-heat. Some of the most commonly used include:

morus leaf (*sang ye*)   chrysanthemum (*ju hua*)
arctium (*niu bang zi*)   mentha (*bo he*)
pueraria (*ge gen*)   cicada (*chan tui*)
soja (*dou chi*)

Morus leaf and chrysanthemum are used for headache and conjunctival congestion, arctium and mentha for sore throats, pueraria for neck rigidity, cicada for hoarseness, and soja for perspiration with persistent fever and anxiety.

Interior-wind Conformations

These conformations involve pathological changes to the internal organs. Either *yin* deficiency in the liver or kidneys or a persistently high fever which consumes body fluids can give rise to interior wind. Symptoms include convulsions of the limbs, rigidity and pain of the neck and head, the upward turning of the eyeballs, opisthotonos, numbness of the limbs, dizziness, vertigo and hemiplegia.

Treatment consists in calming the liver, tranquilizing wind, clearing heat and curtailing *yang*. Common prescriptions are Bupleurum Formula (*yi gan san*) or Gastrodia and Uncaria Combination (*tian ma gou teng yin*) and Antelope Horn and Uncaria Combination (*ling jiao gou teng tang*).

Bupleurum Formula[1]
Yi Gan San
(Restrain the Liver Powder)[2]

Atractylodes, white	*Atractylodis rhizoma*	Bai zhu	4.0
Hoelen	*Poria sclerotium*	Fu ling	4.0
Tang-kuei	*Angelicae radix*	Dang gui	3.0
Cnidium	*Cnidii rhizoma*	Chuan xiong*	3.0
Uncaria stem with hooks	*Uncariae ramulus cum uncus*	Gou teng	3.0
Bupleurum	*Bupleuri radix*	Chai hu	2.0
Licorice	*Glycyrrhizae radix*	Gan cao	1.5

Ligustici rhizoma, also known as *chuan xiong*, may be substituted.

Gastrodia and Uncaria Combination
Tian Ma Gou Teng Yin[3]
(Gastrodia and Uncaria Decoction)[2]

Gastrodia	*Gastrodiae rhizoma*	Tian ma	3.0
Uncaria stem with hooks	*Uncariae ramulus cum uncus*	Gou teng	3.0
Haliotis	*Haliotidis concha*	Shi jue ming	10.0
Gardenia	*Gardeniae fructus*	Zhi zi	3.0
Scute	*Scutellariae radix*	Huang qin	3.0
Eucommia	*Eucommiae cortex*	Du zhong	3.0
Loranthus	*Loranthi ramulus*	Sang ji sheng	3.0
Leonurus	*Leonuri herba*	Yi mu cao	3.0
Fleece-flower stem	*Polygoni multiflori caulis*	Ye jiao teng	5.0
Achyranthes	*Achyranthis radix*	Niu xi	3.0
Fu-shen	*Poria cor*	Fu shen	3.0

Functions: calms the liver; checks excess *yang*; nourishes *yin*; clears heat.

Explanation: Gastrodia, uncaria stem with hooks and haliotis calm the liver, check excess *yang* and tranquilize wind. When combined with gardenia and scute, they clear liver heat and purge pathogenic fire. Eucommia and loranthus invigorate the liver and kidneys, and leonurus and achyranthes move the blood downward, so that *qi* and fire no longer rise with ill effects. Fleece-flower stem and *fu-shen* tranquilize *shen* by nourishing *yin*. When the above-mentioned herbs are combined, they cure the conformation of *yin* deficiency and *yang* excess by transforming fire into interior wind. Experimental studies at Zhong Shan Hospital in Shanghai have concluded that this prescription decreases hypertension in laboratory animals. Clinically, it can be used to treat hypertension and preeclampsia.

Antelope Horn and Uncaria Combination
Ling Jiao Gou Teng Tang[4]
(Antelope Horn and Uncaria Decoction)[2]

Antelope horn	*Antelopis cornu*	*Ling yang jiao*	0.3
Uncaria stem with hooks	*Uncariae ramulus cum uncus*	*Gou teng*	3.0
Morus leaf	*Mori folium*	*Sang ye*	3.0
Fritillaria	*Fritillariae bulbus*	*Chuan bei mu*	1.5
Rehmannia, raw	*Rehmanniae radix*	*sheng di huang*	5.0
Chrysanthemum	*Chrysanthemi flos*	*ju hua*	3.0
Peony, white	*Paeoniae radix alba*	*Bai shao*	3.0
Licorice	*Glycyrrhizae radix*	*Gan cao*	1.0
Fu-shen	*Poria cor*	*Fu shen*	3.0
Bamboo shavings	*Bambusae caulis in taeniis*	*Zhu ru*	5.0

Functions: calms the liver; tranquilizes wind; clears heat; disperses phlegm.

Explanation: The principal herbs--antelope horn, uncaria stem, morus leaf and chrysanthemum--calm the liver and tranquilize wind. Antelope horn used in combination with uncaria stem is more effective than either morus leaf or chrysanthemum in calming the liver, tranquilizing wind, clearing heat and relieving convulsions. Raw rehmannia and white peony nourish *yin* and invigorate the liver. Added to licorice, they become even more effective in nourishing the liver. *Fu-shen* calms the heart and tranquilizes *shen*, while fritillaria and bamboo shavings clear heat and disperse phlegm. When the above-mentioned herbs are combined, they calm the liver, tranquilize wind, clear heat, disperse phlegm, nourish *yin* and tranquilize *shen*. This prescription can be applied to acute infectious diseases at the high fever stage or to wind diseases caused by extreme heat.

Herbs commonly used to expel interior wind are:

antelope horn (*ling yang jiao*)   gastrodia (*tian ma*)
batryticated silkworm   uncaria stem with hooks
   (*jiang can*)   (*gou teng*)
centipede (*wu gong*)   scorpion (*quan xie*)
earthworm (*di long*)

Of all these materia medica, antelope horn is the most efficacious against convulsions accompanied by high fever and headache associated with liver wind. Since antelope are wild animals, their horns are often difficult and expensive to obtain and so sheep's horn (*yang jiao*) is often substituted. Gastrodia and silkworm are mainly used for treating vertigo, headache and convulsions caused by wind-phlegm. Uncaria is less efficacious in calming liver wind and is used chiefly for the compatible application of the herbs. Centipede and scorpion, when combined, are known as *zhi jing san* or anticonvulsive powder. Earthworm is also effective in suppressing convulsions.

Acupuncture and Moxibustion Treatment[5]

Points for Dispelling Wind-cold

- *dazhui* (GV 14)
- *fengfu* (GV 16)

Points for Expelling Wind-heat

- *fengchi* (G 20)
- *fengfu* (GV 16)
- *quchi* (LI 11)
- *hegu* (LI 4)

Points for Expelling Interior Wind

- *fengchi* (G 20)
- ganshu (U 18)
- *taichong* (Liv 3)

Cold

Cold is the prevailing climatic *qi* in winter and can be classified into interior or exterior cold. The latter is cold evil which tightens the skin, thereby preventing *yang qi* from being transmitted to the environment. Interior cold is a reflection of organ dysfunctions or *yang* deficiency.

Cold represents *yin* evil, which tends to inhibit the body's *yang qi*. If the cold evil tightens the skin and if *wei yang* (defensive *yang*) becomes impaired, an aversion to cold will appear. Should the cold evil invade the internal organs, particularly the spleen and stomach, or impair kidney or lung *yang, yang* may be unable to warm and nourish the limbs, digest food, and transport and distribute water and nutrients. Symptoms such as a sensation of cold in the extremities, an aversion to cold, watery diarrhea containing undigested food, clear and profuse urine, and the vomiting of water and thin sputum are then apt to appear. It is stated in *Su Wen* (Plain Questions), in a section titled "A Great Treatise on the Most

Precise and Important Essence," that "thin, clear and watery discharges of the body are all related to a cold conformation."

Cold is further characterized by dormancy, coagulation and the ability to induce pain. Dormancy connotes contraction. If cold stays inside the skin and the interstitial spaces of the muscles, thereby causing the contraction of sweat pores and the stagnation of *wei yang*, fever, anhidrosis and an aversion to cold will appear. If cold remains in the muscles and meridians, rigidity and cold, numb limbs will result.

Coagulation refers to stagnation and impediments. Cold evil causes *qi* and blood to coagulate, stagnate and fail to circulate freely.

Pain appears when there is an obstruction, and cold evil is one factor which poses as an obstruction. When *qi* and blood become coagulated and stagnated because of exterior cold, the body aches all over. If the cold evil attacks the intestines and stomach, a stomachache will occur.

Exterior Cold

Exterior cold tightens the surface of the body so that *wei yang* (defensive *yang*) cannot work itself to the surface. Symptoms such as fever without sweating, an aversion to cold, nasal obstruction, headache, a floating and tense pulse, and a white tongue coating will appear. Treatment dispels cold by relieving the exterior through diaphoresis. *Ma-huang* Combination (*ma huang tang*) can be used.

Ma-huang Combination[1]

Ma Huang Tang
(Ephedra Decoction)[2]

Ma-huang	Ephedrae herba	Ma huang	5.0
Cinnamon twig	Cinnamomi ramulus	Gui zhi	4.0
Apricot seed	Armeniacae semen	Xing ren	5.0
Licorice	Glycyrrhizae radix	Gan cao	1.5

Impairment of the spleen and stomach by the excess intake of cold or raw foods or by catching cold in the abdomen damages the *yang qi* of these organs. Borborygmus, stomachache, vomiting and diarrhea will occur. The pulse is then submerged and slow, and the tongue is light-colored and covered with a white coating.

Proper treatment dispels cold by warming the middle energizer. Ginseng and Ginger Combination (*ren shen tang*) is recommended.

Ginseng and Ginger Combination[1]
Ren Shen Tang*
(Regulate the Middle Pill)[2]

Ginseng	Ginseng radix	Ren shen	3.0
Atractylodes, white	Atractylodis rhizoma	Bai zhu	3.0
Ginger, dry	Zingiberis siccatum rhizoma	Gan jiang	3.0
Licorice, baked	Glycyrrhizae radix	Zhi gan cao	3.0

* also known as *li zhong wan* (Ginseng and Ginger Formula)

Interior Cold

Though affected internal organs exhibit different clinical manifestations, the most prevalent symptoms are an aversion to cold, cold limbs, a pale complexion, listlessness, edema of the face and feet, a swollen tongue with a white, creamy coating, a slow, weak pulse and watery stools or even stools containing undigested food.

Treatment warms and invigorates *yang* with Rehmannia Eight Formula (*ba wei di huang wan*) or Aconite, Ginseng and Ginger Combination (*fu zi li zhong tang*).

Rehmannia Eight Formula[1]

Ba Wei Di Huang Wan

(Eight-ingredient Pill with Rehmannia)[2]

Aconite, prepared	*Aconiti carmichaelii praeparata radix*	*Zhi fu zi*	1.0
Cinnamon twig	*Cinnamomi ramulus*	*Gui zhi*	1.0
Rehmannia, cooked	*Rehmanniae radix*	*Shu di huang*	5.0
Cornus	*Corni fructus*	*Shan zhu yu*	3.0
Dioscorea	*Dioscorea batatis rhizoma*	*Shan yao*	3.0
Alisma	*Alismatis rhizoma*	*Ze xie*	3.0
Hoelen	*Poria sclerotium*	*Fu ling*	3.0
Moutan	*Moutan radicis cortex*	*Mu dan pi*	3.0

Aconite, Ginseng and Ginger Combination[1]

Fu Zi Li Zhong Tang

(Prepared Aconite Pill to Regulate the Middle)[2]

Aconite, prepared	*Aconiti carmichaelii praeparata radix*	*Zhi fu zi*	0.5-1.0
Ginseng	*Ginseng radix*	*Ren shen*	3.0
Atractylodes, white	*Atractylodis rhizoma*	*Bai zhu*	3.0
Ginger, dried	*Zingiberis siccatum rhizoma*	*Gan jiang*	3.0
Licorice, baked	*Glycyrrhizae radix*	*Zhi gan cao*	3.0

Common herbs for dispelling cold are:

prepared aconite (*zhi fu zi*)   cinnamon bark (*rou gui*)

dried ginger (*gan jiang*)   galanga (*gao liang jiang*)

peppertree (*chuan jiao*)   evodia (*wu zhu yu*)

clove (*ding xiang*)   fennel (*xiao hi xiang*)

Sichuan aconite root (*chuan wu*)

All herbs for dispelling cold also restore *yang*, warm the middle energizer and alleviate pain. Specifically, prepared aconite dispels cold throughout the body, while cinnamon bark dispels cold from the lower abdomen. Dried ginger and galanga cure cold pains from the epigastrium. Furthermore, dried ginger warms the lungs, thereby curing chronic coughs accompanied by white, foamy phlegm.

Peppertree invigorates the vital functions of the stomach and is also beneficial in alleviating dyspepsia. Evodia can relieve acid regurgitation, vomiting and diarrhea occurring before dawn, while clove and fennel are generally employed to relieve pain in the lower abdomen and testes, and Sichuan aconite root is helpful in dispelling wind-cold for the treatment of serious rheumatalgia, as well as abdominal pain due to *yang* deficiency.

Acupuncture and Moxibustion Treatment[5]

Exterior Cold

- *dazhui* (GV 14)
- *fengfu* (GV 16)

Interior Cold

- *shenjue* (CV 8)
- *qihai* (CV 6)
- *guanyuan* (CV 4)

Summer Heat

High temperatures can cause acute febrile diseases which are known as summer heat. In "A Treatise on Heat," found in *Su Wen* (Plain Questions), it is stated that "febrile diseases before the summer solstice are called warm diseases and those after the summer solstice are called summer-heat diseases."

Briefly, summer heat belongs to *yang* evil. It is upward and dissipating, tendencies which promote a consumption of fluids and *qi.* Furthermore, it is always complicated by dampness.

Overexposure to Summer Heat

This condition is characterized by fever, perspiration, fidgeting, thirst, general lassitude, a weak and rapid pulse and a thin, white and creamy tongue coating.

Treatment entails the removal of heat. Lotus Stem and Ginseng Combination (*qing shu yi qi tang*) can be used.

Lotus Stem and Ginseng Combination
Qing Shu Yi Qi Tang[6]
(Clear Summer Heat and Augment the *Qi* Decoction)[2]

Watermelon rind, outer	*Citrulli pericarpium*	*Xi gua cui yi*	10.0
Ginseng, American	*Panacis quinquefolic radix*	*Xi yang shen*	2.0
Lotus stem	*Nelumbinis petiolus*	*He geng*	3.0
Dendrobium	*Dendrobii caulis*	*Shi hu*	4.0
Ophiopogon	*Ophiopogonis rhizoma*	*Mai men dong*	3.0
Coptis	*Coptidis rhizoma*	*Huang lian*	0.5
Anemarrhena	*Anemarrhenae rhizoma*	*Zhi mu*	2.0
Lophatherum	*Lophatheri herba*	*Dan zhu ye*	2.0
Licorice	*Glycyrrhizae radix*	*Gan cao*	3.0
Rice	*Oryzae semen*	*Jing mi*	5.0

Heatstroke

In its mild form, heatstroke is accompanied by symptoms of dizziness and nausea. In an acute case, high fever, profuse sweating, unconsciousness or coma, a surging pulse and a thin, white and creamy tongue coating may appear.

A mild case necessitates rest in a cool, dark place. In an acute case, Gypsum Combination (*bai hu tang*) can be used.

Gypsum Combination[1]
Bai Hu Tang
(White Tiger Decoction)[2]

Gypsum	*Gypsum fibrosum*	*Shi gao*	5.0
Anemarrhena	*Anemarrhenae rhizoma*	*Zhi mu*	3.0
Rice	*Oryzae semen*	*Jing mi*	3.0
Licorice, baked	*Glycyrrhizae radix*	*Zhi gan cao*	1.0

Summer Heat-dampness

This condition is manifested in low-grade fever rising in the afternoon, nausea, a feeling of suffocation, general lassitude, poor appetite, loose stools, a thick, yellow, creamy tongue coating and a soft, thready pulse.

Treatment clears summer heat and eliminates dampness. Agastache Formula (*huo xiang zheng qi san*), in combination with Magnolia and Ginger Formula (*ping wei san*), can be used.

Agastache Formula[1]
Huo Xiang Zheng Qi San
(Agastache Powder to Rectify the *Qi*)[2]

Agastache	*Agastache rugosa herba*	*Huo xiang*	1.0
Magnolia bark	*Magnoliae officinalis cortex*	*Hou pu*	2.0
Perilla leaf	*Perillae folium*	*Zi su ye*	1.0
Angelica	*Angelicae dahuricae radix*	*Bai zhi*	1.5
Citrus peel	*Citri pericarpium*	*Chen pi*	2.0
Hoelen	*Poria sclerotium*	*Fu ling*	3.0
Atractylodes, white	*Atractylodis rhizoma*	*Bai zhu*	3.0
Areca peel	*Arecae pericarpium*	*Da fu pi*	1.0
Platycodon	*Platycodi radix*	*Jie geng*	1.5
Pinellia	*Pinellia rhizoma*	*Ban xia*	2.0
Licorice	*Glycyrrhizae radix*	*Gan cao*	1.0
Ginger, dried	*Zingiberis siccatum rhizoma*	*Gan jiang*	1.0
Jujube	*Zizyphi fructus*	*Da zao*	3.0

Magnolia and Ginger Formula[1]

Ping Wei San
(Calm the Stomach Powder)[2]

Atractylodes	*Atractylodis lanceae rhizoma*	*Cang zhu*	4.0
Magnolia bark	*Magnoliae officinalis cortex*	*Hou pu*	3.0
Citrus peel	*Citri pericarpium*	*Chen pi*	3.0
Licorice	*Glycyrrhizae radix*	*Gan cao*	1.0
Ginger, fresh	*Zingiberis rhizoma*	*Sheng jiang*	1.0
Jujube	*Zizyphi fructus*	*Da zao*	2.0

Acupuncture and Moxibustion Treatment[5]

Summer Heat

- *dazhui* (GV 14)
- *quchi* (LI 11)
- *hegu* (LI 4)
- *neiguan* (P 6)

Heatstroke

- *renzhong* (GV 26)
- *shixuan* (EX-UE11)
- *quze* (P 3)
- *weizhong* (B 40)
- *guanyuan* (CV 4)

Summer Heat-dampness

- *quchi* (LI 11)
- *hegu* (LI 4)
- *gongsun* (Sp 4)
- *pishu* (B 20)

Dampness

Dampness can be divided into two kinds: exterior and interior. The former is related to dampness *qi* in the environment, the prevailing climatic factor of late summer. Additionally, working on or in water, wearing wet or damp clothes, living in a damp dwelling or sweating profusely may aggravate dampness evil.

Spleen dysfunctions may lead to water disturbances and fluid transformations, which result in fluid retention. In "A Great Treatise on the Most Precise and Important Essence," a section in *Su Wen* (Plain Questions), it is stated: "Edema and swelling from dampness are all due to splenic disorders."

Dampness evil is always characterized by heaviness, turbidity, sluggishness and aches in the limbs or the entire body. When the head is afflicted with dampness, it feels as if a tight band surrounds it. If dampness resides in the joints, it may produce arthralgia or arthritis with continual pain, heaviness and difficulty in movement. Turbidity is descriptive of secretions and excretions associated with dampness. These include turbid urine; sticky, loose stools; dysentery with pus and mucous; ulcer; eczema; herpes with pus; and, in women, bloody, whitish discharges from the vagina.

By nature, dampness is viscose and stagnant. When dampness evil attacks the body, obstinate diseases such as rheumatism, as well as some infectious febrile diseases, are often the result. Some manifestations of these afflictions are tenesmus, strangury and oliguria.

Dampness belongs to *yin* evil and therefore tends to attack *yang qi*, particularly spleen *yang*. This induces water retention, thereby creating edema, which, in the gastrointestinal tract, results in diarrhea.

Exterior Dampness (Catch-dampness)

Manifestations include an aversion to cold, a fever which is not relieved by perspiration, heavy-headedness, body soreness, a constricted feeling in the chest, no desire to drink, a thin, whitish and slippery tongue coating and a soft and floating pulse.

Treatment alleviates symptoms by removing dampness. Agastache Formula (*huo xiang zheng qi san*) can be used.

Dampness *Bi* (*Zhuo Bi*)

Manifestations include arthralgia or arthritis with fixed pain and heaviness in the joints and numbness of the muscles and skin. For a thorough discussion, see Chapter 4, Section 35.

Interior Dampness

Heavy-headedness, a feeling of oppression in the chest, abdominal distention, a poor appetite, general lassitude, a creamy tongue coating and a thready, soft pulse characterize interior dampness.

Treatment invigorates splenic functioning and eliminates dampness. Magnolia and Hoelen Combination (*wei ling tang*) can be used.

Magnolia and Hoelen Combination[1]

Wei Ling Tang

(Calm the Stomach and Poria Decoction)[2]

Alisma	*Alismatis rhizoma*	*Ze xie*	2.5
Hoelen	*Poria sclerotium*	*Fu ling*	2.5
Polyporus	*Polyporus sclerotium*	*Zhu ling*	2.5
Cinnamon twig	*Cinnamomi ramulus*	*Gui zhi*	2.0
Atractylodes, white	*Atractylodis rhizoma*	*Bai zhu*	2.5
Atractylodes	*Atractylodis lanceae rhizoma*	*Cang zhu*	2.5
Magnolia bark	*Magnoliae officinalis cortex*	*Hou pu*	2.5
Citrus peel	*Citri pericarpium*	*Chen pi*	2.5
Licorice	*Glycyrrhizae radix*	*Gan cao*	1.0
Ginger, fresh	*Zingiberis rhizoma*	*Shen jiang*	1.5
Jujube	*Zizyphi fructus*	*Da zao*	1.5

There are many commonly used herbs for removing dampness. A brief discussion of some of them follows.

Herbs for warming *yang* and removing dampness are:

prepared aconite (*zhi fu zi*)   cinnamon bark (*rou gui*)
cinnamon twig (*gui zhi*)   dried ginger (*gan jiang*)

Cinnamon bark is mainly used for dispelling cold-dampness from the abdomen, while cinnamon twig dispels cold-dampness from the limbs.

Herbs for invigorating the spleen and removing dampness are:

white atractylodes (*bai zhu*)   atractylodes (*cang zhu*)
coix (*yi yi ren*)

White atractylodes functions mainly as a splenic tonic and is more effective at invigorating the spleen and stomach than atractylodes or coix. Atractylodes is an effective herb for drying dampness in the treatment of dyspepsia, rheumatic arthritis and night blindness. Coix is used to improve splenic functioning in the treatment of diarrhea, as well as discharge pus in the treatment of acute appendicitis and lung abscesses. It is also an anti-cancer herb.

Herbs for dispelling wind and checking dampness are:

siler (*fang feng*)   chiang-huo (*qiang huo*)
ma-huang (*ma huang*)   asarum (*xi xin*)

Mild-flavored herbs for dispelling dampness are:

hoelen (*fu ling*)   polyporus (*zhu ling*)
alisma (*ze xie*)   talc (*hua shi*)

The above diuretics are used for the treatment of edema and oliguria. Hoelen is both a stomachic to treat diminished appetite and a sedative. The diuretic effect of polyporus is stronger than those of the other three herbs. In addition, alisma reduces blood cholesterol levels and treats the dizziness associated with Meniere's disease. Talc is the standard treatment for summer heat-dampness and urinary-tract infections.

Fragrant herbs for dispelling dampness are:

cardamom (*suo sha ren*)   cluster (*bai dou kou*)
agastache (*huo xiang*)   eupatorium (*pei lan*)

Cardamom can be used for the treatment of chronic diarrhea and the prevention of miscarriages in women who have a history of spontaneous abortions. Cluster is a stomach-warming and carminative agent for the treatment of gastrointestinal fullness, nausea and vomiting. Agastache dispels summer heat-dampness and is effective against dyspepsia, poor appetite and diarrhea. Eupatorium is a stomachic and an antiemetic agent for the treatment of poor appetite and gastrointestinal fullness due to dampness accumulation.

Bitter, cold-natured herbs for dispelling dampness are:

coptis (*huang lian*)   phellodendron (*huang bo*)
ailanthus root (*bai chun pi*) capillaris (*yin chen hao*)
smilax (*tu fu ling*)

Coptis works in the middle energizer to eliminate heat-dampness from the gastrointestinal tract, while phellodendron acts mainly in the lower energizer to eliminate the heat-dampness from the kidneys and bladder which is often associated with urinary-tract infections. Ailanthus root is effective against diarrhea, chronic dysentery, spontaneous emission and leukorrhea. Capillaris eliminates heat-dampness in the liver and gallbladder, a condition generally associated with jaundice, icteric hepatitis and cholecystitis. Smilax is often used to treat dermatological diseases, leptospirosis and cancer.

Acupuncture and Moxibustion Treatment

Exterior Dampness (Catch-dampness)
- *gongsun* (Sp 4)
- *pishu* (B 20)

Dampness *Bi*
- *zusanli* (S 36)
- *shangqiu* (Sp 5)

(as well as the local points)

Interior Dampness
- *pishu* (B 20)
- *gongsun* (Sp 4)
- *fenglong* (S 40)

Dryness

Autumn is characterized by low humidity. Such dryness can bring on disease. This kind of dryness is called exterior dryness and, as diseases caused by it are mostly seen in autumn, it is also called autumn dryness. Dryness tends to consume body fluids and impair the lungs, since they are tender and closely associated with the skin.

Exterior Dryness

1. Cold-dryness

Manifestations include fever, an aversion to cold, headache, an absence of sweat, a dry mouth and throat, dry skin, a cough with scanty or no sputum and a white, thin and dry tongue coating.

Treatment aims to ventilate the lungs and moisten the tissues. Apricot Seed and Perilla Formula (*xing su san*), to which is added 3 *qian* glehnia (*sha shen*) and 6 *qian* ophiopogon (*mai men dong*), can be effectively employed.

22

Apricot Seed and Perilla Formula[1]

Xing Su San
(Apricot Kernel and Perilla Leaf Powder)[2]

Apricot seed	*Armeniacae semen*	*Xing ren*	6.0
Perilla leaf	*Perillae folium*	*Zi su ye*	3.0
Chih-ko	*Citri fructus*	*Zhi ke*	3.0
Platycodon	*Platycodi radix*	*Jie geng*	3.0
Peucedanum	*Peucedani radix*	*Qian ho*	6.0
Citrus peel	*Citri pericarpium*	*Chen pi*	3.0
Pinellia	*Pinellia rhizoma*	*Ban xia*	6.0
Hoelen	*Poria sclerotium*	*Fu ling*	6.0
Ginger, fresh	*Zingiberis rhizoma*	*Sheng jiang*	1.0
Licorice	*Glycyrrhizae radix*	*Gan cao*	1.5
Jujube	*Zizyphi fructus*	*Da zao*	3.0

2. Heat-dryness

Manifestations include fever; mild chills; headache; a decreased amount of sweat; a dry cough or a cough with scanty sticky or even bloody sputum; a sore, swollen throat; dry skin, nose and throat; thirst; anxiety; a red tongue tip or a red-edged tongue. Treatment clears the lungs and moistens the tissues with Eriobotrya and Ophiopogon Combination (*qing zao jiu fei tang*).

Eriobotrya and Ophiopogon Combination[1]

Qing Zao Jiu Fei Tang
(Eliminate Dryness and Rescue the Lungs Decoction)[2]

Morus leaf	*Mori folium*	*Sang ye*	3.0
Gypsum	*Gypsum fibrosum*	*Shi gao*	10.0
Gelatin	*Asini gelatinum*	*A jiao*	2.4
Ophiopogon	*Ophiopogonis rhizoma*	*Mai men dong*	3.6
Sesame	*Sesami semen*	*Hu ma ren*	2.4
Ginseng	*Ginseng radix*	*Ren shen*	2.0
Apricot seed	*Armeniacae semen*	*Xing ren*	2.0
Eriobotrya	*Eriobotryae folium*	*Pi pa ye*	3.0
Licorice	*Glycyrrhizae radix*	*Gan cao*	2.0

Interior Dryness

This condition is typically the result of high fever and profuse sweating, both of which consume body fluids. Additionally, chronic diseases, or those with a long disease course, can prompt fluid depletion. Interior dryness can also be caused by vomiting, diarrhea or bleeding, all of which reduce fluids and promote conditions under which blood is prevented from nourishing and moistening the tissues. Manifestations of interior dryness include excessive thirst; dry, rough skin; dry, lifeless hair; constipation; emaciation; a dry tongue with no saliva; and a thready, hesitant pulse.

Treatment is aimed at nourishing *yin* and replenishing lost fluids. Ophiopogon and Trichosanthes Combination (*mai men dong yin zi*) or Scrophularia and Ophiopogon Combination (*zeng ye tang*) can be used.

Ophiopogon and Trichosanthes Combination[1]

Mai Men Dong Yin Zi

(Ophiopogon and Trichosanthes Decoction)

Ophiopogon	*Ophiopogonis rhizoma*	*Mai meng dong*	7.0
Pueraria	*Puerariae radix*	*Ge gen*	3.0
Licorice	*Glycyrrhizae radix*	*Gan cao*	1.0
Ginseng	*Ginseng radix*	*Ren shen*	2.0
Rehmannia, raw	*Rehmanniae radix*	*Sheng di huang*	4.0
Trichosanthes root	*Trichosanthis radix*	*Gua lou gen*	2.0
Hoelen	*Poria sclerotium*	*Fu ling*	6.0
Bamboo leaf	*Bambusae folium*	*Zhu ye*	1.0
Anemarrhena	*Anemarrhenae rhizoma*	*Zhi mu*	3.0
Schizandra	*Schizandrae fructus*	*Wu wei zi*	1.0

Scrophularia and Ophiopogon Combination
Zeng Ye Tang[7]
(Increase the Fluids Decoction)[2]

Rehmannia, raw	*Rehmanniae radix*	*Sheng di huang*	3.0
Scrophularia	*Scrophulariae radix*	*Xuan shen*	3.0
Ophiopogon	*Ophiopogonis rhizoma*	*Mai men dong*	3.0

Functions: nourishes *yin*; replenishes body fluids; clears heat; moistens tissues.

Explanation: Raw rehmannia and ophiopogon are cool, sweet herbs that nourish *yin* and replenish body fluids. When combined with bitter, cold-natured scrophularia, rehmannia and ophiopogon can be even more effective in clearing heat and moistening the tissues. Three *qian* dendrobium stem (*shi hu*) and 10 *qian* phragmites (*lu gen*) are generally added to Scrophularia and Ophiopogon Combination (*zeng ye tang*) to enhance effectiveness.

Acupuncture and Moxibustion Points for Dryness

- *shousanli* (LI 10)
- *zusanli* (S 36)

Fire

Fire is usually interior and more harmful than heat and it generally flames upwards. Fire symptoms can be induced either directly by external-heat evil or by the invasion of any of the five evils--namely, wind, cold, summer heat, dampness or dryness--which can transform into fire inside the body. Interior fire results from dysfunctions of the internal organs or from extreme emotional swings. In traditional Chinese medicine it is said: "All five *qi* can transform into fire." And: "All five emotions can give rise to fire." For instance, liver or heart fire are often seen in clinical practice.

Fire symptoms are generally a fever; a flushed face; red eyes; a swollen, sore throat; and redness, swelling, heat and pain from local inflammatory lesions. It has been observed in clinical practice that, when heart fire flames upward, injury to the tongue and oral cavity occurs, and when stomach fire flares upward, the gums swell and bleed. In turn, when liver fire flames upward, the eyes become red, dry and irritated.

Since fire depletes body fluids, fire conformations are also characterized by a dry mouth, a desire for cold drinks and a dry tongue coating with scanty saliva. Furthermore, fire may also force blood to escape from its vessels. Consequently, fire often induces hematemesis, epistaxis and ecchymosis.

Exterior Fire

The onset is often acute, the disease course is short, and the vital *qi* (*zheng qi*) of the body is still abundant. The primary manifestations are fever; an aversion to heat; a flushed face; red eyes; fidgeting or nervousness; thirst with a desire for cold beverages; constipation or diarrhea with foul-smelling, scanty, red urine; a dry, yellow tongue coating; and a rapid, excess pulse. In severe cases, loss of consciousness, delirium, irritability, restlessness, eruption, hematemesis, epistaxis, hematuria or hematochezia may occur.

Treatment is aimed at clearing heat and purging fire. Coptis and Scute Combination (*huang lian jie du tang*) can be used.

Coptis and Scute Combination[1]

Huang Lian Jie Du Tang
(Coptis Decoction to Relieve Toxicity)[2]

Coptis	Coptidis rhizoma	Huang lian	1.5
Scute	Scutellariae radix	Huang qin	3.0
Phellodendron	Phellodendri cortex	Huang bo	1.5
Gardenia	Gardeniae fructus	Zhi zi	2.0

If the patient has constipation, abdominal fullness or distention, or hard stools, Major Rhubarb Combination (*da cheng qi tang*) is recommended.

Major Rhubarb Combination[1]

Da Cheng Qi Tang

(Major Order the *Qi* Decoction)[2]

Rhubarb	Rhei rhizoma	Da huang	2.0
Mirabilitum	Natrium sulfuricum	Mang xiao	2.0
Magnolia bark	Magnoliae officinalis cortex	Hou pu	5.0
Caih-shih	Citri fructus immaturus	Zhi shi	2.0

If bleeding occurs, Rhinoceros and Rehmannia Combination (*xi jiao di huang tang*) can be selected.

Rhinoceros and Rehmannia Combination[1]

Xi Jiao Di Huang Tang

(Rhinoceros Horn and Rehmannia Decoction)[2]

Rhinoceros horn*	Rhinocerotis cornu	Xi jiao	1.0
Rehmannia, raw	Rehmannia radix	Sheng di huang	8.0
Peony, red	Paeoniae rubra radix	Chi shao	3.0
Moutan	Moutan radicis cortex	Mu dan pi	2.0

* Rhinoceros is an endangered species and its import and/or use in the United States is strictly limited to approved scientific studies. Buffalo horn may be substituted in the ratio of 30 *qian* of buffalo horn for each *qian* of rhinoceros horn.

One dose per day is to be decocted twice daily. In severe cases, two doses may be used and decocted four times daily.

Functions: clears and relieves interior heat; cools blood; eliminates blood stasis.

Explanation: This is the most commonly used formula for dispelling heat evil from the blood (*xue*) *fen*. Rhinoceros horn and raw rehmannia cool the blood, relieve interior heat, nourish *yin* and clear heat. Red peony and moutan cool the blood, clear heat, activate blood circulation and eliminate blood stasis. When heat evil invades *xue fen*, blood heat and blood stasis always coexist, so herbs for clearing heat and cooling the blood and those for eliminating blood stasis and activating blood circulation are both used in this formula. With only four herbs, this formula can clear *ying fen* and *xue fen* heat directly, as well as dispel heart heat.

If this formula is given to an unconscious patient with a high fever, Rhinoceros and Antelope Horn Formula (*zi xue dan*) or Bezoar and Curcuma Formula (*an gong niu huang wan*) may be added to help clear heat and revive consciousness.

Rhinoceros and Antelope Horn Formula[1]

Zi Xue Dan

(Purple Snow Special Pill)[2]

Rhinoceros horn	*Rhinocerotis cornu*	*Xi jiao*	1.0
Musk	*Moschus*	*She xiang*	0.5
Antelope horn	*Antelopis cornu*	*Ling yang jiao*	1.0
Aristolochia root	*Aristolochiae radix*	*Qing mu xiang*	9.0
Aquilaria	*Aquilariae lignum*	*Chen xiang*	3.0
Clove	*Caryophylli flos*	*Ding xiang*	3.0
Gypsum	*Gypsum fibrosum*	*Shi gao*	5.0
Calcite	*Glauberitum*	*Han shui shi*	9.0
Loadstone	*Magnetitum*	*Ci shi*	9.0
Talc	*Talcum*	*Hua shi*	9.0
Mirabilitum	*Natrium sulfuricum*	*Mang xiao*	6.0
Niter	*Nitrum*	*Xiao shi*	6.0
Scrophularia	*Scrophulariae radix*	*Xuan shen*	9.0
Cimicifuga	*Cimicifugae rhizoma*	*Sheng ma*	6.0
Licorice	*Glycyrrhizae radix*	*Gan cao*	3.0
Cinnabar	*Cinnabaris*	*Zhu sha*	0.5

Take 0.3-0.5 *qian* three times daily.

When accompanied by bleeding, the following is recommended: 10 *qian* imperata (*bai mao gen*), 5 *qian* of eclipta (*han lian cao*) and 3 *qian* each of sophora (*huai hua*) and sanguisorba (*di yu*). These herbs cool heat and achieve hemostasis. Bezoar Resurrection Pill (*an gong niu huang wan*) is often used for subacute yellow atrophy, hepatic coma, uremia, loss of consciousness and septicemia.

Deficiency Fire

Its onset is slow, its disease course long, and the body's vital energy (*zheng qi*) is already deficient. The main manifestations are those of the conformations of excess interior fire due to *yin* deficiency in the lungs, kidneys, heart, liver and stomach, namely, flushed cheeks, a feverish sensation in the palms, soles and heart area, or a hectic fever, fidgeting, insomnia, night sweats, dry mouth, throat and eyes, a dry cough with little sputum, scanty, reddish urine, a denuded tongue or a red tongue with little coating, and a thready, rapid pulse.

Treatment nourishes *yin* and subdues fire with Anemarrhena, Phellodendron and Rehmannia Formula (*zhi bo ba wei wan*) or *Chin-chiu* and Turtle Shell Formula (*qin jiao bie jia san*).

Anemarrhena, Phellodendron and Rehmannia Formula[1]

Zhi Bo Ba Wei Wan
(Eight-herb Pill, Including Anemarrhena and Phellodendron)

Anemarrhena	*Anemarrhenae rhizoma*	*Zhi mu*	2.0
Phellodendron	*Phellodendri cortex*	*Huang bo*	2.0
Rehmannia, cooked	*Rehmanniae radix*	*Shu di huang*	8.0
Cornus	*Corni fructus*	*Shan zhu yu*	4.0
Dioscorea	*Dioscorea batatis rhizoma*	*Shan yao*	4.0
Alisma	*Alismatis rhizoma*	*Ze xie*	3.0
Moutan	*Moutan radicis cortex*	*Mu dan pi*	3.0
Hoelen	*Poria sclerotium*	*Fu ling*	3.0

Chin-chiu and Turtle Shell Formula[1]

Qin Jiao Bie Jia San
(Gentian *Qinjiao* and Soft-shelled Turtle Shell Powder)[2]

Chin-chiu	Gentianae macro-phyllae radix	Qin jiao	2.0
Ching-hao	Artemisiae ching hao herba	Qing hao	2.0
Mume	Mume fructus	Wu mei	2.0
Anemarrhena	Anemarrhenae rhizoma	Zhi mu	2.0
Tang-kuei	Angelicae radix	Dang gui	3.0
Turtle shell	Amydae carapax	Bie jia	3.0
Bupleurum	Bupleuri radix	Chai hu	3.0
Lycium root bark	Lycii radicis cortex	Di gu pi	3.0
Ginger, fresh	Zingiberis rhizoma	Sheng jiang	1.5

Interior Fire

Uncontrolled emotional outbursts may disturb and stagnate *qi*, thereby transforming the emotions into liver, heart or stomach fire.

Liver fire is characterized by headache, dizziness, a flushed face, red eyes, irritability, restlessness, a bitter taste in the mouth, a dry throat, burning pain in the costal region, constipation, yellow urine, a red tongue with yellow coating and a rapid pulse.

To purge liver fire, Gentian Combination (*long dan xie gan tang*) can be used.

Stomach fire is characterized by burning epigastrium pain; thirst with a preference for cold beverages; the consumption of large amounts of food, but with no alleviation of hunger; acid regurgitation; stomach distress; foul breath; painful or hemorrhaging gums; ulcers; constipation; a red tongue with a creamy, yellow coating; and a rapid, slippery pulse.

To purge stomach fire, Coptis and Rehmannia Formula (*qing wei san*) is recommended.

Gentian Combination[1]

Long Dan Xie Gan Tang

(Gentian *Longdancao* Decoction to Drain the Liver)[2]

Gentian	Gentianae scabre radix	Long dan cao	1.0
Scute	Scutellariae radix	Huang qin	3.0
Gardenia	Gardeniae fructus	Zhi zi	1.0
Alisma	Alismatis rhizoma	Ze xie	3.0
Plantago	Plantaginis semen	Che qian zi	3.0
Akebia	Akebiae caulis	Mu tong	5.0
Rehmannia, raw	Rehmanniae radix	Sheng di huang	5.0
Tang-kuei	Angelicae radix	Dang gui	9.0
Bupleurum*	Bupleuri radix	Chai hu	1.0
Licorice	Glycyrrhizae radix	Gan cao	1.0

* In some books, bupleurum is not included.

Coptis and Rehmannia Formula[1]

Qing Wei San

(Clear the Stomach Powder)[2]

Moutan	Moutan radicis cortex	Mu dan pi	6.0
Tang-kuei	Angelicae radix	Dang gui	6.0
Rehmannia, raw	Rehmanniae radix	Sheng di huang	6.0
Coptis	Coptidis rhizoma	Huang lian	1.0
Cimicifuga	Cimicifugae rhizoma	Sheng ma	1.0

Heart fire is manifested in tongue and mouth ulcers, fidgeting, insomnia, thirst, painful urination, a red tongue tip, a yellow tongue coating and a rapid pulse. In order to purge heart fire, use Rehmannia and Akebia Formula (*dao chi san*) or Lotus Seed Combination (*qing xin lian zi yin*).

Rehmannia and Akebia Formula[1]
Dao Chi San
(Guide Out the Red Powder)[2]

Rehmannia, raw	*Rehmanniae radix*	*Sheng di huang*	15.0
Akebia	*Akebiae caulis*	*Mu tong*	3.0
Lophatherum	*Lophatheri herba*	*Dan zhu ye*	3.0
Licorice, raw	*Glycyrrhizae radix*	*Sheng gan cao*	3.0

Lotus Seed Combination [1]
Qing Xin Lian Zi Yin
(Lotus Seed Decoction to Clear Heart Fire)[2]

Lotus seed	*Nelumbinis semen*	*Lian zi*	4.0
Plantago	*Plantaginis semen*	*Che qian zi*	3.0
Astragalus	*Astragali radix*	*Huang qi*	2.0
Ophiopogon	*Ophiopogonis rhizoma*	*Mai men dong*	4.0
Scute	*Scutellariae radix*	*Huang qin*	3.0
Lycium root bark	*Lycii radicis cortex*	*Di gu pi*	2.0
Hoelen	*Poria sclerotium*	*Fu ling*	4.0
Ginseng	*Ginseng radix*	*Ren shen*	3.0
Licorice	*Glycyrrhizae radix*	*Gan cao*	2.0

Herbs for clearing heat and purging fire are all suitable for the various fire conformations. These herbs can be divided into four groups: febrifugal and detoxicant; heat-clearing and fire-purging; blood heat-clearing; and heat-clearing and damp-ness-drying. Only when interior heat occurs in patients with strong constitutions may these herbs be administered, since many of them have intense antibacterial or antiviral actions.

Febrifugal and detoxicant herbs are used for various infectious diseases, such as furuncle, carbuncle, tonsillitis and pneumonia. Commonly used febrifugal and detoxicant herbs:

lonicera (*jin yin hua*)	forsythia (*lian qiao*)
isatis leaf (*da qing ye*)	isatis root (*ban lan gen*)
dandelion (*pu gong yin*)	houttuynia (*yu xing cao*)
viola (*zi hua di ding*)	oldenlandia (*bai hua she she cao*)
scute (*ban zhi lian*)	stringy stonecrop (*chui pen cao*)
trachea (*zao xiu*)	wild chrysanthemum (*ye jua hua*)

Among the above-cited herbs, lonicera and forsythia are most frequently selected for colds or influenzas with fever, furuncle and carbuncle. Stir-baked lonicera can cure enteritis and dysentery.

Both isatis leaf and isatis root have antibacterial and antiviral actions. Indirubin, an extract of isatis leaf, can be used against leukemia, while dandelion is widely used for general inflammatory diseases and especially for acute mastitis, acute inflammation of the biliary tract and chronic gastritis.

Houttuynia is effective in treating chronic bronchitis, pneumonia and pulmonary abscesses. Viola can counteract poisonous snakebites and acute hemorrhagic enteritis necroticans. Oldenlandia and scute are frequently used for malignant tumors such as carcinomas of the stomach and liver. Stringy stonecrop can prompt drops in glutamic pyruvic transaminase and is often used to combat viral hepatitis. Trachea is used for poisonous snakebites and mumps. Wild chrysanthemum calms the liver and reduces hypertension.

Heat-clearing and fire-purging herbs are used for symptoms of intense heat which transform into fire. Commonly used herbs to clear heat and purge fire:

gypsum (*shi gao*)	anemarrhena (*zhi mu*)
gentian (*long dan cao*)	coptis (*huang lian*)
scute (*huang qin*)	phellodendron (*huang bo*)
prunella (*xia ku cao*)	

Rhubarb (*da huang*) is also a heat-clearing and fire-purging herb, but it is generally classified under herbs for purgation, which are not discussed here.

Gypsum is effective in both cooling *qi* and relieving thirst. When combined with anemarrhena, isatis leaf (*da qing ye*) and isatis root (*ban lan gen*), gypsum can be used for patients with epidemic encephalitis B; while combining gypsum with *ma-huang*, apricot seed (*xing ren*) or licorice (*gan cao*) is effective against pneumonia in its high-fever stage. Periodontal disease, toothache and bleeding teeth can be treated with gypsum in combination with anemarrhena and asarum (*zhi mu*).

When combined with gypsum, anemarrhena deals effectively with high fever and thirst. It can also relieve interior heat due to *yin* deficiency, when combined with rehmannia (*sheng di huang*) and turtle shell (*bie jia*). For treating urinary-tract infections, anemarrhena is most effective when combined with phellodendron (*huang bo*) and cinnamon bark (*rou gui*).

Bitter gentian (*long dan cao*) is especially useful for relieving liver fire and, for this reason, is often prescribed for acute hepatitis, cholecystitis and vulvate eczema.

Though coptis (*huang lian*), scute (*huang qin*) and phellodendron (*huang bo*) are often combined, they also can be used separately to achieve various effects. When combined with morus root bark (*sang bai pi*) and apricot seed (*xing ren*), scute can relieve symptoms associated with pneumonia and bronchitis. If combined with schizonepeta (*jing jie*), rehmannia and peony (*shao yao*), scute can be used to correct shorter-than-normal intervals between menstrual periods. Scute and atractylodes (*bai zhu*) are often used to prevent spontaneous abortions or treat prenatal diseases. Alternating spells of fever and chills can be treated with a combination of scute and bupleurum (*chai hu*).

Coptis (*huang lian*), when combined with saussurea (*mu xiang*), is used for enteritis and dysentery. When combined with evodia (*wu zhu yu*), it eliminates stomach heat and acid regurgitation. Combined with rehmannia and lophatherum (*zhu ye*), coptis relieves insomnia. If it is combined with dried ginger (*gan jiang*) and pinellia (*ban xia*), coptis can alleviate abdominal distention, vomiting and difficulty in swallowing.

Phellodendron (*huang bo*), combined with anemarrhena (*zhi mu*), can quench ministerial fire (fire of the vital gate or *xiang huo*), a condition which affects sexual potency and nocturnal emission. To treat vulvate pruritus and eczema, phellodendron should be combined with atractylodes (*cang zhu*) and achyranthes (*niu xi*), while leukorrhea with a pinkish discharge can be cleared up with phellodendron, sanguisorba (*di yu*) and cuttlebone (*wu zei gu*).

Prunella (*xia ku cao*) can quench liver fire and reduce blood pressure, thus, it is often used for the treatment of conjunctival congestion, photophobia, hypertension, mammary lobular hyperplasia and scrofula (tuberculosis of the cervical lymph nodes).

Herbs which cool blood heat are commonly used to treat dysphemia due to high fever, coma or delirium, or hemorrhagic diseases with febrile symptoms. The most commonly used herbs to cool blood heat:

rhinoceros horn (*xi jiao*)	raw rehmannia (*sheng di huang*)
scrophularia (*xuan shen*)	moutan (*dan pi*)
lithospermum (*zi cao*)	gardenia (*zhi zi*)
lycium bark (*di gu pi*)	cynanchum (*bai wei*)

Among these herbs, rhinoceros horn is by far the most effective, but its import into the United States is strictly prohibited under the Endangered Species Act. For this reason, buffalo horn (*shui niu jiao*) serves as a much cheaper, as well as legal, substitute.

To achieve maximum effectiveness in cooling the blood, rehmannia should be fresh. Salty, cold-propertied scrophularia nourishes *yin* and reduces heat, and so is used to treat sore throats associated with *yin* deficiency. Moutan cools blood heat, clears skin rashes and dissipates blood stasis, making it especially useful in halting hemorrhaging. Because of its anitiviral properties, lithospermum is mainly used to promote eruption in the treatment of measles. Gardenia both cools blood heat and cures icterohepatitis, a wind-heat influenza and urinary-tract infection. Lycium bark is principally used for high fever and night sweats caused by *yin* deficiency. Cynanchum treats lingering, low-grade fevers and puerperal fevers due to deficiency.

Heat-clearing and dampness-drying herbs are usually used for skin diseases, hepatitis and bacillary dysentery caused by heat-dampness. Commonly used heat-clearing and dampness-drying herbs:

sophora root (*ku shen*)	anemone (*bai tou wang*)
fraxinella (*bai xian pi*)	kochia (*di fu zi*)
fraxinus (*qin pi*)	capillaris (*yin chen hao*)

Sophora root alleviates eczema and leukorrhea with reddish discharge, and lately it has been used for relieving various types of premature heartbeat with limited curative effects. Anemone is mainly used for the treatment of various bacillary dysenteries and intestinal amebiasis.

Fraxinella and kochia are recommended for various skin diseases, such as eczema, urticaria and cutaneous pruritus. Fraxinus is mainly used for bacillary dysentery and leukorrhagia, while capillaris is a cholagogue used for icterohepatitis.

Acupuncture and Moxibustion Points for Fire

- *qiangu* (SI 2)
- *zusanli* (S 36)

- *xinshu* (B 15)
- *neiting* (S 44)

Section 2
Phlegm and Fluid Retention

Phlegm and retained fluids are pathological substances resulting from the condensation of normal body fluids, the thicker of which is phlegm and the thinner of which is retained fluids. As soon as they accumulate, these fluids induce new pathological processes in the body and produce a variety of conformations. In fact, phlegm gives rise to so many diseases that traditionally it has been said: "All diseases result from phlegm." And: "Disease treatment should be started with the treatment of phlegm."

Phlegm is both the substance expectorated from the lungs and the cause which induces certain symptoms associated with such expectoration. Diseases caused by phlegm retained in different parts of the body are characterized by different clinical symptoms: phlegm in the lungs produces a cough and abundant expectorations; in the heart, unconsciousness or manic or depressive psychosis; in the stomach, nausea, vomiting and a poor appetite; in the upper body, dizziness, nausea and vomiting; in the limbs, numbness and pain; and in the meridians, scrofula, goiter and subcutaneous nodules.

Phlegm-dampness

Manifestations include a sensation of heaviness, weakness and lassitude; profuse, thin, white expectorations; distress in the chest; a thick, creamy tongue coating; and a soft, slippery pulse.

Treatment eliminates dampness and restores phlegm to its proper state of balance within the body. Citrus and Pinellia Combination (*er chen tang*) can be used.

Citrus and Pinellia Combination[1]

Er Chen Tang

(Two-cured Decoction)[2]

Pinellia	Pinellia rhizoma	Ban xia	5.0
Citrus peel	Citri pericarpium	Chen pi	4.0
Hoelen	Poria sclerotium	Fu ling	5.0
Licorice	Glycyrrhizae radix	Gan cao	1.0

Heat-phlegm

Manifestations include a paroxysmal cough; a flushed face; fidgeting; thick, yellow phlegm; a red tongue with a yellow, creamy coating; and a rapid, slippery pulse.

Platycodon and Fritillaria Combination (*qing fei tang*) should be used to clear heat and dissipate phlegm.

Cold-phlegm

Characteristic manifestations include a weak cough with cold, thick and white or frothy, white discharge; a white, moist tongue coating; and a slow pulse.

The aim of treatment is to warm and dissolve cold-phlegm. Minor Blue Dragon Combination (*xiao qing long tang*) is recommended.

Platycodon and Fritillaria Combination[1]

Qing Fei Tang
(Clear Lung Heat Decoction)

Scute	Scutellariae radix	Huang qin	2.0
Platycodon	Platycodi radix	Jie geng	2.0
Morus bark	Mori radicis cortex	Sang bai pi	2.0
Apricot seed	Armeniacae semen	Xing ren	2.0
Gardenia	Gardenia fructus	Zhi zi	2.0
Asparagus	Asparagi radix	Tian men dong	2.0
Fritillaria	Fritillariae bulbus	Bei mu	2.0
Citrus peel	Citri pericarpium	Chen pi	2.0
Jujube	Zizyphi fructus	Da zao	3.0
Bamboo shavings	Bambusae caulis in taeniis	Zhu ru	3.0
Hoelen	Poria sclerotium	Fu ling	3.0
Tang-kuei	Angelicae radix	Dang gui	3.0
Ophiopogon	Ophiopogonis rhizoma	Mai men dong	3.0
Schizandra	Schizandrae fructus	Wu wei zi	1.0
Licorice	Glycyrrhizae radix	Gan cao	1.0
Ginger, fresh	Zingiberis rhizoma	Sheng jiang	1.0

Minor Blue Dragon Combination[1]

Xiao Qing Long Tang
(Minor Bluegreen Dragon Decoction)[2]

Ma-huang	Ephedrae herba	Ma-huang	1.0
Cinnamon twig	Cinnamomi ramulus	Gui zhi	1.0
Peony	Paeoniae radix	Shao yao	2.0
Ginger, dried	Zingiberis siccatum rhizoma	Gan jiang	1.0
Asarum	Asari herba cum radice	Xi xin	1.0
Licorice, baked	Glycyrrhizae radix	Zhi gan cao	2.0
Schizandra	Schizandrae fructus	Wu wei zi	1.0
Pinellia	Pinellia rhizoma	Ban xia	3.0

Phlegm Invading the Heart

For a discussion of this conformation, see Chapter 3.

Commonly used herbs for dissipating phlegm are classified into four groups: herbs for relieving cough and reducing phlegm; herbs for dissipating phlegm and softening hard masses; herbs for the relief of coughs and asthma; and herbs which eliminate phlegm and restore consciousness.

Herbs for relieving cough and reducing phlegm are suitable for any kind of cough, such as that associated with bronchitis or pneumonia. However, heat should be cleared in case of heat-phlegm, while the patient should be warmed in the case of cold-phlegm.

Herbs for resolving heat-phlegm are:

platycodon (*jie geng*)	trichosanthes peel (*gua lou pi*)
peucedanum (*qian hu*)	bamboo shavings (*zhu ru*)
stemona root (*bai bu*)	benincasa (*dong gua zi*)

Platycodon combined with licorice (*gan cao*) is often used for pharyngitis and with houttuynia (*yu xing cao*), benincasa and phragmites (*lu gen*) for pulmonary abscesses.

Trichosanthes peel is more effective than trichosanthes fruit in the treatment of coughs. In addition, trichosanthes peel relieves chest stuffiness and clears the lungs. When combined with dandelion (*pu gong ying*) and bupleurum (*chai hu*), trichosanthes peel can be used for the treatment of acute mastitis. When combined with bakeri (*xie bai*), pinellia and immature bitter orange (*zhi shi*), or with immature bitter orange alone, trichosanthes peel can relieve angina pectoris.

Peucedanum and bamboo shavings treat a cough with thick sputum, which is characteristic of lung heat. Bamboo shavings can also regulate the stomach and stop vomiting.

In addition to resolving heat, stemona root is an antitussive for whooping cough, however, it should not be used at the early stage of coughing. Benincasa is generally used for removing lung heat and so has a strong curative effect on pulmonary abscesses and bronchiectasis.

Herbs for resolving cold-phlegm are:

pinellia (*ban xia*)	mustard seed (*bai jie zi*)
inula (*xuan fu hua*)	affine cudweed (*fo er cao*)

Of these four herbs, pinellia is the one most commonly selected. It relieves coughs and dissipates white, thick phlegm, as well as regulates and reduces the adverse flow of stomach *qi*, thereby alleviating vomiting. When pinellia, fritillaria (*bei mu*) and prunella (*xia ku cao*) are combined, they are effective against cervical lymphadenectasis; while pinellia with husked sorghum (*shu mi*) and albizzia (*he huan pi*) is a common treatment for insomnia and palpitation. Pinellia with white atractylodes (*bai zhu*) and gastrodia (*tian ma*) is often used to cure dizziness due to dampness.

Mustard seed corrects the profuse expectorations characteristic of chronic bronchitis and hydrothorax, while inula keeps *qi* flowing downward and dissipates sputum, and so it may be used to treat belching, vomiting and chest pain. Affine cudweed is effective in treating asthma.

Herbs for dissipating phlegm and softening hard masses are used for diseases such as lymphnoditis and goiter. Those herbs most commonly used are:

fritillaria (*bei mu*)	seaweed (*hai zao*)
ecklonia (*kun bu*)	ark shell (*wa leng zi*)

There are two kinds of fritillaria: *chuan bei mu* and *zhe bei mu*. The former nourishes the lungs and suppresses coughs, thereby making it a useful treatment for chronic coughs and pulmonary tuberculosis. The latter is mostly used to treat patients at the initial stage of cough due to external pathogenic factors or those with acute bronchitis. Both forms of fritillaria can effectively treat tuberculosis of the lymph nodes, subcutaneous nodules and all kinds of carbuncles and masses. In addition, *chuan bei mu* inhibits the secretion of gastric acid, making it useful against peptic ulcers.

Seaweed and ecklonia function similarly to fritillaria and are often combined to counteract goiter. Ark shell neutralizes gastric acid, and so is often used for patients with acid regurgitation and stomachaches.

Herbs for relieving coughs and asthma are also used for treating chronic asthmatic bronchitis. Those commonly used:

ginkgo (*yin xing*)	apricot seed (*xing ren*)
aster (*zi wan*)	tussilago (*kuan dong hua*)
loquat leaf (*pi pa ye*)	

Since it nourishes the lungs and thereby clears sputum, ginkgo is beneficial in treating asthma and is often used in combination with *ma-huang (ma huang)* and perilla seed (*su zi*).

Apricot seed maintains the downward flow of *qi*, dissipates sputum and moistens the bowels, while aster and tussilago are often used together, though the former is more effective in relieving coughs.

Loquat leaf can relieve asmatic cough, as well as maintain the downward flow of *qi*, thereby alleviating vomiting. It is often combined with angelica (*ban zhi*) and bamboo shavings (*zhu ru*) to achieve an antiemetic effect.

Herbs which eliminate phlegm and restore consciousness are especially effective in quieting phlegmatic sounds in the throat, which are a result of phlegm invading the heart. Those herbs commonly selected:

acorus (*chang pu*)	polygala (*yuan zhi*)
arisaema (*tian nan xing*)	tabasheer (*tian zhu huang*)

Acorus is an aromatic, resurgent herb for resuscitation and the dissipation of phlegm. It is often combined with polygala and angelica (*bai zhi*) to treat patients whose heart meridians are obstructed by phlegm. Arisaema dissolves phlegm, prompting resuscitation, the expulsion of wind evil and relief from convulsions. Tabasheer is used for clearing heat and resolving phlegm, and so is prescribed for epilepsy and coughs due to heat.

Acupuncture and Moxibustion Treatment

Phlegm-dampness

- *gongsun* (Sp 4)
- *fenglong* (S 40)
- *pishu* (B 20)

Heat-phlegm

- *yanglingquan* (G 34)
- *fenglong* (S 40)
- *gongsun* (Sp 4)

Cold-phlegm

- *gongsun* (Sp 4)
- *fenglong* (S 40)
- *zhongwan* (CV 12)

Section 3
Blood Stasis

Blood stasis can either mean that blood flow throughout the body is impeded or that there exist localized sites of blood stagnation or internal hemorrhaging. Generally, stasis blood is a consequence of *qi* stagnancy or *qi* deficiency, both of which can impede blood flow and prompt blood coagulation. Blood stasis can also develop from trauma-induced internal hemorrhaging when the blood fails to disperse or be excreted in a timely manner. In turn, the formation of stagnant blood affects the movement of *qi* and blood throughout the body, giving rise to various pathological changes.

The principal symptoms of a blood stasis conformation are: a persistent, stabbing pain which is aggravated by pressure; tumors, especially hepatosplenomegalies and masses resulting from ruptures during ectopic pregnancies; and hemorrhages which are often dark blue and accompanied by blood clots, especially in the case of menstrual disorders or incessant lochia. Blood stasis also has some general manifestations, such as a dark-tinged complexion; scaly, dry skin; a dark purple tongue or a tongue with ecchymosis and etechiae; and a thready, hesitant pulse. If stagnant blood invades the heart, delirium or insanity may result.

Treatment promotes blood circulation and removes blood stasis with *Tang-kuei* Four Combination (*si wu tang*) and 4 *qian* each of persica (*tao ren*) and carthamus (*hong hua*). The resulting formula is called *Tang-kuei* Four Combination With Carthamus and Persica (*tao hong si wu tang*). *Tang-kuei* Four Combination can also be used with Cinnamon and Hoelen Formula (*gui zhi fu ling wan*), Persica and Rhubarb Combination (*tao he cheng qi tang*) or Persica and Achyranthes Combination (*xue fu zhu yu tang*).

Tang-kuei Four Combination[1]
Si Wu Tang
(Four-substance Decoction)[2]

Rehmannia, cooked	*Rehmanniae radix*	*Shu di huang*	4.0
Tang-kuei	*Angelicae radix*	*Dang gui*	4.0
Cnidium	*Cnidii rhizoma*	*Chuang xiong*	4.0
Peony	*Paeoniae radix*	*Shao yao*	4.0

Cinnamon and Hoelen Formula[1]

Gui Zhi Fu Ling Wan
(Cinnamon Twig and Poria Pill)[2]

Cinnamon twig	Cinnamomi ramulus	Gui zhi	4.0
Hoelen	Poria sclerotium	Fu ling	4.0
Moutan	Moutan radicis cortex	Mu dan pi	4.0
Persica	Persicae semen	Tao ren	4.0
Peony, red	Paeoniae rubra radix	Chi shao	4.0

Persica and Rhubarb Combination[1]

Tao He Cheng Qi Tang
(Peach Pit Decoction to Order the Qi)[2]

Persica*	Persicae semen	Tao ren	5.0
Cinnamon twig	Cinnamomi ramulus	Gui zhi	4.0
Rhubarb	Rhei rhizoma	Da huang	3.0
Mirabilitum	Natrium sulfuricum	Mang xiao	2.0
Licorice, baked	Glycyrrhizae radix	Zhi gan cao	1.5

* also known as peach pit

Persica and Achyranthes Combination

Xue Fu Zhu Yu Tang [8]
(Drive Out Stasis in the Mansion of Blood Decoction)[2]

Persica	Persicae semen	Tao ren	4.0
Carthamus	Carthami flos	Hong hua	3.0
Tang-kuei	Angelicae radix	Dang gui	3.0
Peony, red	Paeoniae rubra radix	Chi shao yao	3.0
Cnidium	Cnidii rhizoma	Chuan xiong*	2.0
Achyranthes	Achyranthis radix	Niu xi	3.0
Bupleurum	Bupleuri radix	Chai hu	2.0
Platycodon	Platycodi radix	Jie geng	2.0
Chih-ko	Citri fructus	Zhi ke	2.0
Rehmannia, raw	Rehmanniae radix	Sheng di huang	3.0
Licorice	Glycyrrhizae radix	Gan cao	2.0

*Ligustici rhizoma, also known as chuan xiong, may be substituted.

Functions: promotes blood circulation by removing blood stasis; promotes *qi* circulation; relieves pain.

Explanation: This formula consists of the main herbs for promoting blood circulation--persica, carthamus, red peony, cnidium and achyranthes--as well as auxiliary herbs for soothing the liver, promoting *qi* circulation and replenishing blood. *Tang-kuei* and raw rehmannia nourish and harmonize blood to prevent any possible impairment during the removal of stasis, while bupleurum, platycodon and *chih-ko* soothe the liver and promote *qi* circulation. Licorice can also benefit *qi* circulation, as well as coordinate the actions of the other ingredients. The movement of *qi* helps blood circulation and thereby reinforces the curative effect of the main herbs.

Herbs commonly used for promoting blood circulation are:

persica (*tao ren*)	carthamus (*hong hua*)
red peony (*chi shao*)	salvia (*dan sheng*)
cnidium (*chuan xiong*)	group beetle (*di bie chong*)
sparganium (*san ling*)	zedoaria (*er zhu*)
turmeric (*yu jin*)	lycopus (*ze lan*)
mugwort (*liu ji nu*)	sappan wood (*su mu*)
vaccaria (*wang bu liu xing*)	frankincense (*ru xiang*)
myrrh (*mo yao*)	pteropus (*wu ling zhi*)
leonurus (*yi mu cao*)	giant knotweed (*hu zhang*)

Of the above, persica and carthamus are the ones most commonly used for promoting blood circulation and removing blood stasis. When they are added to *Tang-kuei* Four Combination (*si wu tang*), the new combination is called *Tang-kuei* Four Combination With Carthamus and Persica (*tao hong si wu tang*), which is the basic formula for all blood circulation-promoting and blood stasis-removing formulas.

Every herb listed above can treat dysmenorrhea, amenorrhea, tumors, trauma, and pain in the chest or abdomen; however, all have other functions as well. For instance, persica can also moisten the bowels to relieve constipation and help the liver recover from fibrosis. Red peony relieves sore throats and severe icterohepatitis, while salvia thins the blood, making it a preventative herb for ischemic apoplexy. Cnidium is mainly used for migraines, while group beetle eliminates ascites due to cirrhosis of the liver, and sparganium and zedoaria are mainly used for hepatosplenomegaly. Turmeric soothes the liver and normalizes the secretion and discharge of bile. Lycopus, mugwort and sappan wood can correct menstrual disorders. Vaccaria promotes lactation and may be used for acute mastitis. Frankincense and myrrh are used as analgesics and, when taken before a meal, can treat patients with peptic ulcers. Pteropus can relieve pain. When it is combined with cattail pollen (*pu huang*), it is called Smiling Powder (*shi xiao san*), which is especially effective for relieving chest and abdominal pains. Leonurns is a diuretic, while giant knotweed is used for patients with arthralgia.

Acupuncture and Moxibustion Treatment

- *xuehai* (Sp 10)
- *sanyinjiao* (Sp 6)
- *pishu* (B 20)
- *geshu* (B 17)

Chapter 2

Conformation Differentiation and Treatment According to the Eight Guiding Principles

In traditional Chinese medicine, the eight guiding principles are the eight criteria by which diseases are differentiated, namely, interior and exterior, cold and heat, deficiency and excess, and *yin* and *yang*. Patient data, such as case history and symptoms and signs collected via the four diagnostic methods, are analyzed according to the patient's *zheng qi* (vital energy), the quantity and quality of the evils in the patient's body and the severity of the disease. Other differential diagnoses, such as differentiation of *zang* and *fu* (the solid and hollow organs) and of etiological conformations, are all based on the eight guiding principles.

Of these eight principles, *yin* and *yang* are the most comprehensive. *Yin* conformations are generally associated with interior, cold and deficiency, while *yang* conformations are allied with exterior, heat and excess. In practice, however, it is not that clear-cut, since opposite manifestations often interact. For example, both exterior and interior are of great importance in the differentiation of febrile diseases due to external evils. Similarly, both cold and heat are important in determining the nature of any given disease, and both serve as the basis for the choice and administration of warming or cooling herbs. Likewise, the severity of the deficiency or excess will determine the patient's *zheng* (resistance) to external evils, which, in turn, will dictate treatment for strengthening *zheng* and/or dispelling the evils.

In short, differentiation by means of the eight guiding principles does not mean that the principles can be considered in isolation from one another. The relationships between them are many and complex. The following discussion attempts to convey this complexity.

Concurrence

By concurrence we mean that two or more principles appear simultaneously. For example, when an exterior conformation is determined during the initial stages of an external feverish disease, it is often necessary to further analyze whether it is an exterior-cold or exterior-heat conformation. Similarly, when a deficiency conformation appears in chronic diseases, it is also necessary to differentiate between deficiency-cold and deficiency-heat. It must be pointed out that when two guiding principles appear, one is usually dominant, and, therefore, they cannot be given equal consideration.

Transformation

By transformation we mean one conformation changes into its opposite. For example, an exterior conformation in the initial stage of a feverish disease is characterized by headache, general pain, fever and an aversion to cold. But if the evil is too strong and the constitution too weak, or if the patient is not properly or promptly treated, the exterior conformation may transform into an interior one.

Combination of Opposites

By combination of opposites we mean the simultaneous appearance of two opposing principles, such as the simultaneous occurrence of a cold syndrome and a heat syndrome, or of deficiency and excess. The apparent, though false, appearance of one principle may occur during the course of a disease, such as the subjective sensation of being extremely cold while manifesting a fever or of the development of cancer (excess) in an AIDS (deficiency) patient. Therefore, in order to prescribe the proper treatment, it is necessary to base a diagnosis on the true syndrome, not on false appearances.

Section 1
Exterior and Interior

Exterior and interior indicate the location and severity of an illness. As encroachment by an external evil is usually from the exterior to the interior, it is necessary to make a differentiation between the two principles.

Exterior Conformations

The exterior location of the disease indicates that the illness is in an early stage and not yet serious. The manifestations are fever, chills, an aversion to wind, headache, general aching, arthralgia of the limbs, a thin, white tongue coating, a floating pulse, a stuffy nose, a sore throat and a cough. Exterior conformations are usually seen in upper respiratory-tract infections, acute infectious diseases and the early stages of other infectious diseases. Treatment is aimed at dispelling pathogenic evils from the exterior.

Since the nature of external evils may be either cold or heat, and since the defensive energy (*wei qi*) of any particular patient to resist these evils may be either strong or weak, exterior conformations can be further divided into conformations of exterior cold, exterior heat, exterior deficiency or exterior excess. Consequently, different therapies should be applied.

Exterior Cold

This conformation is characterized by an acute aversion to cold, a slight fever, headache, general aching, a thin, white, moist tongue coating and a floating, wiry pulse.

Treatment attempts to dispel external evils from the exterior with warm-propertied, pungent sudorifics. *Ma-huang* Combination (*ma huang tang*) or Schizonepeta and Siler Formula (*jing fang bai du san*) can be selected.

Exterior Heat

This conformation is characterized by fever with no significant aversion to cold, a sore throat, a thin, white and dry tongue coating, a red tongue tip and a floating, rapid pulse.

Treatment is designed to dispel external evils with cool-propertied, pungent herbs. Either Lonicera and Forsythia Formula (*yin qiao san*) or Morus and Chrysanthemum Combination (*sang ju yin*) can be selected.

Exterior Deficiency

Patients with this conformation exhibit an aversion to wind, profuse sweating and a floating, rapid pulse.

Treatment attempts to rectify an imbalance of the defensive and constructive energies. Cinnamon Combination (*gui zhi tang*) can be used.

Cinnamon Combination[1]

Gui Zhi Tang

(Cinnamon Twig Decoction)[2]

Cinnamon twig	*Cinnamomi ramulus*	*Gui zhi*	4.0
Peony	*Paeoniae radix*	*Shao yao*	4.0
Licorice	*Glycyrrhizae radix*	*Gan cao*	2.0
Ginger, fresh	*Zingiberis rhizoma*	*Sheng jiang*	4.0
Jujube	*Zizyphi fructus*	*Da zao*	4.0

Exterior Excess

Patients with this conformation display general body aches, an absence of sweat and a tense, floating pulse.

Treatment aims to dispel pathogenic evils from the exterior with warm-propertied, pungent sudorifics. *Ma-huang* Combination (*ma huang tang*) or Schizonepeta and Siler Formula (*jing fang bai du san*) can be used.

Interior Conformations

The appearance of interior conformations may be caused by any one of the following: an attack by one or more of the six external evils, which are transmitted to the interior from the outside; excessive or erratic emotional changes; immoderate diet; or fatigue, which directly affects the viscera, vital energy, blood and body fluids.

An interior conformation associated with a febrile disease caused by an external evil is generally manifested as an excess-heat conformation, though, occasionally, as deficiency-cold. Conformations of interior cold, heat, deficiency and excess are treated through warming, clearing, tonifying and purging, respectively.

Interior Cold

This conformation is manifested in a pale complexion; an aversion to cold; cold limbs; an absence of thirst or a preference for hot drinks; abdominal pain which is relieved by warm, loose stools; clear, profuse urine; a pale tongue with a white, slippery coating; and a submerged, slow pulse.

Treatment attempts to dispel cold and warm the middle energizer. Ginseng and Ginger Combination (*ren shen tang*) or Aconite and G.L. Combination (*si ni tang*) can be used.

Aconite and G.L. Combination[1]

Si Ni Tang
(Frigid Extremities Decoction)[2]

Aconite, prepared	*Aconiti carmichaelii praeparata radix*	*Zhi fu zi*	2.0
Ginger, dried	*Zingiberis siccatum rhizoma*	*Gan jiang*	1.5
Licorice, baked	*Glycyrrhizae radix*	*Zhi gan cao*	2.0

Interior Heat

This conformation is characterized by a flushed face, fever, restlessness, thirst, a desire for cold drinks, oliguria with reddish urine, constipation or foul-smelling diarrhea or bloody stools with pus, a cardinal red tongue with a yellow coating, and a rapid pulse.

The aims of treatment are the clearing of heat and the quieting of nervous behavior. Gypsum Combination (*bai hu tang*) or Coptis and Scute Combination (*huang lian jie du tang*) can be used.

If stools contain pus and blood, Anemone Combination (*bai tou weng tang*) can be used.

Anemone Combination[1]

Bai Tou Weng Tang
(Pulsatilla Decoction)[2]

Anemone	*Pulsatillae radix*	*Bai tou weng*	3.0
Coptis	*Coptidis rhizoma*	*Huang lian*	1.5
Fraxinus	*Fraxini cortex*	*Qin pi*	3.0
Phellodendron	*Phellodendri cortex*	*Huang bo*	3.0

Interior Deficiency

This conformation is generally associated with fatigue, lassitude, shortness of breath, a low voice, dizziness, palpitation, mental stupor, a poor appetite, loose stools, a thick tongue with a thin, white coating, and a weak pulse.

Strengthening *qi* and invigorating the vital functions of the spleen and stomach are the aims of treatment. Four Major Herb Combination (*si jun zi tang*), plus *Tang-kuei* Four Combination (*si wu tang*); or *Tang-kuei* and Ginseng Eight Combination (*ba zhen tang*); or Ginseng and *Tang-kuei* Ten Combination (*shi quan da bu tang*) can be selected.

Four Major Herb Combination[1]

Si Jun Zi Tang
(Four-gentleman Decoction)[2]

Ginseng	*Ginseng radix*	*Ren shen*	4.0
Atractylodes, white	*Atractylodis rhizoma*	*Bai zhu*	4.0
Hoelen	*Poria sclerotium*	*Fu ling*	4.0
Licorice	*Glycyrrhizae radix*	*Gan cao*	1.5

Tang-kuei and Ginseng Eight Combination[1]
Ba Zhen Tang
(Eight-treasure Decoction)[2]

Ginseng	*Ginseng radix*	*Ren shen*	3.0
Atractylodes, white	*Atractylodis rhizoma*	*Bai zhu*	3.0
Hoelen	*Poria sclerotium*	*Fu ling*	3.0
Rehmannia, cooked	*Rehmanniae radix*	*Shu di huang*	3.0
Tang-kuei	*Angelicae radix*	*Dang gui*	3.0
Peony	*Paeoniae radix*	*Shao yao*	3.0
Cnidium	*Cnidii rhizoma*	*Chuan xiong**	3.0
Licorice	*Glycyrrhizae radix*	*Gan cao*	1.5
Ginger, fresh	*Zingiberis rhizoma*	*Sheng jiang*	3.0
Jujube	*Zizyphi fructus*	*Da zao*	2.0

Ginseng and *Tang-kuei* Ten Combination[1]
Shi Quan Da Bu Tang
(All-inclusive Great Tonifying Decoction)[2]

Astragalus	*Astragali radix*	*Huang qi*	3.0
Cinnamon bark	*Cinnamomi cortex*	*Rou Gui*	1.0
Ginseng	*Ginseng radix*	*Ren shen*	3.0
Rehmannia, cooked	*Rehmanniae radix*	*Shu di huang*	3.0
Atractylodes, white	*Atractylodis rhizoma*	*Bai zhu*	3.0
Tang-kuei	*Angelicae radix*	*Dang gui*	3.0
Peony	*Paeoniae radix*	*Shao yao*	3.0
Cnidium	*Cnidii rhizoma*	*Chuan xiong**	3.0
Hoelen	*Poria sclerotium*	*Fu ling*	3.0
Licorice	*Glycyrrhizae radix*	*Gan cao*	1.0

Ligustici rhizoma, also known as *chuan xiong*, may be substituted.

Interior Excess

This conformation is characterized by painful abdominal distention which is aggravated by pressure, constipation, delirium, hydrothorax, ascites, a thick, yellow tongue coating and a submerged, excess pulse.

Treatment involves the use of cold-natured purgatives. Either Major Rhubarb Combination (*da cheng qi tang*) or Minor Rhubarb Combination (*xiao cheng qi tang*) can be selected.

Minor Rhubarb Combination[1]

Xiao Cheng Qi Tang

(Minor Order the *Qi* Decoction)[2]

Rhubarb	*Rhei rhizoma*	*Da huang*	2.0
Magnolia bark	*Magnoliae officinalis cortex*	*Hou pu*	3.0
Chih-shih	*Citri fructus immaturus*	*Zhi shi*	2.0

Half-exterior/Half-interior Conformations

A half-exterior/half-interior conformation entails disturbances between the exterior and the interior. The chief symptoms are: alternating spells of chills and fever, fullness of the chest and the hypochondrium, nausea, vomiting, loss of appetite, a bitter-tasting, dry mouth, a wiry pulse and a white or yellow tongue coating.

Treatment seeks to harmonize the exterior and interior. Minor Bupleurum Combination (*xiao chai hu tang*) can be used.

Minor Bupleurum Combination[1]
Xiao Chai Hu Tang
(Minor Bupleurum Decoction)[2]

Bupleurum	Bupleuri radix	Chai hu	3.0
Scute	Scutellariae radix	Huang qin	3.0
Pinellia	Pinellia rhizoma	Ban xia	2.0
Ginseng	Ginseng radix	Ren shen	3.0
Ginger, fresh	Zingiberis rhizoma	Sheng jiang	2.0
Licorice	Glycyrrhizae radix	Gan cao	1.0
Jujube	Zizyphi fructus	Da zao	3.0

Common Acupuncture and Moxibustion Points

Exterior Cold

- *dazhui* (GV 14)
- *fengfu* (GV 16)

Exterior Heat

- *quchi* (LI 11)
- *fengchi* (G 20)
- *hegu* (LI 4)

Exterior Deficiency or Exterior Excess

- *dazhui* (GV 14)

Interior Cold

- *shenque* (CV 8)
- *qihai* (CV 6)
- *guanyuan* (CV 4)

Interior Heat

- *taixi* (K 3)
- *fuliu* (K 7)

Interior Deficiency

1. Complicated by *qi* deficiency

- *qihai* (CV 6)

2. Complicated by blood deficiency

- *pishu* (B 20)
- *geshu* (B 17)

Interior Excess

- *tianshu* (S 25)
- *daheng* (Sp 15)

Half-exterior/Half-interior

- *dazhui* (GV 14)
- *fengfu* (GV 16)

Section 2
Cold and Heat

Cold and heat refer to the specific nature of an illness. Warming herbs are used to treat cold conformations and cooling herbs to treat heat conformations.

Cold Conformations

Cold conformations are provoked by cold evil or by excess *yin* due to a *yang* deficiency. The manifestations are: an aversion to cold; loss of the sense of taste; an absence of thirst; a pale complexion; cold limbs; clear, profuse urine; loose stools; a pale tongue with a moist, slippery coating; and a slow pulse.

Treatment is designed to warm *yang* and dispel cold. Aconite and G.L. Combination (*si ni tang*) or Aconite, Ginseng and Ginger Combination (*fu zi li zhong tang*) can be used.

Heat Conformations

Heat conformations are the result of excess *yang* due to heat evil or such pathological changes as fire arising from stagnation of other evils. The chief manifestations are: fever; a preference for cold beverages; thirst; a flushed face; congested eyes; fidgeting; restlessness; scanty, dark urine; constipation; a red tongue with a yellow, dry coating; and a rapid, excess pulse.

Treatment attempts to clear heat and purge fire. Forsythia and Rhubarb Formula (*liang ge san*) or Gypsum, Coptis and Scute Combination (*san huang shi gao tang*) can be used.

Forsythia and Rhubarb Formula[1]

Liang Ge San

(Cool the Diaphragm Powder)[2]

Rhubarb	*Rhei rhizoma*	*Da huang*	4.5
Mirabilitum	*Natrium sulfuricum*	*Mang xiao*	3.0
Scute	*Scutellariae radix*	*Huang qin*	3.0
Gardenia	*Gardeniae fructus*	*Zhi zi*	3.0
Forsythia	*Forsythiae fructus*	*Lian qiao*	3.0
Mentha	*Menthae herba*	*Bo he*	2.5
Licorice	*Glycyrrhizae radix*	*Gan cao*	2.5
Bamboo leaf	*Bambusae folium*	*Zhu ye*	1.0

Gypsum, Coptis and Scute Combination[1]

San Huang Shi Gao Tang

(Three-yellow and Gypsum Decoction)[2]

Gypsum	*Gypsum fibrosum*	*Shi gao*	10.0
Scute	*Scutellariae radix*	*Huang qin*	3.0
Coptis	*Coptidis rhizoma*	*Huang lian*	1.5
Phellodendron	*Phellodendri cortex*	*Huang bo*	1.5
Gardenia	*Gardeniae fructus*	*Zhi zi*	2.0
Ma-huang	*Ephedrae herba*	*Ma huang*	3.0
Soja	*Sojae semen praeparatum*	*Dan dou chi*	2.0
Ginger, fresh	*Zingiberis rhizoma*	*Sheng jiang*	1.0
Jujube	*Zizyphi fructus*	*Da zao*	3.0
Tea	*Camelliae folium*	*Cha ye*	1.0

Common Acupuncture and Moxibustion Points

Cold Conformation

- *shenque* (CV 8)
- *qihai* (CV 6)
- *guanyuan* (CV 4)

Heat Conformation

- *taixi* (K 3)
- *fuliu* (K 7)

Section 3
Deficiency and Excess

Deficiency and excess assist the practitioner in determining the patient's resistance (*zheng qi*) to disease and the strength of the pathogenic factors. Generally speaking, deficiency conformations are due to a lack of healthy energy and diminished resistance to disease, while excess conformations are associated with pathogenic evils.

Deficiency Conformations

Deficiency conformations are often due to a lack of proper care of the body, e.g. a lack of exercise, dysfunctions in digestive absorption, a severe or long-standing illness, or lack of proper treatment or the improper treatment of an illness. A deficiency conformation is characterized by listlessness, a pale complexion, lassitude, shortness of breath, an unwillingness to speak, emaciation, palpitation, loose stools, frequent urination, a pale tongue or a thick, tender tongue with little or no coating, and a weak pulse.

Treatment attempts to strengthen the middle energizer and replenish *qi*. Ginseng and Astragalus Combination (*bu zhong yi qi tang)* or Ginseng and *Tang-kuei* Ten Combination (*shi quan da bu tang*) can be used.

Ginseng and Astragalus Combination[1]

Bu Zhong Yi Qi Tang

(Tonify the Middle and Augment the *Qi* Decoction)[2]

Astragalus	Astragali radix	Huang qi	4.0
Ginseng	Ginseng radix	Ren shen	4.0
Atractylodes, white	Atractylodis rhizoma	Bai zhu	4.0
Ginger, fresh	Zingiberis rhizoma	Sheng jiang	2.0
Licorice, baked	Glycyrrhizae radix	Zhi gan cao	1.5
Tang-kuei	Angelicae radix	Dang gui	3.0
Cimicifuga	Cimicifugae rhizoma	Sheng ma	1.0
Bupleurum	Bupleuri radix	Chai hu	2.0
Citrus peel	Citri pericarpium	Chen pi	2.0
Jujube	Zizyphi fructus	Da zao	2.0

Excess Conformations

Excess conformations are the result of either of two conditions: (1) infection by external pathogenic factors or (2) the dysfunctioning of the internal organs or the patient's metabolism, either of which can lead to blood stasis or the accumulation and retention of water or phlegm. An excess conformation is characterized by a sturdy physique, coarse breathing, a loud voice, irritability, chest, hypochondriac and epigastric fullness, abdominal pain and tenderness, a high fever, a flushed face, constipation, a yellow, greasy tongue coating and an excess pulse.

Treatment is aimed at purging excess and eliminating evils. Major Rhubarb Combination (*da cheng qi tang*), Rhubarb and Mirabilitum Combination (*tiao wei cheng qi tang*) or Minor Rhubarb Combination (*xiao cheng qi tang*) can be used.

Rhubarb and Mirabilitum Combination[1]
Tiao Wei Cheng Qi Tang
(Regulate the Stomach and Order the *Qi* Decoction)[2]

Rhubarb	*Rhei rhizoma*	*Da huang*	2.5
Mirabilitum	*Natrium sulfuricum*	*Mang xiao*	1.0
Licorice	*Glycyrrhizae radix*	*Gan cao*	1.0

Common Acupuncture and Moxibustion Points

Qi Deficiency

- *qihai* (CV 6)

Blood Deficiency

- *pishu* (B 20)
- *geshu* (B 17)

Excess Conformation

- *daheng* (Sp 15)
- *tianshu* (S 15)

Section 4
Yin and *Yang*

Generally speaking, exterior, heat and excess fall under the category of *yang*, while interior, cold and deficiency are classified under *yin*. Therefore, every symptom and sign can be classified as associated either with a *yin* or a *yang* conformation. As regards the use of herbs for deficiency-cold or excess-heat conformations, see Sections 2 and 3 above. A discussion of *yin* deficiency, *yang* deficiency, *yin* depletion and *yang* depletion follows.

Yin Deficiency

Yin deficiency refers to an insufficiency of *yin* fluid, which leads to a relative abundance of *yang*, which, in turn, causes deficiency-heat. *Yin* deficiency is characterized by a low-grade fever which rises in the afternoon; night sweats; a flushed malar; a dry throat; a feverish sensation in the palms and soles; fidgeting; insomnia; emaciation; fatigue; dizziness; blurred vision; scanty, dark yellow urine; constipation; a fissured tongue or a red tongue with scant coating; and a weak, rapid pulse.

Treatment aims to nourish *yin* and remove heat. *Chin-chiu* and Turtle Shell Formula (*qin jiao bie jia san*) or Phellodendron Combination (*zi yin jiang huo tang*) can be used.

Phellodendron Combination[1]

Zi Yin Jiang Huo Tang

(Nourish *Yin* and Reduce Fire Decoction)

Tang-kuei	Angelicae radix	Dang gui	2.5
Peony	Paeoniae radix	Shao yao	2.5
Asparagus	Asparagi radix	Tian men dong	2.5
Ophiopogon	Ophiopogonis rhizoma	Mai men dong	2.5
Atractylodes, white	Atractylodis rhizoma	Bai zhu	3.0
Rehmannia	Rehmanniae radix	Di huang	2.5
Citrus peel	Citri pericarpium	Chen pi	2.5
Phellodendron	Phellodendri cortex	Huang bo	1.5
Anemarrhena	Anemarrhenae rhizoma	Zhi mu	1.5
Licorice	Glycyrrhizae radix	Gan cao	1.5

Yang Deficiency

Yang deficiency refers to an insufficiency of *yang qi*, which leads to a relative abundance of *yin*, which, in turn, causes deficiency-cold. *Yang* deficiency is characterized by an intolerance of cold, cold limbs, fatigue, spontaneous perspiration, shortness of breath, an unwillingness to speak, loss of the sensation of taste, an absence of thirst, profuse, transparent urine, loose stools, a pale tongue with a white coating, and a weak pulse. Treatment is designed to warm and tonify *yang*, for which Aconite Combination (*fu zi tang*) can be used.

Aconite Combination[1]
Fu Zi Tang
(Prepared Aconite Decoction)[2]

Aconite, prepared	*Aconiti carmichaelii praeparata radix*	*Zhi fu zi*	1.0
Atractylodes, white	*Atractylodis rhizoma*	*Bai zhu*	5.0
Ginseng	*Ginseng radix*	*Ren shen*	3.0
Hoelen	*Poria sclerotium*	*Fu ling*	4.0
Peony	*Paeoniae radix*	*Shao yao*	4.0

Yin Depletion

Yin depletion is characterized by a sticky, sweet, dry mouth, a desire for cold drinks, irritability, an aversion to heat, fever, warm limbs, a red, prickly and dry tongue and a weak pulse.

Treatment attempts to supplement *qi* and astringe *yin*. Ginseng and Ophiopogon Formula (*sheng mai san*) can be used.

Ginseng and Ophiopogon Formula
Sheng Mai San[11]
(Generate the Pulse Powder)[2]

Ginseng	*Ginseng radix*	*Ren shen*	3.0
Ophiopogon	*Ophiopogonis rhizoma*	*Mai men dong*	3.0
Schizandra	*Schizandrae fructus*	*Wu wei zi*	2.0

Functions: replenishes *qi* to arrest sweating; nourishes *yin* to promote the production of body fluids.

Explanation: Ginseng replenishes *qi* to arrest sweating. Ophiopogon nourishes *yin* and clears heat. Schizandra strengthens *yin* fluid to stop sweating and tonifies heart *qi*. This formula is effective in treating *qi* or *yin* depletion or lung deficiency with a chronic cough.

Yang Depletion

Yang depletion is characterized by cold skin due to profuse sweating, cold limbs, a pathetic expression or listlessness, an absence of thirst or thirst with a desire for hot beverages, a pale tongue and an indistinct pulse. These symptoms usually appear at the "shock stage" of the disease.

Treatment aims to revive depleted *yang*. G.L. and Aconite Combination with Ginseng (*si ni jia ren shen tang*) or Dragon Bone, Oyster Shell, Ginseng and Aconite Combination (*shen ju long mu tang*) can be used.

G.L. and Aconite Combination with Ginseng[1]

Si Ni Jia Ren Shen Tang

(Frigid Extremities Decoction plus Ginseng)[2]

Aconite, prepared	*Aconiti carmichaelii praeparata radix*	Zhi Fu zi	2.0
Ginger, dried	*Zingiberis siccatum rhizoma*	Gan jiang	2.0
Licorice	*Glycyrrhizae radix*	Gan cao	3.0
Ginseng	*Ginseng radix*	Ren shen	2.0

Dragon Bone, Oyster Shell, Ginseng and Aconite Combination

Shen Fu Long Mu Tang

(Dragon Bone, Oyster Shell, Ginseng and Aconite Decoction)

Dragon bone	*Draconis os*	*Long gu*	5.0
Oyster shell	*Ostreae testa*	*Mu li*	10.0
Ginseng	*Ginseng radix*	*Ren shen*	2.0
Aconite, prepared	*Aconiti carmichaelii praeparata radix*	*Zhi fu zi*	2.0

Common Acupuncture and Moxibustion Points

Yin Deficiency

- *taixi* (K 3)
- *fuliu* (K 7)

Yang Deficiency

- *dazhui* (GV 14)
- *taodao* (GV 13)

Yin Depletion

- *sanyinjiao* (Sp 6)

Yang Depletion

- *shenque* (CV 8)

Chapter 3

The Differentiation of Visceral Conformations and Their Treatment with Herbs and Formulas

Known since ancient times as *zang xiang*, the traditional Chinese medicine (TCM) theory of the viscera deals with the physiological activities, pathological changes and interconnectedness of the organs. According to this theory, the heart, liver, spleen, lungs, kidneys and other internal material are not simply anatomical structures, but physiological and pathological concepts as well.

Physiologically and pathologically, the solid and hollow organs are closely related. Additionally, they have an inseparable relationship with the skin, muscles, blood vessels, tendons, bones, nose, mouth, tongue, eyes, ears and external genitalia. Because of this interdependence, TCM theory necessitates an understanding of the human body as a dynamic whole, not a collection of disconnected, independent parts. Similarly, the diagnosis and treatment of the body necessitates such a holistic approach. The determination of conformations, or symptom-complexes, is the strategy by which differentiation is made, while still retaining this holism.

According to TCM theory, the viscera fall into three categories: (1) the six hollow organs; (2) the five solid organs; and (3) the six miscellaneous or curious organs.

The six hollow organs, also known as *fu* or as the *yang* organs, are associated with the exterior guiding principle discussed in the last chapter. The five solid organs are known as *zang* or as the *yin* organs and are associated with the interior guiding principle, which was also discussed in Chapter 2. The solid organs are often paired with the hollow organs as follows: heart and small intestine; lungs and large intestine; spleen and stomach; liver and gallbladder; kidneys and urinary bladder; and the sixth solid organ, the pericardium, which is sometimes paired with the triple energizer.

The six miscellaneous or curious organs, known as *qi heng zhi fu*, are the brain, marrow, bones, blood vessels, uterus and, again, the gallbladder.

Section 1
The Heart and Small Intestine

According to both traditional Chinese and Western medicine, the heart regulates the blood and its circulation throughout the body. It is here, however, that similarity in their viewpoints ends.

While Western medicine contends that the heart governs mental functions and so attributes fainting to an insufficient supply of blood to the brain, TCM maintains that a ruddy complexion signals good blood circulation and a pale complexion is a sign of heart blood deficiency. Palpitation and shortness of breath are attributable to heart deficiency, while heart *qi* deficiency results in *shen* deficiency and heart *qi* excess can bring on manic-depression.

According to TCM theory, the heart's orifice is the tongue, and an erosive, sore, red tongue tip indicates a flaring-up of heart fire. Western physicians point to the relationship between the heart and riboflavin metabolism, noting that insufficient riboflavin induces glossitis.

Diagnosis and Herbal Treatment

Heart *Qi* and Heart *Yang* Deficiencies

Heart *qi* deficiency is generally characterized by a lusterless complexion, dizziness, palpitation, shortness of breath, a stuffy feeling in the chest, a weak or irregular pulse, and a light, thick tongue coating. In addition to these manifestations, heart *yang* deficiency is marked by cold limbs, an aversion to cold, and a dark-gray or bluish-purple complexion. Heart *yang* deficiency is especially common in patients with cardiogenic shock or other diseases in the shock stage.

Treatment is designed to reinforce heart *qi*, nourish the heart and relieve anxiety or stress. Astragalus and Zizyphus Combination (*yang xin tang*) can be used.

If a knotty, intermittent pulse is felt, Baked Licorice Combination (*zhi gan cao tang*) is recommended.

When heart *yang* is deficient, it should be restored to prevent total collapse. G.L. and Aconite Combination with Ginseng (*si ni jia ren shen tang*) is also highly recommended.

Astragalus and Zizyphus Combination[1]

Yang Xin Tang
(Nourish the Heart Decoction)[2]

Astragalus	*Astragali radix*	Huang qi	4.0
Hoelen	*Poria sclerotium*	Fu ling	4.0
Fu-shen	*Poria cor*	Fu shen	4.0
Cnidium	*Cnidii rhizoma*	Chuan xiong*	4.0
Tang-kuei	*Angelicae radix*	Dang gui	4.0
Pinellia	*Pinellia rhizoma*	Ban xia	4.0
Ginseng	*Ginseng radix*	Ren shen	1.0
Biota	*Biotae semen*	Bo zi ren	1.0
Cinnamon bark	*Cinnamomi cortex*	Gui pi	1.0
Schizandra	*Schizandrae fructus*	Wu wei zi	1.0
Polygala	*Polygalae radix*	Yuan zhi	1.0
Licorice, baked	*Glycyrrhizae radix*	Zhi gan cao	0.5
Zizyphus	*Zizyphi spinosi semen*	Suan zao ren	1.0

**Ligustici rhizoma*, also known as *chuan xiong*, may be substituted.

Baked Licorice Combination[1]

Zhi Gan Cao Tang
(Honey-fried Licorice Decoction)[2]

Licorice, baked	*Glycyrrhizae radix*	Zhi gan cao	3.0
Ginseng	*Ginseng radix*	Ren shen	3.0
Rehmannia, raw	*Rehmanniae radix*	Sheng di huang	6.0
Ophiopogon	*Ophiopogonis rhizoma*	Mai meng dong	6.0
Linum	*Cannabis semen*	Ma zi ren	3.0
Gelatin	*Asini gelatinum*	A jiao	2.0
Cinnamon twig	*Cinnamomi ramulus*	Gui zhi	3.0
Ginger, fresh	*Zingiberis rhizoma*	Sheng jiang	3.0
Jujube	*Zizyphi fructus*	Da zao	3.0

Heart Blood and Heart *Yin* Deficiencies

Heart blood deficiency is marked by a pale complexion, palpitation, a poor memory or memory loss, insomnia, drowsiness, anxiety, a light-colored tongue coating, and a rapid or floating and thready pulse.

A deficiency of heart blood should be treated by enriching the blood, nourishing the heart and relieving mental distress. Ginseng and Longan Combination (*gui pi tang*) and Licorice and Jujube Combination (*gan mai da zao tang*) can be used.

Fidgeting, hectic fever, flushed cheeks, a feverish sensation in the palms and soles, night sweats, dry mouth and throat, a red tongue with little saliva, and a thready and rapid pulse are characteristic of heart *yin* deficiency.

To nourish heart *yin*, Ginseng and Zizyphus Formula (*tian wang bu xin dan*) can be used.

Ginseng and Longan Combination[1]
Gui Pi Tang
(Restore the Spleen Decoction)[2]

Ginseng	Ginseng radix	Ren shen	3.0
Astragalus	Astragali radix	Huang qi	2.0
Tang-kuei	Angelicae radix	Dang gui	2.0
Longan aril	Longanae arillus	Long yan rou	3.0
Atractylodes, white	Atractylodis rhizoma	Bai zhu	3.0
Saussurea	Saussureae radix	Mu xiang	1.0
Hoelen	Poria sclerotium	Fu ling	3.0
Polygala	Polygalae radix	Yuan zhi	1.0
Zizyphus	Zizyphi spinosi semen	Suan zao ren	3.0
Licorice, baked	Glycyrrhizae radix	Zhi gan cao	1.0
Ginger, fresh	Zingiberis rhizoma	Sheng jiang	1.0
Jujube	Zizyphi fructus	Da zao	3.0

Licorice and Jujube Combination[1]
Gan Mai Da Zao Tang[10]
(Licorice, Wheat and Jujube Decoction)[2]

Licorice	Glycyrrhizae radix	Gan cao	5.0
Light wheat	Tritici fructus	Fu xiao mai	10.0
Jujube	Zizyphi fructus	Da zao	9.0

Ginseng and Zizyphus Formula[1]

Tian Wang Bu Xin Dan

(Emperor of Heaven's Special Pill to Tonify the Heart)[2]

Rehmannia, raw	*Rehmanniae radix*	*Sheng di huang*	1.2
Scrophularia	*Scrophulariae radix*	*Xuan shen*	1.2
Ophiopogon	*Ophiopogonis rhizoma*	*Mai men dong*	1.2
Asparagus	*Asparagi radix*	*Tian men dong*	1.2
Salvia	*Salviae miltiorrhizae radix*	*Dan shen*	1.2
Tang-kuei	*Angelicae radix*	*Dang gui*	1.2
Hoelen	*Poria sclerotium*	*Fu ling*	1.2
Biota	*Biotae semen*	*Bo zi ren*	1.2
Polygala	*Polygalae radix*	*Yuan zhi*	1.2
Schizandra	*Schizandrae fructus*	*Wu wei zi*	1.0
Zizyphus	*Zizyphi spinosi semen*	*Suan zao ren*	1.2
Platycodon	*Platycodi radix*	*Jie geng*	1.2
Cinnabar	*Cinnabaris*	*Zhu sha*	1.0
Ginseng	*Ginseng radix*	*Ren shen*	1.2

Flaring-up of Heart Fire

Characterized by oral and lingual erosion and pain, fidgeting, insomnia, thirst, dark yellow urine, constipation, a red tongue tip, and a wiry and rapid pulse, heart fire can be extinguished through the use of Coptis and Rhubarb Combination (*san huang xie xin tang*).

Coptis and Rhubarb Combination[1]

San Huang Xie Xin Tang

(Purge Heat from the Heart and Stomach Decoction)[1]

Rhubarb	*Rhei rhizoma*	*Da huang*	1.0
Scute	*Scutellariae radix*	*Huang qin*	1.0
Coptis	*Coptidis rhizoma*	*Huang lian*	1.0

Heart Blood Stagnancy

Heart blood stagnancy manifests itself in palpitation, chest stuffiness, intermittent pain in the heart region, a dark red or purple-spotted tongue, and a weak, hesitant pulse or an irregular or intermittent pulse. In severe cases, there may be cyanosis on the face, lips or fingernails, as well as cold limbs and sweating.

Treatment is aimed at the removal of obstructions to the flow of *qi*, the reinforcement of *yang* and the removal of blood stasis. Appropriate formulas are Trichosanthes, Bakeri and Pinellia Combination (*gua lou xie bai ban xia tang*) and Salvia and Carthamus Combination (*guan xin er hao*).

Trichosanthes, Bakeri and Pinellia Combination[1]

Gua Lou Xie Bai Ban Xia Tang[10]

(Trichosanthes Fruit, Chinese Chive and Pinellia Decoction)[2]

Trichosanthes fruit	*Trichosanthis fructus*	*Gua lou*	3.0
Bakeri*	*Allii chinensis bulbus*	*Xie bai*	4.5
Pinellia	*Pinellia rhizoma*	*Ban xia*	6.0

*also known as Chinese chive

Salvia and Carthamus Combination

Guan Xin Er Hao

(Coronary Heart Disease Formula No. II)

Salvia	*Salviae miltiorrhizae radix*	*Dan shen*	10.0
Carthamus	*Carthami flos*	*Hong hua*	3.0
Peony, red	*Paeoniae rubra radix*	*Chi shao*	3.0
Cnidium	*Cnidii rhizoma*	*Chuan xiong**	2.0
Acronychia	*Acronychiae lignum*	*Jiang xiang*	3.0

Ligustici rhizoma, also known as *chuan xiong*, may be substituted.

Functions: promotes blood circulation in order to remove blood stasis; activates *qi* circulation to relieve pain.

Explanation: The main herbs of this formula--salvia, carthamus, red peony and cnidium--invigorate blood circulation and eliminate blood stasis, while acronychia promotes *qi* circulation. All five herbs augment each other, since blood circulation is stimulated when *qi* circulation is enhanced.

This formula has been proved effective against lingering angina pectoris and acute myocardial infarction by practitioners at Xi Yuan Hospital of the Academy of Traditional Chinese Medicine in Beijing. If chest stuffiness and angina pectoris cannot be relieved, Styrax Formula (*su he xiang wan*) should also be given.

Styrax Formula
Su He Xiang Wan[9]
(Liquid Styrax Pill)[2]

Styrax	*Styrax liquidis*	*Su he xiang*	2.0
Benzoin	*Benzoinum*	*An xi xiang*	4.0
Musk	*Moschus*	*She xiang*	4.0
Aquilaria	*Aquilariae lignum*	*Chen xiang*	4.0
Clove	*Caryophylli flos*	*Ding xiang*	4.0
Aristolochia	*Aristolochiae radix*	*Qing mu xiang*	4.0
Rhinoceros horn	*Rhinocerotis cornu*	*Xi jiao*	4.0
Cyperus	*Cyperi rhizoma*	*Xiang fu*	4.0
Cinnabar	*Cinnabaris*	*Zhu sha*	4.0
Terminalia	*Chebulae fructus*	*Ke zi*	4.0
Santalum	*Santali lignum*	*Tan xiang*	4.0
Piper	*Piperis fructus*	*Pi bo*	4.0
Borneol	*Borneolum*	*Bing pian*	2.0
Frankincense	*Olibanum*	*Ru xiang*	2.0

Styrax Formula is administered in 3-*qian* boluses which are taken one at a time by breaking into pieces and swallowing with warm water.

Functions: aids in the restoration of consciousness; eliminates heart fire; alleviates depression.

Explanation: A great number of active aromatic herbs are gathered in this formula in order to enhance *qi* circulation and restore consciousness. Especially useful are styrax oil, benzoin, musk and borneol. They are supplemented by aquilaria, aristolochia, santalum, cyperus, frankincense, clove and piper to correct stagnant *qi* and blood in the viscera and to reinforce the resuscitative actions of the aromatic herbs. Rhinoceros horn can lessen virulence and clear heart fire. Cinnabar acts as a sedative, while terminalia both disintegrates evil *qi* and astringes vital *qi*.

Traditionally, this formula was used to treat coma due to apoplexy or pestilent diseases. More recently, it has been found effective in the treatment of angina pectoris.

Heart Confused by Phlegm

Typical manifestations are mental confusion, unconsciousness, the vomiting of phlegm or phlegmatic sounds in the throat, speech difficulties due to a stiff tongue, a white, creamy tongue coating and a slippery pulse.

Treatment is aimed at removing phlegm, regulating *qi* circulation and restoring consciousness. Either Hoelen and Bamboo Combination (*wen dan tang*), combined with 6 *qian* each of arisaema with bile (*dan nan xing*), acorus (*chang pu*) and ginseng (*ren shen*); or Hoelen and Bamboo Combination with 3 *qian* coptis (*huang lian*) can be selected.

Hoelen and Bamboo Combination[1]

Wen Dan Tang

(Warm the Gallbladder Decoction)[2]

Pinellia	Pinellia rhizoma	Ban xia	3.0
Citrus peel	Citri pericarpium	Chen pi	2.5
Hoelen	Poria sclerotium	Fu ling	6.0
Chih-shih	Citri fructus immaturus	Zhi shi	1.5
Bamboo shavings	Bambusae caulis in taeniis	Zhu ru	2.0
Licorice	Glycyrrhizae radix	Gan cao	1.0
Jujube	Zizyphi fructus	Da zao	3.0

Disturbance of Phlegm-fire in the Heart

This condition is typically characterized by mental confusion, unprovoked laughing and weeping, mania, erratic or uncontrolled behavior, a flushed face, short and rapid breathing, thirst, red-tinged urine, a creamy, yellow tongue coating, and a slippery, rapid and excess pulse.

Lapis and Scute Formula (*meng shi gun tan wan*) can be used to remove phlegm and purge fire.

Lapis and Scute Formula

Meng Shi Gun Tan Wan[11]

(Phlegm-dispelling Pill)[9]

Rhubarb	Rhei rhizoma*	Da huang	180.0
Chlorite schist	Lapis chloriti**	Meng shi	30.0
Scute	Scutellariae radix	Huang qin	30.0
Aquilaria	Aquilariae lignum	Chen xiang	15.0

* steam with wine
** char until brittle

The above ingredients are smashed to make a powder, which is then mixed with water and prepared in pill form. The recommended dose is one pill swallowed with warm water, though the number of pills may be increased to reflect the severity of the patient's condition.

Functions: reduces fire; removes phlegm.

Explanation: Rhubarb, scute and aquilaria clear fire, purge excess, suppress phlegm fire and, indeed, eliminate the source of fire and phlegm. They are aided by chlorite schist, which also serves to counteract and dispel chronic, insidious and stubborn phlegm. In short, all the herbs affect the descent of phlegm and fire, thereby diminishing fire and dispelling phlegm.

Excess Heat in the Small Intestine

As a *yang* organ, the heart relates to the exterior, while the small intestine, as a *yin* organ, is associated with the interior. Since these two are paired, flaring fire in the heart can migrate to the small intestine and result in excess heat. This morbid condition is manifested by dark urine, short and painful urination or even hematuria, fidgeting, a painful tongue, oral erosion, a red tongue with a yellowish coating, and a rapid pulse.

Purging heart fire and clearing fire from the small intestine through the use of diuretics are the main treatment principles for this conformation. Rehmannia and Akebia Formula (*dao chi san*), plus 1.5 *qian* coptis (*huang lian*), can be used.

Summary of Herbs for Heart Disease

Herbs for Reinforcing Heart *Qi*

ginseng (*ren shen*)	codonopsis (*dang shen*)
lotus seed (*lian zi*)	pseudostellaria root (*tai zi shen*)

Herbs for Warming Heart *Yang*

prepared aconite (*zhi fu zi*)	cinnamon twig (*fu zhi*)

Herbs for Removing Obstructions to Vital Energy and Reinforcing Vital Functions of Heart *Yang*

trichosanthes fruit (*gua lou*)   bakeri (*xie bai*)

Herbs for Enriching Heart Blood

tang-kuei (*dang gui*)   cooked rehmannia (*shu di huang*)
gelatin (*a jiao*)

Herbs for Nourishing Heart *Yin*

ophiopogon (*mai men dong*)   egg yolk (*ji zi huang*)
light wheat (*fu xiao mai*)

Herbs for Clearing Heart Fire

coptis (*huang lian*)   picrorrhiza (*hu huang lian*)
forsythia center (*lian qiao xin*) lotus embryo (*lian zi xin*)
lophatherum (*dan zhu ye*)

Herbs for Reducing Anxiety

zizyphus (*suan zao ren*)   polygala (*yuan zhi*)
biota (*bo zi ren*)   longan aril (*long yan rou*)
fu-shen (*fu shen*)   albizzia (*he huan pi*)
juncus (*deng xin cao*)

Herbs for Restoring Consciousness

rhinoceros horn (*xi jiao*)   cow gallstone (*niu huang*)
acorus (*shi cang pu*)   turmeric (*yu jin*)
arisaema with bile (*dan nan xing*)

Common Acupuncture and Moxibustion Points

For Reinforcing Heart *Qi*

- *tanzhong* (CV 17) - *shengjue* (CV 8, moxibustion)

For Warming Heart *Yang*

- *jujue* (CV 14) - *tongli* (H 5)

For Nourishing Heart Blood

- *xinshu* (B 15) - *geshu* (B 17)

For Nourishing Heart *Yin*

- *shenmen* (H 7)
- *daling* (P 7)

For Clearing Heart Fire

- *qiangu* (SI 2)
- *xinshu* (B 15)

For Relief of Anxiety and Tension

- *shaohai* (H 3)
- *tongli* (H 5)
- *neiguan* (P 6)

For Restoring Consciousness

- *baihui* (GV 20)
- *renzhong* (GV 26)

Treatment Method

1. The reducing method should be used in the case of an excess conformation, while the reinforcing method, or moxibustion, is recommended for the treatment of deficiency conformations.

2. Treat once or twice daily for 10-20 days.

3. These general guidelines hold for conformations discussed in the following sections as well.

Section 2
The Liver and Gallbladder

According to TCM theory, blood is stored in the liver. Consequently, TCM practitioners attribute hemoptysis, nose bleeds and menorrhalgia to the liver's inability to store blood. In contrast, Western medical science contends that blood is not stored anywhere in the body, but is rather in constant motion. A Western practitioner, therefore, cites the liver and spleen as temporary reservoirs for the blood which is being purified.

While TCM holds that the liver controls the hypochondrium and the tendons, Western medicine makes the lesser claim that the liver and spleen are merely located in hypochondrium. A conventional practitioner sees the liver as related to vitamin A metabolism and the proper functioning of neurotransmitters, while the Chinese doctor points to the eyes as the liver's orifices. For this reason, liver deficiency manifests itself in blurry vision, night blindness and red eyes.

Other TCM-diagnosed ailments include liver *qi* stagnation, which causes hypochondriac and chest pain; liver wind, which results in convulsions and spasms; and liver heat, which induces mastitis. Furthermore, as the liver meridians pass through the vertex, throat, eyes, chest and genitals, their function may possibly be related to the nervous and endocrine systems, and, consequently, heat-dampness in the liver meridians results in itching and pain of the vulva or leukorrhea with reddish discharge.

Diagnosis and Herbal Treatment
Deficiencies of Liver *Yin* and Liver Blood

Dizziness, blurred vision, dry eyes, night blindness, numbness of the limbs, tendon spasms, a dry mouth and throat, pain in the hypochondriac region, irregular menstruation, a red tongue with scant coating, and a thready, wiry and rapid pulse characterize deficiencies of liver *yin* and liver blood.

Treatment attempts to nourish liver *yin* or liver blood. Glehnia and Rehmannia Combination (*yi guan jian*), plus 3 *qian* ligusticum (*nu zhen zi*), can be selected for this purpose.

Glehnia and Rehmannia Combination
Yi Guan Jian[12]
(Linking Decoction)[2]

Glehnia	*Glehniae radix cum rhizoma*	Sha shen	3.0
Ophiopogon	*Ophiopogonis rhizoma*	Mai men dong	3.0
Tang-kuei	*Angelicae radix*	Dang gui	3.0
Rehmannia, raw	*Rehmanniae radix*	Sheng di	6.0
Lycium fruit	*Lycii fructus*	Gou qi zi	3.0
Melia	*Meliae toosendan fructus*	Chuan lian zi	6.0

Functions: nourishes liver *yin* and liver blood.

Explanation: As a general rule, liver *qi* stagnation may be relieved by pungent and aromatic herbs, however, if both liver and kidney deficiencies are present, these herbs can damage *qi* and *yin* alike.

In such a case, Glehnia and Rehmannia Combination is recommended as a means of safely and effectively nourishing liver blood and liver *yin*. In this formula, a delicate balance between relieving *qi* and tonifying *yin* is achieved. Without such a balance, those herbs which promote *qi* circulation would also tend to deplete body fluids, thereby diminishing *yin*.

Glehnia and ophiopogon nourish *yin* and promote the secretion of saliva and body fluids, while *tang-kuei*, rehmannia and lycium nourish liver *yin*, blood, the liver and the kidneys. Melia has a cold, bitter flavor and can soothe and harmonize liver *qi* in such a way that it does not adversely affect *yin*. When combined, these herbs harmonize liver *qi* and replenish body fluids, thereby relieving *yin* deficiency and *qi* stagnancy.

Because of the nourishing herbs in this formula, it is contraindicated for patients with weak spleens or stomachs, or those with phlegm or dampness stagnation.

Liver *Qi* Stagnancy

Depression, irritability, a distended pain in the hypochondrium, chest stuffiness, poor appetite, eructation, abdominal distention, abnormal bowel movements, and the sensation of an obstruction in the throat characterize liver *qi* stagnancy. In women, irregular menstruation, dysmenorrhea, premenstrual soreness of the breasts, a thin, white tongue coating and a wiry pulse may also be present. If *qi* stagnancy is complicated by blood stasis, twinges in the hypochondrium (or possibly hepatosplenomegaly), a dark purple tongue with petechiae or ecchymoses along the edges, and a wiry, hesitant pulse are frequently observed.

In general, treatment is aimed at soothing the liver and regulating *qi*. *Tang-kuei* and Bupleurum Formula (*xiao yao san*) can be used. When the patient complains of the sensation of a throat obstruction, this is known as *mei he qi* (plum pit *qi*) and can be treated with Pinellia and Magnolia Combination (*ban xia hou pu tang*) to regulate *qi* and dissipate sputum.

Tang-kuei and Bupleurum Formula[1*]

Xiao Yao San
(Rambling Powder)[2]

Bupleurum	*Bupleuri radix*	Chai hu	3.0
Tang-kuei	*Angelicae radix*	Dang gui	3.0
Peony	*Paeoniae radix*	Shao yao	3.0
Atractylodes	*Atractylodis rhizoma*	Bai zhu	3.0
Hoelen	*Poria sclerotium*	Fu ling	3.0
Mentha	*Menthae herba*	Bo he	1.0
Ginger, fresh	*Zingiberis rhizoma*	Sheng jiang	2.0
Licorice, baked	*Glycyrrhizae radix*	Zhi gan cao	1.5

* also known as Bupleurum and *Tang-kuei* Formula

When both *qi* and blood are stagnant, the aims of treatment are the regulation of *qi*, the activation of blood circulation and the removal of blood stasis. These objectives can be achieved with the administration of Persica and Achyranthes Combination (*xue fu zhu yu tang*).

Pinellia and Magnolia Combination[1]

Ban Xia Hou Pu Tang
(Pinellia and Magnolia Bark Decoction)[2]

Pinellia	*Pinellia rhizoma*	Ban xia	4.0
Magnolia bark	*Magnoliae officinalis cortex*	Hou pu	3.0
Perilla leaf	*Perillae folium*	Zi su ye	2.0
Hoelen	*Poria sclerotium*	Fu ling	5.0
Ginger, fresh	*Zingiberis rhizoma*	Sheng jiang	2.0

Flaring-up of Liver Fire

Distending pain in the head, dizziness, a flushed face, red eyes, irritability, a bitter taste in the mouth, a dry throat, a burning pain in the costal region, tinnitus, hearing loss, dark yellow urine, constipation, hematemesis, epistaxis, a red tongue with a yellow coating, and a wiry, rapid pulse are all characteristic of liver fire.

Liver fire can be quenched with *Tang-kuei*, Gentian and Aloe Formula (*dang gui long hui wan*).

Tang-kuei, Gentian and Aloe Formula
Dang Gui Long Hui Wan[9]
(*Tang-kuei*, Gentian *Longdancao* and Aloe Pill)[2]

Tang-kuei	Angelicae radix	Dang gui	30.0
Gentian	Gentianae scabrae radix	Long dan cao	30.0
Scute	Scutellariae radix	Huang qin	30.0
Coptis	Coptidis rhizoma	Huang lian	30.0
Phellodendron	Phellodendri cortex	Huang bo	30.0
Gardenia	Gardeniae fructus	Zhi zi	30.0
Rhubarb	Rhei rhizoma	Da huang	15.0
Aloe	Aloe	Lu hui	15.0
Indigo, natural	Indigo naturalis	Qing dai	15.0
Saussurea	Saussureae radix	Mu xiang	7.5
Musk	Moschus	She xiang	3.0

The above herbs are ground into a powder, mixed with *shen-chu* (*shen qu*) and water to form a paste and then made into 2-*qian* pills, which are taken two to three times daily with warm water.

Functions: quenches liver fire; purges heat; clears the bowels.

Explanation: *Tang-kuei*, Gentian and Aloe Formula is based on Coptis and Scute Combination (*huang lian jie du tang*), which is composed of scute, coptis, phellodendron and gardenia. Combined with rhubarb, aloe and indigo, these herbs can clear the bowels and purge heat and fire. Thus, the formula has strong curative effects on liver and gallbladder fire, which is marked by dizziness, headache, anxiety, convulsions, palpitation and constipation.

The primary difference between this formula and Gentian Combination (*long dan xie gan tang*) is that, while the latter purges excess heat of the liver and gallbladder through the urine, the former does so through the feces.

Heat-dampness in the Liver and Gallbladder

A distending pain in the costal region; jaundice; scanty, red-tinged urine or yellow, turbid urine; yellow, foul-smelling leukorrhea; an itching of the vulva or a burning pain in the testes; a yellow, creamy tongue coating; and a rapid, wiry pulse characterize heat-dampness in the liver and gallbladder.

Treatment is designed to remove heat-dampness, for which Gentian Combination (*long dan xie gan tang*) or Major Bupleurum Combination (*da chai hu tang*) can be used.

Major Bupleurum Combination[1]

Da Chai Hu Tang
(Major Bupleurum Decoction)[2]

Bupleurum	*Bupleuri radix*	Chai hu	6.0
Scute	*Scutellariae radix*	Huang qin	3.0
Chih-shih	*Citri fructus immaturus*	Zhi shi	2.0
Rhubarb	*Rhei rhizoma*	Da huang	1.0
Pinellia	*Pinellia rhizoma*	Ban xia	3.0
Peony	*Paeoniae radix*	Shao yao	3.0
Ginger, fresh	*Zingiberis rhizoma*	Sheng jiang	2.0
Jujube	*Zizyphi fructus*	Da zao	3.0

Excess Liver *Yang*

Headache, dizziness, irritability, a flushed face, a wiry and rapid pulse, and a thin, white tongue coating characterize an excess of liver *yang*. If dry eyes, mouth and throat; insomnia; dream-disturbed sleep; fidgeting; a feverish sensation in the chest, palms and soles; tinnitus; hearing loss; a wiry, thready and rapid pulse; and a red tongue with a thin, white coating are also observed, the patient not only has an excess of liver *yang*, but a deficiency of liver *yin* as well.

To treat excess liver *yang* in isolation, use Gastrodia and Uncaria Combination (*tian ma gou teng yin*).

Excess liver *yang* complicated by a deficiency of liver *yin* can be treated with Lycium, Chrysanthemum and Rehmannia Formula (*qi ju di huang wan*), plus 5 *qian* each of haliotis (*shi jue ming*) and oyster shell (*mu li*).

Lycium, Chrysanthemum and Rehmannia Formula[1]

Qi Ju Di Huang Wan

(Lycium Fruit, Chrysanthemum and Rehmannia Pill)[2]

Lycium fruit	Lycii fructus	Gou qi zi	2.0
Chrysanthemum	Chrysanthemi flos	Ju hua	1.0
Rehmannia, cooked	Rehmanniae radix	Shu di huang	4.0
Cornus	Corni fructus	Shan zhu yu	3.0
Dioscorea	Dioscorea batatis rhizoma	Shan yao	3.0
Alisma	Alismatis rhizoma	Ze xie	3.0
Moutan	Moutan radicis cortex	Mu dan pi	3.0
Hoelen	Poria sclerotium	Fu ling	3.0

Liver *Yang* Turning into Wind

Dizziness, headache, numbness or trembling of the limbs, tongue tremors, a red tongue with scant coating, and a rapid, wiry pulse, or even sudden lapses of consciousness, dysphasia due to rigidity of the tongue, mouth and eyes awry, and hemiplegia characterize liver *yang* turning into wind.

Subduing the liver and internal wind is achieved by using 5 *qian* haliotis (*shi jue ming*), 3 *qian* gastrodia (*tian ma*) and Antelope Horn and Uncaria Combination (*ling jiao gou teng tang*).

Cold Stagnancy in the Liver Meridians

A distending pain in the lower abdomen; a pressing and distending sensation in the testes which is aggravated by cold, or a scrotal contraction and pain radiating to the lower abdomen; a white tongue coating; and a submerged, wiry pulse are characteristic of cold stagnancy in the liver meridians.

Treatment attempts to warm the liver and dispel cold. Evodia Combination (*wu zhu yu tang*), to which has been added 1 *qian* fennel (*xiao hui xiang*) and 0.5 *qian* cinnamon bark (*rou gui*), is suitable to achieve this end.

Evodia Combination[1]

Wu Zhu Yu Tang

(Evodia Decoction)[2]

Evodia	*Evodiae fructus*	*Wu zhu yu*	3.0
Ginseng	*Ginseng radix*	*Ren shen*	3.0
Ginger, fresh	*Zingiberis rhizoma*	*Sheng jiang*	4.0
Jujube	*Zizyphi fructus*	*Da zao*	3.0

Gallbladder Stagnancy and Excess Phlegm

Dizziness, a bitter taste in the mouth, nausea, vomiting, insomnia, excessive fear, irritability, chest stuffiness, a smooth and greasy tongue coating, and a wiry and slippery pulse are typical signs and symptoms of this conformation.

Hoelen and Bamboo Combination (*wen dan tang*) can be used for removing phlegm and regulating *qi*.

Herbs for Liver and Gallbladder Disorders

Herbs for Soothing Liver *Qi*

bupleurum (*chai hu*)   turmeric (*yu jin*)
cyperus (*xiang fu zi*)   immature citrus peel (*qing pi*)
white mume flower (*lu e mei*)   magnolia bark (*hou pu*)
perilla stem (*su gen*)

Herbs for Clearing Liver Fire

gentian (*long dan cao*)   gardenia (*zhi zi*)
prunella (*xia ku cao*)   scute (*huang qin*)

Herbs for Removing Liver Heat and Improving Eyesight

pipewort (*gu jing cao*)   buddleia (*mi meng hua*)
celosia (*qing xiang zi*)   equisetum (*mu zei*)

Herbs for Calming the Liver and Subduing Liver *Yang*

haliotis (*shi jue min*)   cowry (*bei ci*)
oyster shell (*mu li*)   cassia seed (*jue ming zi*)
tribulus (*ji li*)

Herbs for Subduing Internal Wind and Liver Hyperactivity

antelope horn (*ling yang jiao*)   goat horn (*shan yang jiao*)
gastrodia (*tian ma*)   uncaria stem with hooks (*gou tang*)
chrysanthemum (*ju hua*)   Chinese holly (*ku ding cha*)
scorpion (*quan xie*)   centipede (*wu gong*)
cicada (*chan tui*)

Herbs for Nourishing Liver *Yin*

turtle shell (*bie jia*)   lycium fruit (*gou qi zi*)
eclipta (*han lian cao*)   ligustrum (*nu zhen zi*)

Herbs for Warming Liver Cold

fennel (*xiao hui xiang*)   evodia (*wu zhu yu*)
litchi seed (*li zhi he*)   citrus seed (*ju he*)

Herbs Which Act as Cholagogues

capillaris (*yin chen huo*)   desmodium (*jin qian cao*)
corn stigma (*yu mi xu*)   turmeric (*yu jin*)
raw crataegus (*shen shan zha*)

Herbs for Relieving Pain in the Liver

cherokee rose (*jin ying zi*)   corydalis (*yan hu suo*)
fraxinus (*qing pi*)   cyperus (*xiang fu zi*)
dry stinkbug (*jiu xiang chong*)

Common Acupuncture and Moxibustion Points

For Soothing Liver *Qi*

- *xingjiang* (Liv 2)   - *ganshu* (B 18)
- *fengchi* (G 20)

For Clearing Liver Fire and Subduing Excess Liver *Yang*

- *xingjian* (Liv 2)   - *ganshu* (B 18)
- *shenshu* (B 23)

For Removing Liver Heat and Improving Eyesight

- *ganshu* (B 18)   - *tongziliao* (G 1)
- *fengchi* (G 20)

For Subduing Internal Wind and Liver Hyperactivity

- *fengchi* (G 20)   - *ganshu* (B 18)
- *taicong* (Liv 3)

For Nourishing Liver *Yin*

- *sanyinjiao* (Sp 6)   - *ganshu* (B 20)
- *shenshu* (B 23)

For Serving as a Cholagogue

- *xingjian* (Liv 2)   - *danshu* (B 19)
- *xuanzhong* (G 39)

Section 3
The Spleen and Stomach

According to a TCM understanding, the spleen, which also includes the pancreas of Western medicine, controls digestion, regulates muscle tone and muscle control, and prevents hemorrhaging. Given this, the proper absorption and digestion of food keep the limbs and muscles strong. Spleen *qi* deficiency, then, can result in lassitude and edema of the limbs.

The spleen's orifice is the mouth, while the lips are the mirror of the spleen. Ruddy, lustrous lips are the by-product of good absorption and digestion of ingested food, while pale, lusterless lips can be attributed to splenic malfunction. Furthermore, spleen deficiency causes diarrhea, edema, and abdominal distention and fullness. In contrast, a Western perspective views the spleen as related to the quality and quantity of platelets in the blood.

As regards the stomach, both TCM and Western medicine consider this organ as primarily responsible for the acceptance and digestion of ingested food. Briefly, food enters the stomach, the pylorus closes, food is transformed into chyme, and the chyme moves into the small intestine. Dyspepsia, foul belching and sour regurgitation result from the retention of food in the stomach.

Diagnosis and Herbal Treatment

Spleen *Qi* Deficiency

A sallow complexion, a gaunt appearance, general lassitude, feeble breathing, apathy, poor appetite, abdominal fullness, diarrhea, a pale tongue with a thin coating, and a slow, weak pulse characterize spleen *qi* deficiency.

Treatment attempts to reinforce *qi* and tonify the spleen. The suggested formulas are Ginseng and Atractylodes Formula (*shen ling bai zhu san*) and Four Major Herb Combination (*si jun zi tang*).

Ginseng and Atractylodes Formula[1]

Shen Ling Bai Zhu San

(Ginseng, Poria and Atractylodes Macrocephala Powder)[2]

Ginseng	*Ginseng radix*	*Ren shen*	3.0
Lotus seed	*Nelumbinis semen*	*Lian zi rou*	4.0
Dioscorea	*Dioscorea batatis rhizoma*	*Shan yao*	3.0
Atractylodes, white	*Atractylodis rhizoma*	*Bai zhu*	3.0
Hoelen	*Poria sclerotium*	*Fu ling*	3.0
Dolichos	*Dolichoris semen*	*Bai pian dou*	4.0
Coix	*Coicis semen*	*Yi yi ren*	5.0
Cardamom	*Amoni semen*	*Sha ren*	2.0
Platycodon	*Platycodi radix*	*Jie geng*	2.0
Licorice, baked	*Glycyrrhizae radix*	*Zhi gan cao*	1.5

Spleen *Yang* Deficiency

In addition to those manifestations listed above for spleen *qi* deficiency, spleen *yang* deficiency is also characterized by the following symptoms: cold and pain in the abdomen or stomach region which is relieved by pressure or the regurgitation of warm, clear fluids; cold limbs; watery leukorrhea; and a "bearing-down" sensation in the urethral region and lower abdomen. Moreover, the patient will have a pale tongue with a white coating, and a submerged, slow pulse.

Ginseng and Ginger Combination (*li zhong tang*) can be used to warm the middle energizer and dispel cold. If the patient feels very cold, Aconite, Ginseng and Ginger Combination (*fu zi li zhong tang*) should be selected.

Descent of Spleen *Qi*

Prolapse of the uterus, rectum or other internal organs; a sallow complexion; dizziness; lassitude; difficulty in breathing; apathy; taciturnity; distention and a "bearing-down" sensation in the lower abdomen; poor appetite; abdominal fullness after meals; pale tongue; and weak pulse characterize the descent of spleen *qi*. Ginseng and Astragalus Combination (*bu zhong yi qi tang*) strengthens spleen *qi* and promotes its ascent.

Edema Due to Spleen Deficiency

Edema which is especially severe in the waist and lower extremities; oliguria; cold limbs; poor appetite; distention and fullness in the stomach region and abdomen; diarrhea; a pale tongue with a white, slippery coating; and a slow, submerged pulse are characteristic of edema caused by spleen deficiency.

Treatment is centered about strengthening the spleen to alleviate water retention. Magnolia and Atractylodes Combination (*shi pi yin*) can be used to achieve this end.

Magnolia and Atractylodes Combination
Shi Pi Yin[13]
(Bolster the Spleen Decoction)[2]

Magnolia bark	*Magnoliae officinalis cortex*	Hou pu	2.0
Aconite, prepared	*Aconiti carmichaelii praeparata radix*	Zhi fu zi	2.0
Hoelen	*Poria sclerotium*	Fu ling	2.0
Licorice	*Glycyrrhizae radix*	Gan cao	1.0
Areca peel	*Arecae pericarpium*	Da fu pi	2.0
Atractylodes, white	*Atractylodis rhizoma*	Bai zhu	3.0
Chaenomeles	*Chaenomelis fructus*	Mu gua	3.0
Saussurea	*Saussureae radix*	Mu xiang	2.0
Tsao-ko	*Amomi tsaoko fructus*	Cao guo	2.0
Ginger, fresh	*Zingiberis rhizoma*	Sheng jiang	1.0
Ginger, dried	*Zingiberis siccatum rhizoma*	Gan jiang	1.0
Jujube	*Zizyphi fructus*	Da zao	3.0

Functions: warms and strengthens spleen *yang*; promotes *qi*; alleviates water retention.

Explanation: This is the most commonly used formula for warming *yang*, strengthening the spleen and alleviating water retention. Aconite, *tsao-ko*, white atractylodes and both forms of ginger warm the middle energizer and strengthen the spleen to help the flow of body fluids. Hoelen, areca seed, chaenomeles and fresh ginger alleviate water retention, while magnolia bark, licorice and saussurea promote *qi* to resolve dampness. Areca peel corrects diuresis, while jujube and licorice reinforce the spleen to regulate the middle energizer and also coordinate the actions of the other ingredients.

If the patient has a *qi* deficiency in addition to edema due to spleen deficiency, accompanied by feeble breathing and a weak voice, 3 *qian* ginseng (*ren shen*) should be substituted for the magnolia bark and the *tsao-ko* in Magnolia and Atractylodes Combination.

Cold-dampness Invading the Spleen

Fullness and distention of the epigastrium and abdomen; poor appetite; absence of thirst; stickiness in the mouth; an aversion to cold; heavy-headedness; sluggishness; edema in the face and limbs; diarrhea; oliguria; a white, greasy tongue coating; and a floating, soft and slow pulse are the signs and symptoms generally associated with cold-dampness invading the spleen.

Treatment is aimed at warming the middle energizer and dispelling dampness. Magnolia and Hoelen Combination (*wei ling tang*) can be used to achieve these ends.

Heat-dampness in the Spleen and Stomach

This conformation is marked by a loss of appetite; an aversion to oily foods; nausea; vomiting; fullness and distention of the epigastrium and abdomen; a sticky feeling and a sweet taste in the mouth; a general heaviness and sluggishness; scanty, dark yellow urine; and any of the following: (1) fetid stools with tenesmus, (2) a bright yellow cast to the skin and the whites of the eyes (*yang* jaundice), or (3) thick, yellow leukorrhea, a yellow, greasy tongue coating and a soft, weak, slippery and rapid pulse.

Treatment is aimed at removing heat-dampness, tonifying the spleen and regulating the stomach. Capillaris and Hoelen Five Formula (*yin chen wu ling san*) can be selected.

Stomach *Yin* Deficiency

Dry mouth and lips, belching, nausea, stomachache and gastric discomfort with acid regurgitation, dry stools, a red tongue which is denuded in the center and has very little saliva, and a thready and rapid pulse are characteristic of stomach *yin* deficiency.

Treatment attempts to nourish stomach *yin*. Glehnia and Ophiopogon Combination (*yi wei tang*) and Ophiopogon Combination (*mai men dong tang*) are particularly well-suited to achieving this end.

Glehnia and Ophiopogon Combination
Yi Wei Tang[7]
(Benefit the Stomach Decoction)[2]

Glehnia root	Glehniae radix	Sha shen	10.0
Ophiopogon	Ophiopogonis rhizoma	Mai men dong	5.0
Polygonatum	Polygonati officinalis rhizoma	Yu zhu	5.0
Rehmannia, raw	Rehmanniae radix	Sheng di huang	10.0

Add granulated sugar to the above formula prior to administration.

Functions: nourishes the stomach to promote the secretion of body fluids.

Explanation: Since all the herbs in Glehnia and Ophiopogon Combination are sweet and cold, this formula is highly recommended for nourishing stomach *yin*. It has good curative effects on impaired stomach fluids following a febrile disease and insufficient stomach fluids due to either *yin* deficiency or stomach heat.

Ophiopogon Combination[1]

Mai Men Dong Tang

(Ophiopogon Decoction)[2]

Ophiopogon	*Ophiopogonis rhizoma*	*Mai men dong*	10.0
Pinellia	*Pinellia rhizoma*	*Ban xia*	5.0
Ginseng	*Ginseng radix*	*Ren shen*	2.0
Rice	*Oryzae semen*	*Jing mi*	5.0
Licorice	*Glycyrrhizae radix*	*Gan cao*	2.0
Jujube	*Zizyphi fructus*	*Da zao*	5.0

Stomach Fire

A burning pain in the stomach region; thirst with a preference for cold beverages; a feeling of being hungry, despite having recently eaten; acid regurgitation; gastric discomfort; vomiting; foul-smelling breath; gingival swelling and pain or ulceration and bleeding; constipation; a red tongue with a yellow coating; and a slippery, rapid pulse characterize stomach fire.

Coptis and Rehmannia Formula (*qing wei san*) is effective at purging stomach fire.

Cold Stagnancy in the Stomach Region

Cold and pain in the stomach region which are aggravated by cold and relieved by warmth, belching, watery vomit, a white, slippery tongue coating, and a slow pulse characterize cold stagnancy in the stomach region.

Minor Cinnamon and Peony Combination (*xiao jian zhong tang*), to which has been added 3 *qian* each of *tang-kuei* (*dang gui*) and astragalus (*huang qi*), is suitable for warming the stomach and dispelling cold.

Minor Cinnamon and Peony Combination[1]
Xiao Jian Zhong Tang
(Minor Construct the Middle Decoction)[2]

Cinnamon twig	*Cinnamomi ramulus*	*Gui zhi*	4.0
Peony	*Paeoniae radix*	*Shao yao*	6.0
Licorice, baked	*Glycyrrhizae radix*	*Zhi gan cao*	2.0
Ginger, fresh	*Zingiberis rhizoma*	*Sheng jiang*	4.0
Maltose	*Saccharum granorum*	*Jiao yi*	20.0
Jujube	*Zizyphi fructus*	*Da zao*	4.0

Food Retention in the Stomach

Distention, fullness or pain in the stomach region and abdomen after immoderate eating and/or drinking; foul belching; sour regurgitation; vomiting; foul intestinal flatulence; constipation or diarrhea; a thick, greasy, yellow tongue coating; and a slippery pulse are often seen in patients who retain food in their stomachs.

Treatment promotes digestion and removes food stagnancy. Citrus and Crataegus Formula (*bao he wan*) can do both.

Citrus and Crataegus Formula[1]

Bao He Wan

(Preserve Harmony Pill)[2]

Crataegus	*Crataegi fructus*	*Shan zha*	12.0
Shen-chu	*Massa medicata fermentata*	*Shen qu*	4.0
Pinellia	*Pinellia rhizoma*	*Ban xia*	6.0
Hoelen	*Poria sclerotium*	*Fu ling*	6.0
Citrus peel	*Citri pericarpium*	*Chen pi*	2.0
Raphanus	*Raphani semen*	*Lai fu zi*	2.0
Forsythia	*Forsythiae fructus*	*Lian qiao*	2.0

The above herbs are prepared for administration by grinding into a powder, which is then made into 2-to-3-*qian* pills or tablets. One pill is taken, two to three times daily with warm water. If the formula is prepared in granular form, 3 *qian* is taken three times daily.

Functions: promotes digestion and regulates stomach functioning to remove food stagnancy.

Explanation: Crataegus is effective at eliminating food retention, and *shen-chu* corrects the retention of stagnant liquids and food. Pinellia and hoelen, which can eliminate dampness, are adjuvant herbs for the elimination of phlegm, dampness and stagnant *qi* caused by the retention of food. Citrus peel is aromatic and can enliven the spleen and regulate *qi*. Raphanus removes wheat-based foods from the stomach and alleviates adverse *qi* flow to relieve distention. When supplemented with forsythia to clear heat, all these herbs can achieve the effect of correcting food retention.

Herbs for Spleen and Stomach Disorders

Herbs for Reinforcing Spleen *Qi*

codonopsis (*dang shen*)   pseudostellaria root (*tai zi shen*)
atractylodes, white (*bai zhu*)   dioscorea (*shan yiao*)
licorice (*gan cao*)   jujube (*da zao*)

Herbs for Warming the Middle Energizer

dried ginger (*gan jiang*)   galanga root (*gao liang jiang*)
evodia (*wu zhu yu*)   cinnamon twig (*gui zhi*)
cinnamon bark (*rou gui*)

Herbs for Strengthening Spleen *Qi*

cimicifuga (*sheng ma*)   bupleurum (*chai hu*)
bitter orange (*zhi ke*)

Herbs for Eliminating Spleen Dampness

atractylodes (*cang zhu*)   magnolia bark (*hou pu*)
coix (*yi yi ren*)

Aromatic Herbs for Stimulating the Spleen

agastache (*huo xiang*)   eupatorium (*pei lan*)
amomum fruit (*sha ren*)   cluster (*bai dou kou*)

Herbs for Promoting the Descent of Adverse Stomach *Qi*

clove (*ding xiang*)   kaki (*shi di*)
bamboo shavings (*zhu ru*)   inula (*xuan fu hua*)
hematite (*dai zhe shi*)

Herbs for Clearing Stomach Heat

coptis (*huang lian*)   gypsum (*shi gao*)
anemarrhena (*zhi mu*)   rhubarb (*da huang*)

Herbs to Nourish the Stomach and Promote Fluid Secretion

dendrobium (*shi hu*)   trichosanthes root (*tian hua fen*)
phragmites (*lu gen*)   ophiopogon (*mai men dong*)

Herbs for Eliminating Food Retention

raphanus (*lai fu zi*)	shen-chu (*shen qu*)
malt (*mai ya*)	crataegus (*shan zha*)
germinated rice (*gu ya*)	chicken gizzard lining (*ji nei jin*)

Herbs for Moistening the Large Intestine

linum (*ma zi ren*)	plum seed (*yu li ren*)
biota (*bo zi ren*)	trichosanthes seed (*gua lou ren*)
sesame seed (*hei zhi ma*)	honey (*feng mi*)

Common Acupuncture and Moxibustion Points

For Reinforcing Spleen *Qi*

- *pishu* (B 20)
- *sanyinjiao* (Sp 6)

For Warming the Middle Energizer (with moxibustion)

- *shenjue* (CV 8)
- *qihai* (CV 6)
- *guanyuan* (CV 4)

For Strengthening Spleen *Qi* (with moxibustion)

- *baihui* (GV 20)

For Eliminating Spleen Dampness

- *gongsun* (Sp 4)
- *fenglong* (S 40)

For Strengthening the Spleen

- *pishu* (B 20)
- *weishu* (B 21)
- *daheng* (Sp 15)
- *tianshu* (S 25)

For Promoting the Descent of Adverse Stomach *Qi*

- *neiguan* (P 6)
- *zhongwan* (CV 12)
- *weishu* (B 21)

For Clearing Stomach Heat

- *neiting* (S 44)
- *zusanli* (S 36)

For Eliminating Food Retention

- *weishu* (B 21)
- *zusanli* (S 36)
- *zhongwan* (CV 12)
- *xiawan* (CV 10)

For Moistening the Large Intestine

- *tianshu* (S 25)
- *dachangshu* (B 25)
- *yanglingquan* (G 34)
- *daheng* (Sp 15)
- *zhigou* (TE 6)

Section 4
The Lungs and Large Intestine

While Western medicine ascribes to the lungs the primary task of respiration, TCM adds the function of governing *qi* circulation. Because of the lungs' vital importance in inhalation and exhalation, cough or shortness of breath mark a lung disorder. In TCM, coughs and watery nasal discharges are attributed to a *qi* obstruction in the lungs, and lung heat is deemed responsible for inflamed nasal passages, since the nose is the specific orifice of the lungs. Western medicine, too, notes that colds and coughs are often accompanied by nasal obstructions.

TCM further notes that the lungs govern the healthy functioning of the hair and skin. This is why lung *qi* deficiency results in spontaneous sweating, thereby causing the skin to become cold and, consequently, increasing the affected person's risk of catching a cold.

Since all blood vessels converge in the lungs, stagnant *qi* and blood in the lungs can cause cyanosis. Similarly, Western medical science has long noted that blood flows through the lungs, where the exchange of O_2 and CO_2 takes place.

As regards the lungs' paired organ, the large intestine, both TCM and Western medicine agree that the latter is responsible for the excretion of feces. TCM further notes that stools with pus and/or blood appear when heat-dampness is present in the large intestine, while insufficient fluids make excretion difficult, thereby resulting in constipation.

Diagnosis and Herbal Treatment

Lung *Qi* Deficiency

A feeble cough; asthma; thin sputum; weak, gasping breathing; apathy; taciturnity; a feeble voice; an aversion to cold; spontaneous sweating; a propensity to catch colds easily; pallor; lassitude; a pale tongue with a thin, white coating; and a weak pulse characterize lung *qi* deficiency.

Treatment is designed to reinforce lung *qi* with Astragalus and Aster Combination (*bu fei tang*).

Astragalus and Aster Combination
Bu Fei Tang[15]
(Tonify the Lungs Decoction)[2]

Ginseng	Ginseng radix	Ren shen	2.0
Astragalus	Astragali radix	Huang qi	3.0
Rehmannia, cooked	Rehmanniae radix	Shu di huang	3.0
Schizandra	Schizandrae fructus	Wu wei zi	1.0
Morus bark	Mori radicis cortex	Sang bai pi	3.0
Aster	Asteris radix et rhizoma	Zi wan	3.0

Following decoction in water, the above herbs are mixed with a little honey and taken by mouth.

Functions: strengthens the lungs; relieves coughing.

Explanation: Ginseng and astragalus strengthen spleen *qi*, which in turn strengthens the lungs. In this way, reinforcing the mother organ (in this case, the spleen) aids in treating a son deficiency (here, lung deficiency).

Rehmannia tonifies kidney *yin*, schizandra astringes lung *qi*, and morus bark clears lung fire so that fire will not impair *qi*, while aster moistens the lungs to relieve coughing.

Lung *Yin* Deficiency

A dry cough or a cough with sticky or blood-tinged sputum; dryness in the mouth and throat; hoarseness; hectic fever; night sweats; a flushed face; a feverish sensation in the palms, soles and heart region; a dry, red tongue; and a thready, rapid pulse characterize lung *yin* deficiency. Lily Combination (*bai he gu jin tang*) is recommended for nourishing *yin* and moistening the lungs.

Lily Combination[1]

Bai He Gu Jin Tang

(Lily Bulb Decoction to Preserve the Metal)[2]

Lily	Lilii bulbus	Bai he	4.0
Rehmannia, cooked	Rehmanniae radix	Shu di huang	4.0
Rehmannia, raw	Rehmanniae radix	Sheng di huang	4.0
Ophiopogon	Ophiopogonis rhizoma	Mai men dong	6.0
Peony	Paeoniae radix	Shao yao	3.0
Scrophularia	Scrophulariae radix	Xuan shen	3.0
Fritillaria	Fritillariae bulbus	Bei mu	3.0
Tang-kuei	Angelicae radix	Dang gui	4.0
Platycodon	Platycodi radix	Jie geng	2.0
Licorice	Glycyrrhizae radix	Gan cao	1.0

Invasion of the Lungs by Wind-cold

Coughing or asthma; thin, white sputum; an absence of thirst; nasal obstruction with watery discharges; fever; an aversion to cold; an absence of perspiration; headache; general aches; a thin, white tongue coating; and a tense, floating pulse are indications of an invasion of the lungs by wind-cold.

Apricot Seed and Perilla Formula (*xing su san*) is an appropriate remedy for dispelling wind-cold and ventilating the lungs to relieve coughing.

Invasion of the Lungs by Wind-heat

A cough; difficulty in expectorating thick, yellow sputum; thirst; a sore throat; headache; fever; an aversion to wind; undue sweating; a thick, yellow tongue coating; and a rapid, floating pulse are indicative of an invasion of the lungs by wind-heat.

Morus and Chrysanthemum Combination (*sang ju yin*) is effective at dispelling wind-heat and ventilating the lungs to relieve coughing.

Invasion of the Lungs by Heat-dryness

A dry cough or a cough with sticky or blood-tinged sputum; chest pain due to a severe cough; dryness in the nose and throat; a sore throat; a dry, red tongue with a thin, yellow coating; and a thready, rapid pulse are common indications of an invasion of the lungs by heat-dryness.

Eriobotrya and Ophiopogon Combination (*qing zao jiu fei tang*) is recommended for clearing and moistening the lungs.

Retention of Heat-phlegm in the Lungs

Coughing; asthma; coarse breathing; flaring of the nostrils; expectoration of thick, yellow sputum, blood-tinged sputum or foul-smelling sputum with pus and blood; fever; chest pain; thirst; dark yellow urine; constipation; a red tongue with a greasy, yellow coating; and a rapid, slippery pulse are characteristic of retention of heat-phlegm in the lungs.

Treatment attempts to clear the lungs in order to resolve sputum and relieve asthma. *Ma-huang* and Apricot Seed Combination (*ma xing gan shi tang*) can be used. If pulmonary abscesses have formed, Phragmites Combination (*wei jing tang*), plus 10 *qian* houttuynia (*yu xing cao*), is recommended for clearing lung heat, resolving phlegm and draining pus.

Ma-huang and Apricot Seed Combination[1]
Ma Xing Gan Shi Tang*
(Ephedra, Apricot Kernel, Gypsum and Licorice Decoction)[2]

Ma-huang**	Ephedrae radix	Ma huang	2.0
Apricot seed	Armeniacae semen	Xing ren	3.0
Gypsum	Gypsum fibrosum	Shi gao	10.0
Licorice	Glycyrrhizae radix	Gan cao	2.0

*also known as *ma xing gan shi tang*
**also commonly known as ephedra

Phragmites Combination
Wei Jing Tang
(Reed Decoction)[2]

Phragmites	Phragmitis rhizoma	Lu gen	4.0
Coix	Coicis semen	Yi yi ren	8.0
Benincasa	Benincasae semen	Dong gua zi	8.0
Persica	Persicae semen	Tao ren	3.0

Functions: clears heat; drains pus.

Explanation: Sweet, cold-natured phragmites clears lung heat and regulates lung *qi*. As adjuvant herbs, coix and benincasa drain pus and resolve phlegm, while persica promotes blood circulation to remove stasis. No sooner have heat, blood stasis and pus been removed and *qi* ventilated than the pulmonary abscesses are healed.

Blockage of the Lungs by Phlegm-dampness

A cough with copious amounts of white, sticky sputum which is easily expectorated; chest fullness; asthma; a greasy, white tongue coating; and a slippery pulse are indicators of a blockage of the lungs by phlegm-dampness.

Treatment is aimed at drying dampness and clearing phlegm. Either Atractylodes and Hoelen Combination (*ling gui zhu gan tang*) or Citrus and Pinellia Combination (*er chen tang*) can be employed for this purpose.

Atractylodes and Hoelen Combination[1]*

Ling Gui Zhu Gan Tang

(Poria, Cinnamon, Atractylodes and Licorice Decoction)

Hoelen	*Poria sclerotium*	*Fu ling*	3.0
Cinnamon twig	*Cinnamomi ramulus*	*Gui zhi*	2.0
Atractylodes, white	*Atractylodis rhizoma*	*Bai zhu*	2.0
Licorice	*Glycyrrhizae radix*	*Gan cao*	1.0

* also known as Hoelen and Atractylodes Combination

Retention of Cold Fluids in the Lungs

Coughing; asthma; difficulty in lying supine; stuffiness in the chest; expectoration of copious amounts of thin, white, frothy sputum; an aversion to cold; and a cough which is aggravated by cold are symptomatic of the retention of cold fluids in the lungs. When present in exterior conformations, a white, slippery, greasy tongue coating and a wiry and slippery or floating pulse will also be observed.

Minor Blue Dragon Combination (*xiao qing long tang*) is effective in warming the lungs and dissipating fluid retention.

Heat-dampness in the Large Intestine

Abdominal pain; diarrhea with foul, sticky stools or dysentery with pus and blood; tenesmus; a burning sensation in the anus; small quantities of red-tinged urine; fever with thirst; a greasy, yellow tongue coating; and a rapid pulse are characteristic of this conformation.

Pueraria, Coptis and Scute Combination (*ge gen huang lian huang qin tang*) can be used for eliminating heat-dampness.

Pueraria, Coptis and Scute Combination[1]
Ge Gen Huang Lian Huang Qin Tang
(Pueraria, Coptis and Scutellaria Decoction)

Pueraria	Puerariae radix	Ge gen	3.0
Scute	Scutellariae radix	Huang qin	3.0
Coptis	Coptidis rhizoma	Huang lian	1.5
Licorice, baked	Glycyrrhizae radix	Zhi gan cao	2.0

Fluid Deficiency in the Large Intestine

Constipation; dry stools or hard, knotty stools; difficulty in defecating; dry mouth and throat; a dry, red tongue with a dry, yellow coating; and a thready pulse are common signs and symptoms of a fluid deficiency in the large intestine.

Linum and Rhubarb Combination (*run chang tang*) may be used for moistening the large intestine to relieve constipation.

Linum and Rhubarb Combination[1]
Run Chang Tang
(Moisten the Intestines Pill)[2]

Tang-kuei	Angelicae radix	Dang gui	3.0
Rehmannia, cooked	Rehmanniae radix	Shu di huang	3.0
Rehmannia, raw	Rehmanniae radix	Sheng di huang	3.0
Scute	Scutellariae radix	Huang qin	2.0
Persica	Persicae semen	Tao ren	2.0
Magnolia bark	Magnoliae officinalis cortex	Hou pu	2.0
Linum	Cannabis semen	Ma zi ren	2.0
Rhubarb	Rhei rhizoma	Da huang	2.0
Apricot seed	Armeniacae semen	Xing ren	2.0
Licorice	Glycyrrhizae radix	Gan cao	1.5
Chih-ko	Citri fructus	Zhi ke	2.0

Herbs for Diseases of the Lungs and Large Intestine

Herbs for Warming Lung Cold

ma-huang (ma huang)　　　cinnamon twig (*gui zhi*)
asarum (*xi xin*)

Herbs for Clearing Lung Heat

scute (*huang qin*)　　　morus bark (*sang bai pi*)
scrophularia (*xuan shen*)　　dayflower (*ya zhi cao*)

Herbs for Strengthening Lung *Qi*

schizandra (*wu wei zi*)　　codonopsis (*dan shen*)
pseudostellaria root (*tai zi shen*)

Herbs for Nourishing Lung *Yin*

glehnia root (*bei sha shen*)　　ophiopogon (*mai men dong*)
asparagus (*tian men dong*)　　polygonatum (*huang jin*)
cordyceps (*dong chong xia cao*)

Herbs for Clearing Deficiency Fire

lycium bark (*di gu pi*)　　ching-hao (*qing hao*)
pai-wei (bai wei)　　　stellaria root (*yin chai hu*)
turtle shell (*bie jia*)

Herbs for Clearing Nasal Passages

xanthium (*cang er zi*)　　magnolia flower (*xin yi*)
angelica (*bai zhi*)　　　wasp's nest (*lu feng fang*)

Herbs for Promoting the Descent of Lung *Qi*

ma-huang (ma huang)　　apricot seed (*xing ren*)
ginkgo (*yin xing*)　　　earthworm (*di long*)
perilla seed (*zi su zi*)　　peucedanum root (*qian hu*)
lepidium (*ting li zi*)

Herbs for Cough Relief

eriobotrya (*pi pa ye*)　　tussilago (*kuan dong hua*)
stemona (*bai bu*)　　　aristolochia (*ma dou ling*)
nandina (*tian zhu zi*)　　metaplexis (*tian jiang ke*)
Sichuan fritillaria (*chuan bei mu*)

Herbs to Relieve Constipation

linum (*ma zi ren*)   persica (*tao ren*)

biota (*bo zi ren*)   cassia (*wang jiang nan*)

walnut (*hu tao rou*)   trichosanthes seed (*guo lou ren*)

Common Acupuncture and Moxibustion Points

For Warming Lung Cold

- *lieque* (L 7)
- *tanzhong* (CV 17)
- *feishu* (B 13)

For Clearing Lung Heat

- *chize* (L 5)
- *hegu* (LI 4)

For Reinforcing Lung *Qi*

- *lieque* (L 7)
- *feishu* (B 13)
- *zhongfu* (L 1)

For Nourishing Lung *Yin* and Clearing Deficiency Fire

- *taiyuan* (B 9)
- *feishu* (B 13)

For Clearing the Nasal Passages

- *heliao* (LI 19)
- *hegu* (LI 4)
- *yingxiang* (LI 20)

For Promoting the Descent of Lung *Qi*

- *dingchuan* (Ex B1)
- *lieque* (L 7)

For Cough Relief

- *taiyuan* (L 9)
- *feishu* (B 13)

For Moistening the Large Intestine to Relieve Constipation

- *tianshu* (S 25)
- *dachangshu* (B 25)
- *yanglingquan* (G 34)
- *daheng* (Sp 15)
- *zhigou* (SI 6)

Section 5
The Kidneys and Urinary Bladder

Chinese medicine sees the kidneys as the source of congenital *qi* and the storehouse of vital essence. As such, the kidneys are associated with growth, development and maturation.

The kidneys are related to the reproductive system and are known to have adrenocortical functions. Emission, impotence or infertility can result from kidney deficiency. Kidney deficiency can also cause hypomnesis, dysplasia, osteoporosis, hyperosteogeny, odontosis, lower back pain, frequent urination, edema and pre-dawn diarrhea. In addition, kidney *yang* deficiency may induce aplastic anemia.

TCM views the kidneys as the site of bone-marrow production and, as such, the regulators of bone and teeth formation. Western medicine also maintains that there is a relationship between the kidneys and the bones. Specifically, the kidneys secrete erythropoietin, a hormone that regulates the production of red blood cells. Additionally, the kidneys are associated with calcium and phosphorus metabolism, which is necessary for the formation of strong, healthy bones and teeth.

TCM points to the ears as the kidneys' specific orifice, and Western medicine realizes the close relationship that exists between the kidneys and the inner ear. Kidney deficiency, therefore, can manifest itself in hearing loss or tinnitus.

As regards general theory concerning the urinary bladder, TCM and Western medicine are in agreement. Both cite the primary function of the urinary bladder as the storage of urine before it is eliminated from the body, and both hold that urinary bladder disorders are marked by urgent, frequent or incontinent urination.

Diagnosis and Herbal Treatment

Kidney *Yang* Deficiency

Pallor, chills, cold limbs, lower back pain, weak knees, dizziness, tinnitus, general lassitude, spontaneous sweating, impotence or infertility, a pale tongue with a white coating, and a submerged, slow pulse that is weak in *chi mai* are characteristic of a kidney deficiency.

Treatment attempts to warm and reinforce kidney *yang*. Rehmannia Eight Formula (*ba wei di huang wan*) or Eucommia and Rehmannia Formula (*you gui wan*) can be used.

Eucommia and Rehmannia Formula

You Gui Wan[11]

(Restore the Right Pill)[2]

Rehmannia, cooked	Rehmanniae radix	Shu di huang	3.0
Cornus	Corni fructus	Shan zhu yu	3.0
Dioscorea	Dioscorea batatis rhizoma	Shan yao	3.0
Eucommia	Eucommiae cortex	Du zhong	3.0
Lycium fruit	Lycii fructus	Gou qi zi	3.0
Cuscuta	Cuscutae semen	Tu si zi	3.0
Tang-kuei	Angelicae radix	Dang gui	3.0
Antler gelatin	Colla cornus cervi colla	Lu jiao jiao	1.0
Aconite, prepared	Aconiti carmichaelii praeparata radix	Zhi fu zi	1.0
Cinnamon bark	Cinnamomi cortex	Gui pi	0.5

Functions: warms and strengthens kidney *yang*; nourishes vital essence and blood.

Explanation: Since kidney *yang* and kidney *yin* are interdependent, the ancient TCM practitioner Zhang Jing-yue said, "Nourishing *yin* to help *yang* is a skillful way to strengthen *yang*." In both Rehmannia Eight Formula and Eucommia and Rehmannia Formula, rehmannia, cornus and dioscorea nourish kidney *yin*, thereby strengthening kidney *yang*. Since all the herbs in the latter formula are tonics, Eucommia and Rehmannia Formula is only suitable for kidney *yang* deficiency or deficiency of fire in the gate of life (*ming men zhi huo*), the latter of which is characterized by chills, cold limbs, impotence, spermatorrhea, lower back pain and weak knees, but no indications of retained dampness or phlegm.

As regards the other ingredients, eucommia strengthens the kidneys and waist, while lycium fruit and cuscuta warm the kidneys and replenish *yang*. *Tang-kuei* nourishes the blood, antler gelatin warms the kidneys and nourishes the *dumai* (GV), and aconite and cinnamon bark warm and strengthen kidney *yang*.

Unconsolidated Kidney *Qi*

Lower-back pain; weak knees; frequent, profuse urination or enuresis and incontinence in urination or "dribbling" following urination; spermatorrhea; cold, watery leukorrhea; a pale tongue with a white coating; and a submerged, weak pulse characterize unconsolidated kidney *qi*. Mantis Formula (*sang piao xiao san*) or Lotus Stamen Formula (*jin suo gu jing wan*) can be used to consolidate kidney *qi*.

Mantis Formula[1]

Sang Piao Xiao San
(Mantis Egg Case Powder)[2]

Mantis	*Mantidis ootheca*	*Sang piao xiao*	3.0
Dragon bone	*Draconis os*	*Long gu*	5.0
Ginseng	*Ginseng radix*	*Ren shen*	3.0
Fu-shen	*Poria cor*	*Fu shen*	3.0
Acorus	*Acori rhizoma*	*Chang pu*	3.0
Polygala	*Polygalae radix*	*Yuan zhi*	3.0
Tang-kuei	*Angelicae radix*	*Dang gui*	3.0
Tortoise shell	*Testudinis plastrum*	*Gui ban*	3.0

Lotus Stamen Formula[1]

Jin Suo Gu Jing Wan
(Metal Lock Pill to Stabilize the Essence)[2]

Astragalus seed	Astragali semen	Sha yuan zi	6.0
Euryale	Euryalis semen	Qian shi	6.0
Lotus seed	Nelumbinis semen	Lian zi rou	3.0
Lotus stamen	Nelumbinis stamen	Lian xu	3.0
Dragon bone	Draconis os	Long gu	5.0
Oyster shell	Ostreae testa	Mu li	5.0

Kidneys' Failure to Regulate *Qi*

Dyspnea, shortness of breath, exhalation of *qi* more pronounced than inhalation, asthmatic breathing with physical exertion, cough with sweating, cold limbs, a puffy face, a pale tongue, and a weak and floating pulse characterize the failure of the kidneys to control inhalation *qi*.

Ginseng and Walnut Combination (*ren shen hu tao tang*) can be used for warming the kidneys and improving inhalation.

Ginseng and Walnut Combination[1]

Ren Shen Hu Tao Tang[13]
(Ginseng and Walnut Decoction)[2]

Ginseng	Ginseng radix	Ren shen	2.0
Walnut	Juglandis semen	Hu tao rou	10.0
Ginger, fresh	Zingiberis rhizoma	Sheng jiang	3.0
Jujube	Zizyphi fructus	Da zao	5.0

Decoct the above ingredients in water and take after meals while still warm.

Functions: nourishes the deficiency to relieve asthma; reinforces the lungs and kidneys.

Explanation: Combined lung and kidney deficiency results in the kidneys' failure to receive air (*qi*), as well as a reversal in the flow of lung *qi*, the latter of which is marked by asthma and difficulty in lying supine. The proper way to relieve asthma and reinforce both the lungs and the kidneys is to resolve the deficiency.

Ginseng reinforces vital *qi* and is especially useful in treating *qi* deficiency of the spleen and lungs. Both walnut and ginseng are effective in resolving the deficiency and preventing asthma. Walnut is sweet and warm-natured when it takes affect in the lung and kidney meridians. There it nourishes and moistens the lungs and invigorates kidney *qi*, thereby improving inspiration. Invigorating kidney *qi* and astringing adverse *qi* in the lungs relieves asthma. Ginger and jujube harmonize the stomach and spleen.

Modified Ginseng and Gecko Formula (*ren shen ge jie san jia wei*) can also be used. It consists of 5 *qian* of ginseng and a pair of geckos (*ge jie*), crushed into powder. Three *qian* are taken twice daily. Many consider this latter formula more effective than Ginseng and Walnut Combination.

Edema Due to Kidney Deficiency

General pitting edema which is especially severe in the lower limbs; abdominal distention and fullness; oliguria; lower back pain; weak knees; chills; cold limbs; palpitation; dyspnea; asthma; coughing; wheezing; a pale, corpulent tongue with a white coating; and a submerged, thready pulse are characteristic of edema due to kidney deficiency.

Vitality Combination (*zhen wu tang*) warms *yang* and alleviates water retention.

Vitality Combination[1]

Zhen Wu Tang

(True Warrior Decoction)[2]

Aconite, prepared	*Aconiti carmichaelii praeparata radix*	*Zhi fu zi*	1.0
Atractylodes, white	*Atractylodis rhizoma*	*Bai zhu*	3.0
Hoelen	*Poria sclerotium*	*Fu ling*	4.0
Peony	*Paeoniae radix*	*Bai shao yao*	3.0
Ginger, fresh	*Zingiberis rhizoma*	*Sheng jiang*	3.0

Kidney *Yin* Deficiency

Dizziness; a poor memory or memory loss; lower back pain; weak knees; hearing loss; tinnitus; a flushed face; a feverish sensation in the palms, soles and heart area; night sweats; dryness in the mouth and throat; insomnia; drowsiness; baldness; odontosis; pain in the heels; or seminal emission, infertility, metrorrhagia or metrostaxia; amenorrhea; a red tongue; and a thready, rapid pulse are the two sets of conditions which can characterize kidney *yin* deficiency. Treatment is aimed at nourishing kidney *yin*, for which either Rehmannia Six Formula (*liu wei di huang wan*) or Achyranthes and Rehmannia Formula (*zuo gui wan*) can be used.

Rehmannia Six Formula[1]

Liu Wei Di Huang Wan

(Six Herbs, Including Rehmannia, Pill)

Rehmannia, raw	*Rehmanniae radix*	*Sheng di huang*	6.0
Cornus	*Corni fructus*	*Shan zhu yu*	3.0
Dioscorea	*Dioscorea batatis rhizoma*	*Shan yao*	3.0
Alisma	*Alismatis rhizoma*	*Ze xie*	3.0
Hoelen	*Poria sclerotium*	*Fu ling*	3.0
Moutan	*Moutan radicis cortex*	*Mu dan pi*	3.0

Achyranthes and Rehmannia Formula
Zuo Gui Wan[11]
(Restore the Left Pill)[2]

Rehmannia, cooked	*Rehmanniae radix*	*Shu di huang*	5.0
Dioscorea	*Dioscorea batatis rhizoma*	*Shan yao*	3.0
Lycium fruit	*Lycii fructus*	*Gou qi zi*	3.0
Cornus	*Corni fructus*	*Shan zhu yu*	3.0
Cuscuta	*Cuscutae semen*	*Tu si zi*	3.0
Achyranthes	*Achyranthis radix*	*Niu xi*	3.0
Antler gelatin	*Cervi cornus colla*	*Lu jiao jiao*	1.5
Tortoise shell gelatin	*Plastrum testudinis colla*	*Gui ban jiao*	1.5

Functions: nourishes *yin*; reinforces the kidneys.

Explanation: Rehmannia and cornus nourish kidney *yin*, dioscorea stops sweating and arrests seminal emission, and lycium fruit replenishes the vital essence of the kidneys and liver, as well as improves eyesight. Cuscuta acts with achyranthes to strengthen the lower back and knees.

Antler and tortoise shell gelatins are more effective when used in combination than when used alone. As they can pass through both the *dumai* (GV) and the *renmai* (CV), antler gelatin reinforces kidney *yang* and tortoise shell gelatin nourishes kidney *yin*. Together, they give credence to Chang Jiang-yue's theory: "Reinforcing *yang* to help *yin* is a skillful way to tonify *yin*."

Considered as a whole, all the herbs of this formula are effective in replenishing and nourishing kidney *yin*, and so can be used in the treatment of lower back pain, seminal emission, infertility and diabetes mellitus.

Heat-dampness in the Urinary Bladder

Frequent urination accompanied by an urgent, painful, burning sensation, difficult urination or dribbling after urination; turbid urine, hematuria or urinary disturbances associated with the presence of urinary calculi; distention and fullness in the lower abdomen; a yellow, greasy tongue coating; and a slippery pulse characterize heat-dampness in the urinary bladder. Either Dianthus Formula (*ba zheng san*) or Gardenia and Hoelen Formula (*wu ling san*) can be selected to clear heat, eliminate dampness and treat strangury.

Dianthus Formula[1]
Ba Zheng San
(Eight Herb Powder for Rectification)[2]

Dianthus	*Dianthi herba*	Qu mai	3.0
Polygonum	*Polygoni avicularis herba*	Bian xu	3.0
Akebia	*Akebiae caulis*	Mu tong	1.0
Talc	*Talcum*	Hua shi	4.0
Plantago	*Plantaginis semen*	Che qian zi	3.0
Gardenia	*Gardeniae fructus*	Zhi zi	3.0
Rhubarb	*Rhei rhizoma*	Da huang	1.0
Licorice	*Glycyrrhizae radix*	Gan cao	1.5

Gardenia and Hoelen Formula[1]
Wu Lin San
(Five Ingredient Powder with Poria)[2]

Hoelen	*Poria sclerotium*	Fu ling	6.0
Peony, red	*Paeoniae rubra radix*	Chi shao yao	2.0
Tang-kuei	*Angelicae radix*	Dang gui	3.0
Gardenia	*Gardeniae fructus*	Zhi zi	3.0
Licorice	*Glycyrrhizae radix*	Gan cao	1.0

Herbs for Diseases of the Kidneys and Urinary Bladder

Herbs to Nourish Kidney *Yin*

rehmannia, cooked (*shu di huang*)
oyster shell (*mu li*)
loranthus (*sang ji sheng*)
cibotium (*gou ji*)

tortoise shell (*gui ban*)
cornus (*shan zhu yu*)
dipsacus (*xu duan*)

Herbs to Clear Kidney Fire

anemarrhena (*zhi mu*)

phellodendron (*huang bo*)

Herbs to Reinforce Kidney *Qi*

gecko (*ge jie*)
walnut (*hu tao rou*)

human placenta (*zi he che*)
schizandra (*wu wei zi*)

Herbs to Warm Kidney *Yang*

curculigo (*xian hao*)
eucommia (*du zhong*)
cynomorium (*suo yang*)
antler (*lu jiao*)
cinnamon bark (*gui pi*)

actinolite (*yang qi shi*)
cistanche (*rou cong rong*)
fenugreek seed (*hu lu ba*)
prepared aconite (*zhi fu zi*)

Herbs to Consolidate Kidney *Jing*

cherokee rose (*jing ying zi*)
euryale (*qian shi*)
leek (*jiu zi*)
dragon bone (*long gu*)

cuscuta (*tu si zi*)
astragalus seed (*sha yuan zi*)
lotus stamen (*lian xu*)

Herbs to Arrest Enuresis

rubus (*fu pen zi*)
mantis (*sang piao xiao*)

alpinia fruit (*yi zhi ren*)

Herbs to Promote Diuresis

polyporus (*zhu ling*)
plantago (*che qian zi*)
tokoro (*bi xie*)

hoelen (*fu ling*)
alisma (*ze xie*)
talc (*hua shi*)

Herbs to Remove Urinary Calculi to Treat Strangury

desmodium (*jin qian cao*)   lygodium (*hai jin shan*)

pyrrosia leaf (*shi wei*)   abutilon (*dong kui zi*)

polygonum (*bian xu*)

Common Acupuncture and Moxibustion Points

Kidney Tonification

- *fuliu* (K 7)   • *taixi* (K 3)
- *shenshu* (B 23)   • *zhishi* (B 52)

Clearing Kidney Fire

- *rangu* (K 2)

Consolidating Kidneys to Arrest Spontaneous Emission

- *qihai* (CV 6)   • *guanyuan* (CV 4)

Arresting Enuresis

- *baihui* (GV 20)   • *renzhong* (GV 26)
- *qihai* (CV 6)   • *sanyinjiao* (Sp 6)

Diuresis

- *qihai* (CV 6)   • *sanyinjiao* (Sp 6)
- *yinlingquan* (Sp 9)

Removing Urinary Calculi to Treat Strangury

- *qihai* (CV 6)   • *guanyuan* (CV 4)
- *sanyinjiao* (Sp 6)   • *qihaishu* (B 24)
- *ciliao* (B 32)

Section 6
Disorders Involving Two Organs

The body is an organic whole and, as such, its constituent parts are connected through complex meridional, *qi*, *yin* and *yang* systems. In a healthy person, the organs function in a harmonious unity with the rest of the body. Should a patient suffer from a chronic disorder, however, the health-care provider must determine which organ is the primary source of illness and if and to what extent the imbalance in one organ has affected the proper functioning of other organs.

Diagnosis and Herbal Treatment

Heart and Lung *Qi* Deficiency

A chronic cough, labored breathing, palpitation which is aggravated by exercise, pallor, blue or purple lips, a pale tongue, and a thready, weak pulse characterize *qi* deficiency of the heart and lungs.

Treatment is aimed at tonifying the heart and lungs, for which Astragalus, Ginseng and Cinnamon Combination (*bao yuan tang*) can be used.

Astragalus, Ginseng and Cinnamon Combination
Bao Yuan Tang[9]
(Preserve the Basal Decoction)[2]

Ginseng	Ginseng radix	Ren shen	2.0
Astragalus	Astragali radix	Huang qi	3.0
Licorice	Glycyrrhizae radix	Gan cao	1.0
Cinnamon bark	Cinnamomi cortex	Gui pi	0.5

The above four ingredients are decocted in water with a pinch of glutinous rice (*nuo mi*).

Function: tonifies the heart and lungs.

Explanation: Ginseng is the chief herb for nourishing *qi*. This is enhanced by the addition of astragalus and licorice. Combined with a little cinnamon bark, they tonify the heart and lungs by warming *yang* and promoting the circulation of *qi* and blood.

Heart and Lung Deficiency

Palpitation which is sometimes accompanied by unwarranted fear, insomnia, drowsiness, a poor memory or a loss of memory, poor appetite, abdominal distention, loose stools, general lassitude and a sallow complexion; or subcutaneous hemorrhaging, light-colored uterine bleeding, a pale tongue with a white coating, and a thready, weak pulse are the two sets of signs and symptoms which generally characterize a deficiency of the heart and lungs.

Ginseng and Longan Combination (*gui pi tang*) can be used for nourishing the heart and lungs.

Imbalance Between the Heart and Kidneys

This conformation is generally caused by a *yin* deficiency of the heart and kidneys. It is marked by insomnia, palpitation, a poor memory or a loss of memory, dizziness, tinnitus, a dry throat, lower back pain, weak knees, drowsiness, spermatorrhea, a red tongue with a thin coating, and a thready, rapid pulse.

Treatment attempts to restore the coordination between the heart and the kidneys. Coptis and Cinnamon Formula (*jiao tai wan*) or Coptis and Gelatin Combination (*huang lian a jiao tang*) can be selected.

Coptis and Cinnamon Formula
Jiao Tai Wan[16]
(Grand Communication Pill)[2]

| Coptis | Coptidis rhizoma | Huang lian | 1.0 |
| Cinnamon bark | Cinnamomi cortex | Gui pi | 0.5 |

Functions: restores the proper balance between the heart and kidneys; treats anxiety, insomnia and cold limbs caused by kidney *yang* deficiency.

Explanation: Coptis purges excess heart *yang*, thereby restoring the coordination between the heart (fire) and the kidneys (water). As fire and water become balanced, anxiety and insomnia are relieved. Meanwhile, cinnamon bark warms kidney *yang* to help kidney *yin* ascend and so nourish heart *yin*.

Coptis and Gelatin Combination[1]

Huang Lian A Jiao Tang*

(Coptis and Ass Hide Gelatin Decoction)[2]

Coptis	*Coptidis rhizoma*	*Huang lian*	3.0
Gelatin	*Asini gelatinum*	*A jiao*	3.0
Scute	*Scutellariae radix*	*Huang qin*	2.0
Peony	*Paeoniae radix*	*Shao yao*	2.5
Egg yolk	*Gallus*	*Ji zi huang*	1 yolk

*also spelled *huang lian e jiao tang*

Liver and Kidney *Yin* Deficiency

Dizziness; tinnitus; pain in the hypochondriac region; lower back pain; weak knees; a dry throat; a flushed face; night sweats; a feverish sensation in the palms, soles and heart area; spermatorrhea or irregular menstruation; a red tongue with no coating; and a thready, rapid pulse are characteristic of *yin* deficiency of the liver and kidneys.

Lycium, Chrysanthemum and Rehmannia Formula (*qi ju di huang wan*) can be selected for nourishing the liver and kidneys.

Disharmony Between the Liver and Spleen

Distending pain and fullness in the hypochondrium; depression or irritability; a poor appetite; distention and fullness in the stomach region and abdomen; borborygmus; flatulence; bowel-movement disorders; a white tongue coating; and a wiry, slow pulse characterize a disharmony between the liver and spleen.

Treatment attempts to tonify the spleen and restore normal functioning to the liver. Bupleurum Formula (*xiao yao san*) is suitable for this purpose.

Disharmony Between the Liver and Stomach

Distention and pain in the hypochondrium and stomach region; belching; acid regurgitation; nausea; vomiting; a thin, yellow tongue coating; and a wiry pulse characterize this conformation.

Treatment restores the normal functioning of the liver, which, in turn, restores the stomach to its normal functioning. Bupleurum and *Chih-shih* Formula (*si ni san*), along with Magnolia and Ginger Formula (*ping wei san*), can be used.

Bupleurum and *Chih-shih* Formula[1]
Si Ni San
(Frigid Extremities Powder)[2]

Bupleurum	Bupleuri radix	Chai hu	3.0
Chih-shih	Citri fructus immaturus	Zhi shi	2.0
Peony	Paeoniae radix	Bai shao	4.0
Licorice	Glycyrrhizae radix	Gan cao	1.5

Invasion of the Lungs by Liver Fire

A burning pain in the chest and hypochondrium; paroxysmal cough; difficult expectoration of yellow sputum or even the coughing up of blood; impatience; irritability; dysphoria with a sensation of heat; a dry, bitter-tasting mouth; dizziness; conjunctival congestion; a red tongue with a thin coating; and a wiry, rapid pulse characterize this conformation.

Treatment is aimed at clearing and purging lung fire. Morus and Lycium Formula (*xie bai san*), together with 1 *qian* natural indigo (*qing dai*) and 3 *qian* cyclina (*hai ge fen*), is recommended. The resulting formula is known as Powder of Natural Indigo and Cyclina (*dai ge san*).

Morus and Lycium Formula[1]
Xie Bai San
(Drain the White Powder)[2]

Lycium bark	*Lycii radicis cortex*	Di gu pi	4.0
Morus bark	*Mori radicis cortex*	Sang bai pi	4.0
Licorice, baked	*Glycyrrhizae radix*	Gan cao	2.0
Rice	*Oryzae semen*	Jing mi	2.0

Spleen and Lung *Qi* Deficiency

Chronic cough; shortness of breath; general lassitude; copious, thin sputum; a poor appetite; abdominal distention; loose stools; a pale tongue with a white coating; and a thready, weak pulse are characteristic of this conformation.

Treatment is aimed at tonifying the spleen and lungs. Six Major Herb Combination (*liu jun zi tang*) can be used.

Six Major Herb Combination[1]
Liu Jun Zi Tang
(Six Gentleman Decoction)[2]

Ginseng	*Ginseng radix*	Ren shen	2.0
Atractylodes, white	*Atractylodis rhizoma*	Bai zhu	3.0
Hoelen	*Poria sclerotium*	Fu ling	4.0
Citrus peel	*Citri pericarpium*	Chen pi	2.0
Pinellia	*Pinellia rhizoma*	Ban xia	3.0
Licorice, baked	*Glycyrrhizae radix*	Gan cao	3.0

Lung and Kidney *Yin* Deficiency

Cough with scanty sputum or blood, lower back pain, weak knees, a gaunt appearance, hectic fever, dry mouth and throat, night sweats, a flushed face, seminal emission, a red tongue with a smooth coating and a thready, rapid pulse characterize this conformation.

Treatment moistens and tonifies the lungs and kidneys with Rehmannia and Schizandra Formula (*qi wei du qi wan*), plus 3 *qian* ophiopogon (*mai men dong*). The resulting formula is known as Pills for a Long Life (*mai wei di huang wan*).

Rehmannia and Schizandra Formula[1]

Qi Wei Du Qi Wan

(Pill of Seven Ingredients, Including Rehmannia)

Schizandra	*Schizandrae fructus*	Wu wei zi	1.0
Rehmannia, cooked	*Rehmanniae radix*	Shu di huang	4.0
Cornus	*Corni fructus*	Shan zhu yu	3.0
Dioscorea	*Dioscorea batatis rhizoma*	Shan yao	3.0
Alisma	*Alismatis rhizoma*	Ze xie	3.0
Hoelen	*Poria sclerotium*	Fu ling	3.0
Moutan	*Moutan radicis cortex*	Mu dan pi	3.0

Spleen and Kidney *Yang* Deficiency

Chills, cold limbs, lower back pain, weak knees, a pale or sallow complexion, shortness of breath, apathy, lack of energy to speak, lassitude, a poor appetite, loose stools or diarrhea before dawn, puffiness of the face, edematous of the extremities or even ascites, a pale, swollen tongue with a white, slippery coating and a submerged, weak pulse characterize *yang* deficiency of the spleen and kidneys. Vitality Combination (*zhen wu tang*) can be used for warming and tonifying the spleen and kidneys.

Common Acupuncture and Moxibustion Points

Heart and Lung *Qi* Deficiency

- *qihai* (CV 6)
- *tangzhong* (CV 7)

Heart and Lung Deficiency

- *xinshu* (B 15)
- *feishu* (B 13)
- *geshu* (B 17)

Imbalance Between the Heart and Kidneys

- *xinshu* (B 15)
- *shenshu* (B 23)
- *dalin* (P 7)
- *taixi* (K 3)

Liver and Kidney *Yin* Deficiency

- *sayinjiao* (Sp 6)
- *ganshu* (B 18)
- *shenshu* (B 23)

Disharmony Between the Liver and Spleen

- *taicong* (Liv 3)
- *zhongwan* (CV 12)

Invasion of the Lungs by Liver Fire

- *xinglian* (Liv 2)
- *hegu* (LI 4)
- *taiyuan* (Lu 9)

Spleen and Lung *Qi* Deficiency

- *feishu* (B 13)
- *pishu* (B 20)
- *lieque* (Lu 9)

Lung and Kidney *Yin* Deficiency

- *taixi* (B 13)
- *shenshu* (B 23)
- *taiyuan* (Lu 9)
- *feishu* (B 13)

Spleen and Kidney *Yang* Deficiency

- *sanyinjiao* (Sp 6)
- *yinlingquan* (Sp 9)
- *mingmen* (GV 4)
- *pishu* (B 20)
- *shenshu* (B 23)

Chapter 4

Differentiation and Treatment of Common Conformations

Section 1
Fever

Fever is one of the most common disease symptoms. The first discussion of fever in traditional Chinese medical literature is seen in *Su Wen* (Plain Questions) in its "Treatise on Fever": "A fever develops when one catches cold." The TCM theories of febrile diseases and fever due to internal injuries offer a means of differentiating between conformations. In treating fever, TCM practices are not inferior to the use of antibiotics, and this should be acknowledged by Western health-care providers.

Fevers have various causes, and their clinical manifestations are also complicated. In general, they may be divided into two types: those due to external pathogens and those which arise as a result of injuries.

Fever Due to External Pathogens

The six evils, or six excesses, associated with the six climatic factors act upon the surface of the body. *Zhen qi*, or healthy energy, struggles against the evils and attempts to subdue them. The six evils usually invade the body from the exterior to the interior, from the skin and hair to the meridians, collaterals, internal organs and tissues.

At the initial stage, a fever is known as an exterior fever. When pathogenic heat is both exterior and interior, it is referred to as a half-exterior/half-interior fever. If pathogenic heat invades the interior, it is then known as interior fever. In Western medicine, fevers caused by influenza and epidemic diseases belong to the TCM classification of fevers caused by external pathogens.

Exterior Fever

1. Fever due to wind-cold

Fever due to wind-cold can manifest itself as either of two constellations of symptoms: (1) an aversion to cold; fever; headache; an absence of sweat; arthralgia; a stuffy nose; watery nasal discharge; continual sneezing and coughing; and an itchy sore throat; or (2) profuse, thin sputum; a thin, white tongue coating; and a floating or/and tense pulse.

Treatment is aimed at the relief of the exterior conformation with pungent, warm-natured herbs to dispel wind and disperse cold. Schizonepeta and Siler Formula (*jing fang bai du san*) can be administered.

If an acute headache occurs, add 6 *qian* angelica (*bai zhi*).

If there is also profuse sputum, add 6 *qian* each of pinellia (*ban xia*) and citrus peel (*chen pi*).

2. Fever due to wind-heat

This type of fever is generally accompanied by the following signs and symptoms: a slight aversion to wind and cold; perspiration; headache; general aching; coughing; scant amounts of thick, yellow sputum; a dry mouth and a feeling of being somewhat thirsty; a red, swollen, sore throat; a thin, yellow tongue coating; and a rapid, floating pulse.

Treatment seeks to relieve exterior symptoms with pungent, cool-natured herbs which expel wind and clear heat. Lonicera and Forsythia Formula (*yin qiao san*) is recommended.

If the conformation is aggravated by a severe headache, add 3 *qian each of* morus leaf (*san ye*) and chrysanthemum (*ju hua*).

If the patient has a severe cough, add 3 *qian* apricot seed (*xing ren*) and 4 *qian* peucedanum (*qian hu*).

If the patient has a high fever and a dry mouth, add 3 *qian* each of scute (*huang qin*) and anemarrhena (*zhi mu*) and 5 *qian* raw gypsum (*shi gao*).

If the patient's throat is swollen and sore, add 3 *qian* each of scrophularia (*xuan shen*) and subprostrata (*shan dou gen*).

During the summer months, wind-heat is known as summer heat, the external evil that causes summer influenza. Symptoms include an absence of or decrease in the amount of sweat, restlessness, thirst, fullness in the head, a sensation of a weight on the chest, general aching, dark yellow urine, a yellow tongue coating and a soft, rapid pulse.

Summer influenza may be treated by clearing summer heat and removing dampness through diuresis--aims for which Elsholtzia Combination (*xiang ru yin*) is highly recommended.

If a more potent effect is desired, add 3 *qian* each of lonicera (*jin yin hua*), hoelen (*fu ling*), plantago (*che qian zi*), forsythia (*lian qiao*), agastache (*huo xiang*) and eupatorium (*pei lan*), as well as 5 *qian* each of lotus leaf (*he ye*) and the patent medicine *liu yi san*. The latter consists of talc (*hua shi*) and licorice (*gan cao*) in a 5:1 ratio.

Elsholtzia Combination[1*]
Xiang Ru Yin[1]
(Elsholtzia Powder)[2]

Elsholtzia	Elsholtziae herba	Xiang ru	6.0
Dolichos	Dolichoris semen	Bai bian dou	6.0
Magnolia bark	Magnoliae officinalis cortex	Hou pu	3.0

*also known as *xiang ru san*

If the conformation of wind-heat with dampness is manifested by heavy-headedness, lassitude, a sensation of oppression in the chest, nausea, dark yellow urine, and a greasy, yellow tongue coating, add 3 *qian* each of atractylodes (*cang zhu*), pinellia (*ban xia*), plantago (*che qian zi*) and hoelen (*fu ling*).

3. Fever due to heat-dampness accumulation

A lingering fever, a sensation of heaviness throughout the body, an oppressed feeling in the epigastrium, loss of appetite, nausea, loose stools, a red tongue with a yellow coating, and a soft, floating and rapid or slippery and rapid pulse characterize fever due to an accumulation of heat-dampness.

Treatment aims to clear heat and dissolve dampness with Talc and Scute Formula (*gan lu xiao du dan*).

Talc and Scute Formula

Gan Lu Xiao Du Dan

(Sweet Dew Special Pill to Eliminate Toxin)[2]

Talc	Talcum	Hua shi	45.0
Capillaris	Artemisiae capillaris herba	Yin chen hao	33.0
Scute	Scutellariae radix	Huang qin	33.0
Acorus	Acori rhizoma	Chang pu	18.0
Akebia	Akebiae caulis	Mu tong	15.0
Fritillaria	Fritillariae bulbus	Bei mu	15.0
Belamcanda	Belamcandae rhizoma	She gan	12.0
Forsythia	Forsythiae fructus	Lian qiao	12.0
Mentha	Menthae herba	Bo he	12.0
Cluster	Amomi rotundi fructus	Bai dou kou	12.0
Agastache	Agastache rugosa herba	Huo xiang	12.0

The above ingredients are ground into a powder and administered in 3- or 5-*qian* dosages once daily with water. The formula may be supplemented with a 2- or 3-*qian* dose of *shen-chu* (*shen qu*), taken once or twice daily.

Functions: dissolves turbid evil; drains dampness; clears heat; detoxifies.

Explanation: Talc, capillaris and akebia drain dampness and alleviate water retention, while scute and forsythia clear heat and detoxify. Acorus, fritillaria and belamcanda resolve phlegm and alleviate dampness. Mentha induces diaphoresis and eliminates dampness, and cluster and agastache are aromatic herbs which dissolve dampness.

Half-exterior/Half-interior Fever

Alternating attacks of chills and fever, a bitter taste in the mouth, a dry throat, dizziness, fullness and discomfort in the chest and hypochondrium, fidgeting, nausea, loss of appetite, taciturnity, a thin, white tongue coating, and a wiry pulse characterize half-exterior/half-interior fever conformation.

Treatment is aimed at abating the fever with Minor Bupleurum Combination (*xiao chai hu tang*).

If the patient is also very thirsty, add 3 *qian* trichosanthes root (*gua lou gen*).

Should the patient have an aversion to cold, add 2 *qian* cinnamon twig (*gui zhi*).

If the patient is experiencing abdominal pain, add 3 *qian* peony (*shao yao*) to Minor Bupleurum Combination.

Interior Fever

1. Heat in *qi fen*

A high fever, an aversion to heat, panting, thirst with a preference for cold beverages, a red tongue with a yellow coating, and a surging, rapid pulse characterize heat in *qi fen*.

Treatment attempts to clear *qi* and abate fever with Gypsum Combination (*bai hu tang*), to which is added 3 *qian* each of lonicera (*jin yin hua*) and forsythia (*lian qiao*), as well as 5 *qian* phragmites (*lu gen*) and 2 *qian* lophatherum (*dan zhu ye*).

If the patient complains of an acute sensation of tightness in the chest, add 3 *qian* each of magnolia bark (*hon pu*) and *chih-ko* (*zhi ke*).

If an inward transmission of pathogenic heat occurs, accompanied by the consumption of body fluids, the following manifestations may be observed: high fever or afternoon tidal fever; constipation; distention, fullness and pain in the abdomen; loss of consciousness; delirium; a dry tongue with a thick, yellow coating, or a gray or black, prickled tongue; and a submerged, excess pulse or a submerged, rapid and excess pulse. The fever is treated through purging heat with bitter, cold-natured herbs. Major Rhubarb Combination (*da cheng qi tang*) can be used.

If pathogenic heat impairs *yin*, add 3 *qian* each of raw rehmannia (*sheng di huang*), scrophularia (*xuan shen*) and ophiopogon (*mai men dong*) to Major Rhubarb Combination. The resulting formula is known as Scrophularia and Rhubarb Combination (*zeng ye cheng qi tang*).

If the patient is producing only small amounts of dark yellow urine, add 3 *qian* hoelen (*fu ling*) and 4 *qian* each of plantago (*che qian zi*) and coix (*yi yi ren*).

If dampness is acute and heat is only mild, the symptoms are headache, a sensation of heaviness in the torso and limbs, a slightly yellow complexion, a feeling of oppression in the chest, a loss of appetite, afternoon fever, a loss of the sense of taste, no desire to drink, a white tongue coating, and a soft, floating pulse. Apricot, Coix and Cluster Combination (*san ren tang*) can be used to treat these symptoms.

Apricot, Coix and Cluster Combination
San Ren Tang[7]
(Three Nut Decoction)[2]

Apricot seed	*Armeniacae semen*	*Xing ren*	3.0
Talc	*Talcum*	*Hua shi*	5.0
Pinellia	*Pinellia rhizoma*	*Ban xia*	2.0
Tetrapanax	*Tetrapanacis medulla*	*Tong cao*	2.0
Coix	*Coicis semen*	*Yi yi ren*	6.0
Lophatherum	*Lophatheri herba*	*Dan zhu ye*	2.0
Magnolia bark	*Magnoliae officinalis cortex*	*Hou pu*	2.0
Cluster	*Amomi rotundi fructus*	*Bai kou ren*	1.0

Functions: dissolves dampness; purges heat; disperses excess *qi*.

Explanation: Apricot seed promotes lung *qi* in the upper *jiao* (upper energizer), while cluster resolves dampness in the middle *jiao*. Pinellia aids apricot seed and cluster in coordinating and/or correcting the functioning of the upper and middle *jiao*. Coix, talc, tetrapanax, lophatherum and magnolia bark clear heat-dampness from the lower *jiao*. This prescription is especially recommended for heat-dampness conformation when dampness is more acute than heat.

2. *Ying fen* and blood *fen* invaded by heat

Fever which is more intense at night, fidgeting, a red tongue, skin rashes, hemoptysis, bloody stools and a rapid pulse characterize this conformation. When the patient is very ill, delirium or coma may also occur.

Treatment aims to clear *ying* and blood, as well as remove heat toxins and nourish *yin* with Rhinoceros and Scrophularia Combination (*qing ying tang*).

Rhinoceros and Scrophularia Combination

Qing Ying Tang[7]

(Clear Heat in *Ying Fen* Decoction)

Rhinoceros horn*	*Rhinocerotis cornu*	*Xi jiao*	0.2
Rehmannia, raw	*Rehmanniae radix*	*Sheng di huang*	5.0
Bitter bamboo leaf	*Pleioblasti folium*	*Zhu ye xin*	3.0
Lonicera	*Lonicerae flos*	*Jin yin hua*	3.0
Forsythia	*Forsythiae fructus*	*Lian qiao*	3.0
Coptis	*Coptidis rhizoma*	*Huang lian*	1.0
Scrophularia	*Scrophulariae radix*	*Xuan shen*	3.0
Ophiopogon	*Ophiopogonis rhizoma*	*Mai men dong*	3.0
Salvia	*Salviae miltiorrhizae radix*	*Dan shen*	5.0

* grind to a powder and take with warm water

For mild cases, decoct the standard dose and administer twice daily. For acute cases, double the dose and administer four times daily.

Functions: removes heat from *ying fen* and blood *fen*; detoxifies; nourishes *yin*.

Explanation: Rhinoceros horn, rehmannia and salvia clear, cool and detoxify *ying* and blood. Bitter bamboo leaf, lonicera, coptis and forsythia play supporting roles in detoxification and the clearing of heat. Scrophularia and ophiopogon nourish *yin* and clear heat.

If pathogenic heat penetrates deeply into blood *fen*, Rhinoceros and Rehmannia Combination (*xi jiao di huang tang*) can be used.

If the patient has a tendency to bleed, add 4 *qian* biota top (*ce bo ye*) and 3 *qian* each of lithospermum (*zi cao*), madder (*qian cao gen*), Japanese thistle (*da ji*) and field thistle (*xiao ji*).

For unconscious or delirious patients, add aromatic herbs to restore consciousness. For example, Bezoar and Curcuma Formula (*an gong niu huang wan*) can be taken twice or three times daily, depending on the patient's condition.

Bezoar and Curcuma Formula[1]

An Gong Niu Huang Wan

(Calm the Palace Pill with Cattle Gallstone)[2]

Cow gallstone	*Bovis bezoar*	Niu huang	4.0
Turmeric	*Curcumae rhizoma*	Yu jin	4.0
Rhinoceros horn	*Rhinocerotis cornu*	Xi jiao	4.0
Coptis	*Coptidis rhizoma*	Huang lian	4.0
Realgar	*Realgar*	Xiong huang	4.0
Gardenia	*Gardeniae fructus*	Zhi zi	4.0
Cinnabar	*Cinnabaris*	Zhu sha	4.0
Borneol	*Borneolum*	Bing pian	1.0
Musk	*Moschus*	She xiang	1.0
Pearl	*Margarita*	Zhen shu	2.0
Scute	*Scutellariae radix*	Huang qin	4.0

The ingredients are ground into powder and made into boluses by mixing with honey. Each bolus weighs 3 *qian* and is coated in gold foil and sealed in wax. For oral administration, one bolus is taken once daily after dissolution in warm water.

Functions: clears heat; detoxifies; restores consciousness; calms delirium.

Explanation: Cow gallstone, rhinoceros horn, coptis and gardenia clear heart fire and detoxify. Turmeric, cinnabar, pearl and gold foil have a tranquilizing affect, while realgar alleviates fetidness and detoxifies. Borneol and musk restore consciousness by promoting *qi* circulation. This prescription may be used for encephalitis B, epidemic cerebrospinal meningitis, severe hepatitis, coma and convulsions due to infections.

Fever Due to Internal Injury

Such fevers are the result of injury to *qi* and blood in the viscera, a disorder between *yin* and *yang*, or a disharmony between *ying* (nutrients) and defensive *qi*. If a person's mind is not at ease, *qi* will stagnate and transform into fire. Likewise, if blood stasis is present, *qi* will transform into heat. Sometimes *yin* or *yang* deficiencies cause this type of disease as well. Fever which accompanies tuberculosis, tumors and chronic infectious diseases in Western medicine belongs to the TCM classification of fever due to internal injury.

1. Fever due to *yin* deficiency

A fever which rises in the afternoon or at night, red cheeks, fidgeting, night sweats, insomnia, drowsiness, a dry mouth and throat, constipation, small amounts of dark yellow urine, a dry, red tongue with fissures and little or no coating, and a thready, rapid pulse characterize fever due to *yin* deficiency.

This syndrome is treated by nourishing *yin* and clearing heat with *Chin-chiu* and Turtle Shell Formula (*qin jiao bie jia san*).

If the *yin* deficiency is acute, add 5 *qian* raw rehmannia (*sheng di huang*) and 4 *qian* scrophularia (*xuan shen*).

If the patient also has blood deficiency, add 3 *qian* tang-kuei (*dang gui*) and 5 *qian* cooked rehmannia (*shu di huang*).

For insomnia, add 2 *qian* zizyphus (*suan zao ren*) and 4 *qian* biota (*bo zi ren*).

For night sweats, add 4 *qian* light wheat (*fu xiao mai*) and 10 *qian* each of oyster shell (*mu li*) and glutinous rice root (*nuo dao gen*).

2. Fever due to *qi* deficiency

Fever which is aggravated by fatigue, a soft voice, shortness of breath, no sensation of taste, an aversion to wind, spontaneous sweating, a pale, teeth-marked tongue with a thin coating, and a weak pulse characterize fever due to *qi* deficiency.

Treatment is aimed at relieving fever with warm, sweet-flavored herbs, specifically, Ginseng and Astragalus Combination (*bu zhong yi qi tang*).

3. Heat stagnancy in the liver meridians

This conformation is characterized by occasional fever; fidgeting; a propensity to become easily angered; a feeling of fullness in the head; tinnitus that becomes more serious when the patient is ill at ease; fullness in the chest and hypochondrium; excessive sighing; a bitter taste in the mouth; nausea; a red tongue with a thin, yellow coating; and a wiry, rapid and thready pulse.

Treatment is aimed at soothing the liver and clearing heat with *Tang-kuei* and Bupleurum Formula (*xiao yao san*).

If there is a high fever, Bupleurum and Peony Formula (*jia wei xiao yao san*) may be administered. Bupleurum and Peony

Formula is Bupleurum and *Tang-kuei* Formula plus 3 *qian* each of moutan (*mu dan pi*) and gardenia (*zhi zi*).

If the patient complains of pain in the hypochondriac region, add 4 *qian* turmeric (*yu jin*) and 3 *qian* each of melia (*chuan lian zi*) and corydalis (*yan hu suo*) to Bupleurum and Peony Formula.

Bupleurum and Peony Formula[1]

Jia Wei Xiao Yao San

(Rambling Powder plus Moutan and Gardenia)

Bupleurum	*Bupleuri radix*	Chai hu	3.0
Mentha	*Menthae herba*	Bo he	1.0
Tang-kuei	*Angelicae radix*	Dang gui	3.0
Peony	*Paeoniae radix*	Shao yao	3.0
Atractylodes, white	*Atractylodis rhizoma*	Bai zhu	3.0
Hoelen	*Poria sclerotium*	Fu ling	3.0
Licorice	*Glycyrrhizae radix*	Gan cao	2.0
Ginger, dried	*Zingiberis siccatum rhizoma*	Gan jiang	1.0
Moutan	*Moutan radicis cortex*	Mu dan pi	2.0
Gardenia	*Gardeniae fructus*	Zhi zi	2.0

4. Fever due to blood stasis

Fever in the afternoon or at night, a dry mouth and throat, body aches and pains, an abdominal mass, squamous and dry skin, cyanosed lips, a dark purple complexion, a purple tongue with petechiae, and a thready, hesitant pulse characterize blood stasis.

This conformation is treated by promoting blood circulation, dissolving stasis, regulating the flow of *qi* and activating the meridians with Persica and Rhubarb Combination (*tao he cheng qi tang*).

Acupuncture and Moxibustion Treatment

Common Points

- *dazhui* (GV 14)
- *fengchi* (G 20)
- *fengmen* (B 12)
- *hegu* (LI 4)
- *quchi* (LI 11)

Treatment Method

Use the above points or employ the 12 *jing* (well) points in addition to bloodletting.

Section 2
Cough

A cough is one of the principal symptoms of pulmonary diseases. Clinically, it can be classified into two groups: a cough which is caused by an attack of external pathogens on the lungs or one which is the result of a functional imbalance of the internal organs. As the section "Treatise on the Cough" in *Su Wen* (Plain Questions) points out: "Cough is induced by disorders of the internal organs." Generally speaking, coughs can be observed in upper respiratory tract infections, bronchitis, pneumonia, pulmonary tuberculosis and bronchiectasis.

A differentiation must be made before the onset of treatment as to whether the cough is due to external pathogens or internal injury. The former is considered an excess conformation, while the latter is a deficiency conformation or a deficiency complicated by an excess conformation.

Generally speaking, a cough due to external pathogens is a symptom indicating an acute, sudden disease following the patient's encounter with wind or cold. Such a disease is often accompanied by the following symptoms: a stuffy nose, nasal discharge, sneezing, itchiness and pain in the throat, distention and pain in the head, general soreness, an aversion to wind and cold, and fever.

On the other hand, coughs due to internal injuries indicate chronic diseases. Such diseases are often the result of visceral and bowel disorders, and are characterized by the following symptoms: lassitude, poor appetite, loose stools, and pain and fullness in the chest and hypochondrium. Patients with coughs due to internal injuries tend to be easily affected by external pathogens, which further exacerbate the coughs. This is especially common when the weather is cold. In such a case, the cough is said to be caused by both external pathogens and internal injury.

Coughs Due to External Pathogens

When external wind, cold, heat or dryness invade the lungs, obstruction of lung *qi* results, which, in turn, brings on a cough. Since the lungs are delicate organs, directly linked to the nose and associated with the skin and hair, they tend to be quite vulnerable to attack by external pathogens, particularly wind-cold, wind-heat and heat-dryness.

Cough Due to Wind-cold

A cough with thin, white sputum; nasal discharge; sneezing; an aversion to cold; an absence of sweat; arthralgia; distention and pain in the head; a thin, white tongue coating; and a floating or normal pulse characterize a cough brought about by wind-cold.

If dampness is also present, an absence of the sensation of taste, a sticky mouth and a thin, greasy tongue coating may be observed.

Treatment is aimed at dispelling wind-cold and ventilating lung *qi*, for which *Ma-huang*, Licorice and Apricot Seed Combination (*san ao tang*) can be given.

If the exterior cold manifestations are severe and accompanied by an aversion to cold, an absence of sweat and arthralgia, 3 *qian* cinnamon twig (*gui zhi*) or 3 *qian* each of schizonepeta (*jing jie*) and siler (*fang feng*) should be added to *Ma-huang*, Licorice and Apricot Seed Combination.

If the patient is troubled by sputum which is difficult expectorate, 4 *qian* each trichosanthes peel (*gua lou pi*) and benincasa (*dong gua zi*) should be added.

Ma-huang, Licorice and Apricot Seed Combination[1]

San Ao Tang

(Three Unbinding Decoction)[2]

Ma-huang	Ephedrae radix	Ma huang	3.0
Apricot seed	Armeniacae semen	Xing ren	3.0
Licorice	Glycyrrhizae radix	Gan cao	3.0

Cough Due to Wind-heat

A cough with yellow sputum which is thick or difficult to expectorate, thirst, a sore throat, yellowish nasal discharge, fever with sweating, an aversion to wind, headache, general soreness, a thin, yellow or thin, white tongue coating and a floating, rapid pulse characterize a cough due to wind-heat.

Treatment aims to dispel wind-heat and ventilate lung *qi*. Morus and Chrysanthemum Combination (*sang ju yin*) can be given to achieve these ends.

If a high fever is present, 10 *qian* each of houttuynia (*yu xing cao*) and cymosum (*kai jin suo*) should be added.

If the patient has a sore throat, add 5 *qian* isatis leaf (*da qing ye*) and 3 *qian* scrophularia (*xuan shen*).

If the sputum is profuse, 3 *qian* each of peucedanum (*qian hu*) and fritillaria (*bai mu*) should be added, while if the sputum is difficult to expectorate, 5 *qian* each of trichosanthes peel (*gua lou pi*) and benincasa *dong gua zi*) should be added.

If the patient is plagued by severe thirst, add 6 *qian* gypsum (*shi gao*) and 5 *qian* trichosanthes root (*gua lou gen*).

Cough Due to Heat-dryness

A dry cough or a cough with sputum which is difficult to expectorate; a dry nose and throat; chest pain during severe coughing fits; an aversion to cold; fever; a red tongue tip; a thin, yellow tongue coating; and a weak, rapid pulse characterize a cough due to heat-dryness.

Treatment aims to clear the lungs and moisten dryness. Morus and Apricot Seed Combination (*sang xing tang*) can be used.

Morus and Apricot Seed Combination
Sang Xing Tang[7]
(Mulberry Leaf and Apricot Kernel Decoction)[2]

Morus leaf	*Mori folium*	Sang ye	3.0
Apricot seed	*Armeniacae semen*	Xing ren	3.0
Glehnia	*Glehniae radix cum rhizoma*	Bei sha shen	2.0
Soja	*Sojae semen praeparatum*	Dan dou chi	3.0
Fritillaria	*Fritillariae bulbus*	Bei mu	3.0
Gardenia	*Gardeniae fructus*	Zhi zi	2.0
Pear peel	*Pyri fructus*	Li pi	2.0

Functions: clears heat; moistens dryness.

Explanation: This formula is good for treating the conformation of lungs attacked by heat-dryness. Morus leaf and soja are used to ventilate the lungs and dispel external evils, while apricot seed promotes the circulation of lung *qi*. Glehnia, fritillaria and pear peel moisten the lungs and relieve coughing, while gardenia clears heat from the chest.

If the patient's throat is dry and itchy, 9 *qian* each of scrophularia (*xuan shen*) and ophiopogon (*mai men dong*) should be added to Morus and Apricot Seed Combination.

If heat-dryness is severe, 10 *qian* gypsum (*shi gao*) and 3 *qian* lycium bark (*di gu pi*) should be added.

If there is oppressive chest pain, 3 *qian* each of tussilago (*kuan dong hua*) and inula (*xuan fu hua*) should be added.

For a persistant cough caused by external pathogens and accompanied by an itchy throat and difficulty in expectorating sputum, or for a recurring cough or one which persists after the external pathogens have been eliminated, Platycodon and Schizonepeta Formula (*zhi sou san*) can be used.

Coughs Due to Internal Injury

Such coughs are either caused by lung deficiency or a disorder of another organ which affects the lungs (as, for example, phlegm-dampness invading the lungs or liver fire attacking the lungs). As regards lung deficiency, it may be divided into lung *yin* deficiency and lung *qi* deficiency.

The differentiation and treatment of the cough can be made according to the organs of the upper, middle and lower body. Treating coughs associated with the upper body means treating the lungs. Treating the mid-section centers around the treatment of the spleen, which includes tonifying the spleen to resolve sputum. Treating chronic coughs which emanate from the lower body and are associated with a shortness of breath necessitates treating the kidneys with the patent medicine Ginseng and Concha Formula (*shen ge san*), to which has been added cooked rehmannia (*shu di huang*) and schizandra (*wu wei zi*).

Lung *Yin* Deficiency

Lung *yin* deficiency develops slowly. The cough may be with or without sputum. When present, this sputum is sometimes mixed with blood. The patient has a gaunt appearance, a dry mouth and throat, afternoon hectic fever, a flushed malar, a feverish sensation in the palms and soles, insomnia, night sweats, a red tongue and a thready, rapid pulse.

Treatment attempts to nourish *yin*, clear heat, resolve phlegm and suppress the cough. Lily Combination (*bai he gu jin tang*) can be used.

Lung *Qi* Deficiency

In this case, a cough accompanied by a shortness of breath or a cough with thin sputum; pallor; insufficient strength to speak or a low, weak voice; an aversion to cold; spontaneous sweating; a susceptibility to influenza; asthma; a pale, tender tongue; and a weak pulse may be observed.

Six Major Herb Combination (*liu jun zi tang*), to which is added 3 *qian* each of astragalus (*huang qi*) and schizandra (*wu wei zi*) and 2 *qian* siler (*fang feng*), can be used.

Lungs Attacked by Liver Fire

The liver meridian runs through the chest and hypochondrium to the lungs. If *qi* stagnancy in the liver is transformed into fire, it will ascend into the lungs, resulting in a cough.

This condition is characterized by a cough due to the ascent of lung *qi*; a flushed face; a dry throat; pain in the hypochondrium which is aggravated by coughing; bloody sputum; a dry, thin, yellow tongue coating; and a rapid, wiry pulse.

Treatment attempts to purge lung and liver fire. Morus and Lycium Formula (*xie bai san*), to which has been added 3 *qian* each of gardenia (*zhi zi*) and apricot seed (*xing ren*) and 1 *qian* licorice (*gan cao*), can be given.

If there is fidgeting, insomnia, a dry mouth and a red tongue, 1 *qian* coptis (*huang lian*) and 2 *qian* lophatherum (*dan zhu ye*) should be added.

If there is thick, yellow sputum, add Indigo and Concha Formula (*dai ge san*), as well as 5 *qian* benincasa (*dong gua zi*) and 10 *qian* houttuynia (*yu xing cao*).

Indigo and Concha Formula

Dai Ge San

(Indigo and Concha Powder)

Indigo, natural	*Indigo Naturalis*	Qing dai	1.5
Cyclina	*Cyclinae concha*	Hai ge fen	1.5

Phlegm-dampness Invading the Lungs

This condition is characterized by a cough with profuse, white sputum; a feeling of oppression in the chest; a white, greasy tongue coating; and a soft, floating and slippery pulse.

A deficient spleen fails to appropriately transport and transform nutrients and fluids, the latter of which accumulate and turn into phlegm. When stored in the lungs, phlegm can prevent lung *qi* from descending, and so produce a cough. A TCM saying offers this: "The spleen is the source of phlegm and the lungs are its container."

Treatment aims to remove dampness and tonify the spleen in order to resolve phlegm. Citrus and Pinellia Combination (*er chen tang*), to which is added 3 *qian* each of perilla (*zi su zi*), brassica (bai jie zi), aster (*zi wan*), apricot seed (*xing ren*) and inula (*xuan fu hua*), can be used.

If the patient coughs up yellow sputum and has a fever and a bitter taste in his mouth, brassica should be deleted from the above formula and 3 *qian* scute (*huang qin*) and 10 *qian* houttuynia (*yu xing cao*) should be added.

Acupuncture and Moxibustion Treatment

Cough Due to External Evils

- *feishu* (B 13)
- *lieque* (L 7)
- *hegu* (LI 4)

Cough Due to Internal Injury

1. Phlegm-dampness invading the lungs

- *feishu* (B 13)
- *taiyuan* (L 9)
- *zhangmen* (Liv 13)
- *taibai* (Sp 3)
- *fenglong* (S 40)

2. Liver fire attacking the lungs

- *feishu* (B 13)
- *chize* (L 5)
- *yanglingquan* (G 34)
- *taicong* (Liv 3)

Section 3
Asthmatic Dyspnea

Asthmatic dyspnea is marked by a shortness of breath, bronchial wheezing, breathing through the mouth and difficulty in lying down. Some TCM literature differentiates between asthma and dyspnea. As *Yi Xue Xin Wu* (The Medical Compendium) points out: "Dyspnea refers to a disorder of breathing rhythm, while asthma refers to the presence of abnormal sounds during respiration." Shortness of breath, then, is associated with dyspnea, while bronchial wheezing is an asthmatic symptom. Clinically, both dyspnea and asthma can be observed at the same time, thus they will be discussed together in this section.

Asthmatic dyspnea can appear in bronchial asthma, asthmatic bronchitis, pulmonary emphysema and pulmonary heart disease. Asthmatic dyspnea may result from either external pathogens or internal injury. Clinically, it is due to either an excess of pathogens or a deficiency of vital energy; the former is called excess asthmatic dyspnea and the latter, deficient asthmatic dyspnea.

Differentiation between excess and deficiency should first be made in order to design an appropriate treatment. The main manifestations of the excess type are deep inhalation and difficult exhalation, harsh breathing, a rapid, excess pulse and a sudden onset. It should be treated by relieving the asthma and resolving phlegm.

The deficient type is marked by a shortness of breath following any exertion, a weak voice, a submerged and thready or large, floating pulse, and a slow onset. This disease can become serious, especially when aggravated by fatigue. It should be treated by reinforcing and consolidating kidney *qi*.

Both deficiency and excess cases are often seen together in the clinic. In excess cases, a deficiency of vital energy may be present, while in deficiency cases, the disease is usually aggravated by external pathogens.

Deficiency complicated by excess should be treated by strengthening the body's resistance against pathogenic factors. While the disease is in the exacerbation stage, it should be d by expelling the external pathogens, and when it is in remission, vital energy should be strengthened.

Excess Asthmatic Dyspnea

An excess of pathogens is related to external pathogens and turbid phlegm. Turbid phlegm develops from a deficiency of the spleen, kidney *yang*, or lung or kidney *yin*. If the spleen is deficient, fluids cannot be properly transported and transformed; if kidney *yang* is deficient, fluid retention cannot be resolved; and if lung or kidney *yin* is deficient, heat develops inside the body, thereby consuming fluids.

All of the above conditions produce phlegm, which is stored in the lungs. When phlegm and *qi* obstruct the collateral branch of the lungs and thereby impair their clearing function, as well as the function of directing *qi* downward, dyspnea, wheezing and asthma develop. Phlegm can also be induced by improper diet, emotional problems or fatigue. Based on clinical manifestations, there are two types of excess asthmatic dyspnea--cold and heat.

Cold Asthmatic Dyspnea

This variation is characterized by paroxysm induced by cold; shortness of breath or wheezing; a cough with thin, white sputum; watery nasal discharge; an aversion to cold; fever; headache; an absence of perspiration; a pale tongue with a thin, white coating; and a floating or floating and tense pulse.

Treatment focuses on warming the lungs and resolving phlegm to relieve asthma. Minor Blue Dragon Combination (*xiao qing long tang*) can be given.

Heat Asthmatic Dyspnea

This type is manifested by a shortness of breath; wheezing; a cough with yellow sputum; fidgeting; a sensation of oppression in the chest; thirst with a preference for cold beverages; dark yellow urine; a red tongue with a yellow, greasy coating; and a rapid pulse. In addition, some symptoms which are associated with the exterior, such as fever, a slight aversion to cold, headache, an absence of sweat and a floating pulse, may also be present.

Treatment is aimed at clearing lung heat and resolving phlegm to relieve asthma. *Ma-huang* and Apricot Seed Combination (*ma xing shi gan tang*), to which is added 3 *qian* perilla seed (*zi su zi*) and 4 *qian* earthworm (*di long*), can be used.

Deficient Asthmatic Dyspnea

This form of dyspnea is associated with vital energy deficiency, especially *qi* deficiency in the lungs and kidneys. The lungs control *qi*, while the kidneys are the source of *qi*. Both the lungs and kidneys control the inhalation and exhalation of air. If the lungs are deficient, they will be unable to properly control *qi*, and *qi* will reverse its flow, moving upward and thus causing dyspnea.

Kidney deficiency has an even greater affect on asthma than does lung deficiency. If kidney *yang* is too weak to regulate *qi*, fluids and abnormal, ascending *qi* will invade the heart and lungs, thereby inducing asthma.

Lung Deficiency

Lung deficiency is characterized by a shortness of breath, a weak voice, a weak cough, spontaneous sweating, an aversion to cold and a weak pulse.

Treatment attempts to tonify the spleen, replenish *qi* and relieve asthma. Six Major Herb Combination (*liu jun zi tang*) can be used.

If the patient also manifests some *yin* deficiency symptoms, such as pain in the throat, a dry mouth and a flushed face, 5 *qian* glehnia (*bei sha shen*) and 3 *qian* ophiopogon (*mai men dong*) should be added.

If the patient is troubled by severe spontaneous sweating, 3 *qian* astragalus (*huang qi*), 5 *qian* light wheat (*fu xiao mai*) and 10 *qian* glutinous rice root (*nuo dao gen*) can be added.

Kidney Deficiency

Kidney deficiency is manifested by lingering asthma, gasping breathing which is aggravated by physical exertion, listlessness, shortness of breath, sweating, cold limbs, an aversion to cold, a pale tongue with a white coating, and a submerged pulse.

Treatment is focused on warming the kidneys and improving inhalation by invigorating kidney *qi*. Rehmannia Eight Formula (*ba wei di huang wan*) can be used.

If shortness of breath is acute, add 3 *qian* each of codonopsis (*dang shen*) and walnut (*hu tao rou*), as well as 2 *qian* schizandra (*wu wei zi*).

In summary, asthmatic dyspnea is a chronic recurrent conformation. Strengthening the body's natural resistance should be affected during the initial stage, while the elimination of external pathogens is the recommended strategy during the paroxysmal stage. Thus, asthmatic dyspnea should be treated with herbs to relieve acute symptoms in emergency cases, but when these symptoms are relieved, the fundamental cause should be treated.

Acupuncture and Moxibustion Treatment

Paroxysmal Stage

1. Points of first choice

- *tiantu* (CV 22)
- *taiyuan* (L 9)
- *fenglong* (S 40)

2. Reserved points

- *feishu* (B 13)
- *dingchuan* (EX-B1)
- *dazhui* (GV 14)

Remission

1. Points of first choice

- *dazhui* (GV 14)
- *feishu* (B 13)
- *shenshu* (B 23)
- *pishu* (B 20)

2. Reserved points

- *guanyuan* (CV 4)
- *qihai* (CV 6)
- *taiyuan* (L 9)
- *fenglong* (S 40)

Treatment Method

1. Treat once or twice daily in the paroxysmal stage.

2. During remission, treat once daily or once every other day for a total of 10 treatments.

Section 4
Phlegm and Fluid Retention

Phlegm and fluid retention causes dysfunctions in the transportation, transformation and distribution of body fluids, which are then retained in various regions of the body cavity. Generally speaking, if the sputum is sticky, it is called phlegm; if it is clear and thin, it is called fluid retention.

Clinically, however, chronic bronchitis, bronchial asthma, exudative pleuritis, pyloric obstruction, intestinal obstruction and other hydropsy diseases which are associated with fluid retention are treated as phlegm-retention syndrome by TCM practitioners.

In ancient times, this syndrome was classified as either interior or exterior fluid retention, though the two are often present simultaneously. The former results from *yang qi* deficiency, particularly a deficiency of spleen *yang* in the middle energizer, which then loses its ability to properly transport and transform nutrients. Exterior fluid retention is induced by prolonged invasion of cold-dampness, poor dietary habits or fatigue, all of which can result in *yang qi* stagnation and the poor flow of *qi*.

Phlegm and fluid retention, induced by either an exterior or interior cause, is associated with the lungs, spleen and kidneys. Normally, absorption, transportation and excretion of body fluids are a coordinated effort between *qi*; the lungs, which maintain proper water transportation; the spleen, which transforms fluids; and the kidneys, which control the transportation of fluids. If dysfunctions occur in any of these organs, body fluids stagnate, resulting in fluid retention.

Yang deficiency of the spleen and kidneys is the main culprit in the formation and retention of phlegm. Indeed, phlegm retention is generally regarded as the conformation of *yang* deficiency and *yin* excess. Its origin is *yang* deficiency of the spleen and kidneys, while its exterior manifestation is interior stagnation of water and other fluids.

Diagnosis and Herbal Treatment

Differentiation should be made according to the location and severity of the fluid retention and the nature of the deficiency or excess. Because the accumulation of phlegm and fluids is a *yin* evil induced by cold, treatment is aimed at warming *yin* and resolving phlegm. *Jin Kui Yao Lue* (Synopsis of Prescriptions of the Golden Chamber) points out: "Cases of fluid and phlegm retention should be treated with warm herbs."

In general, if fluids are retained in the exterior, warm herbs should be accompanied by herbs for dispelling evils and resolving fluid retention; whereas if the fluid retention is in the interior, diuresis is the recommended treatment. In addition, hydragogue herbs should be administered to ward off excess evils, and if there is a spleen or kidney *yang* deficiency, tonifying herbs are most effective. External evils accompanied by a deficiency of body resistance are treated by using both dispelling and tonifying herbs, while the retention of cold fluids and heat evils are treated simultaneously. As regards emergency cases, the acute symptoms should be alleviated first. Only then should the fundamental cause be addressed.

Retained Fluids Invading the Lungs and Chest

This condition is characterized by the following signs and symptoms: cough; asthma; chest fullness; difficulty in breathing while lying supine; profuse, white, frothy sputum; paroxysm induced by cold; exterior chills; fever; and general soreness. In the lingering stage, edema of the face, a white, greasy tongue coating and a wiry, tense pulse may also be observed.

Treatment is aimed at warming the lungs, resolving fluid retention and relieving asthma and cough. Minor Blue Dragon Combination (*xiao qing long tang*) can be given.

If there is heat stagnancy marked by asthma, fidgeting and thin, white or yellow, frothy sputum, add 5 *qian* gypsum (*shi gao*).

If cough, asthma and profuse sputum are present without prominent exterior cold symptoms, add 3 *qian* each of lepidium (*ting li zi*) and perilla seed (*zi su zi*).

Fluid Retention in the Gastrointestinal Tract

Abdominal distention and fullness; a dry mouth and tongue; a splashing sound in the stomach; borborygmus; alternating constipation and diarrhea; small quantities of dark yellow urine; a thick, yellow tongue coating; and a submerged, slippery pulse characterize fluid retention in the gastrointestinal tract.

Treatment focuses on purging and dispelling retained fluids. Stephania and Lepidium Formula (*ji jiao li huang wan*) can be given.

Stephania and Lepidium Formula
Ji Jiao Li Huang Wan[10]
(Stephania, Zanthoxylum, Descurainia and Rhubarb Pill)[2]

Stephania	*Aristolochiae fangchi radix*	*Fang ji*	3.0
Zanthoxylum	*Zanthoxyli fructus*	*Shan jiao*	2.0
Lepidium	*Lepidii semen**	*Ting li zi*	3.0
Rhubarb	*Rhei rhizoma*	*Da huang*	2.0

**Descurainiae semen* may be substituted.*

Functions: dispels retained fluids; affects diuresis; alleviates constipation.

Explanation: Stephania and zanthoxylum are diuretics, while lepidium purges lung pathogens, facilitates the downward movement of *qi*, and dispels phlegm and fluid retention. Rhubarb is a purgative. Together these four herbs correct fluid retention in both the urine and the stools.

If the patient has a gaunt appearance, a poor appetite, loose stools, dizziness, palpitation and shortness of breath, use Atractylodes and Hoelen Combination (*ling gui zhu gan tang*) for warming *yang* and expelling retained fluids.

Fluid Retention in the Chest and Hypochondrium

Distention and pain in the chest and hypochondrium which are aggravated by coughing, difficulty in breathing, shortness of breath, a white tongue coating and a wiry pulse characterize this type of fluid retention.

Treatment attempts to purge retained fluids with Lepidium and Brassica Seed Combination (*si zi tang*).

Lepidium and Brassica Seed Combination*

Si Zi Tang

(Four Seed Decoction)

Lepidium	Lepidii semen	Ting li zi	8.0
Jujube	Zizyphi fructus	Da zao	5.0
Raphanus	Raphani semen	Lai fu zi	4.0
Perilla seed	Perillae semen	Zi su zi	3.0
Brassica	Sinapis semen	Bai jie zi	2.0
Atractylodes, white	Atractylodis rhizoma	Bai zhu	5.0
Hoelen peel	Poria cortex	Fu ling pi	4.0

*This formula has proved effective through years of clinical practice, though it is not included in most medical texts.

Fluid Retention in the Limbs

General body aches and heaviness; an absence of sweat; an absence of thirst; coughing; asthma; white, frothy sputum; a white tongue coating; and a wiry, tense pulse frequently signal fluid retention in the limbs.

Treatment is aimed at warming and dissipating fluid retention. Minor Blue Dragon Combination (*xiao qing long tang*) can be given.

Should stagnant cold transform into heat marked by fever, fidgeting, a white tongue coating and yellow sputum, Major Blue Dragon Combination (*da qing long tang*) should be given.

Acupuncture and Moxibustion Treatment

Please consult the sections in this chapter on cough, edema, asthma and chest pain.

Section 5
Chest Pain

Chest pain is often associated with the heart and lungs. Painful symptoms may be related to respiratory tract infections, pneumonia, pleuritis, coronary heart disease or intercostal neuralgia. In this section, treatments are given for precordial pain, angina pectoris and precordial pain with cold limbs-- terms recorded throughout the ages in TCM literature. In Western medicine, these diseases are called coronary heart disease, angina pectoris and cardiac infarction, respectively. A discussion of the causes of these three conditions follows.

Causes of Chest Pain

Impairment of the Interior by the Seven Emotions

Prolonged anxiety or mental stress results in *qi* stagnancy in the heart and liver, which, in turn, results in the condensation of water and fluids into phlegm. *Qi* stagnancy may also result in the formation of fire, which consumes body fluids and transforms them into phlegm. *Qi* stagnancy and phlegm accumulation may induce pain, dysfunctions of the heart and blockage of the blood vessels and meridians.

Intemperate Eating or Drinking

Excessive consumption of fatty foods, meats or alcoholic beverages impairs the spleen and stomach, thereby resulting in dysfunctions in the transportation and transformation of nutrients. As a result, phlegm is produced in the interior, blood vessels are obstructed, *yang qi* in the chest fails to circulate and chest pain occurs.

Old Age or Infirmity

When a person is over 50, kidney *qi* declines. Since the kidneys are the source of congenital *qi*, should the kidneys be deficient, other viscera will also become deficient.

If there is a deficiency of kidney *yang*, deficiency of heart *yang* and an obstruction of *yang* in the chest will also occur, resulting in chest pain. Likewise, if kidney *yin* is deficient, excess heart fire will result. Excess fire, in turn, impairs fluids, prompts phlegm accumulation and induces chest pain.

If a person is feeble and does not exercise, *qi* and blood cannot circulate freely. As long as blood vessels in the heart are blocked, chest *yang* will not circulate properly and chest pain will develop.

Diagnosis and Herbal Treatment

Chest pain is treated according to the conformation with which it is associated. Furthermore, differentiation must be made on the basis of the etiology of the pain, the accompanying symptoms and whether the condition is marked by deficiency or excess. In general, symptoms associated with the paroxysmal stage are treated first and the source of the pain is dealt with afterwards.

Since chest pain is associated with both phlegm retention and blood stasis, treatment is usually aimed at activating *yang* to dissipate phlegm and improving blood circulation to remove stasis.

Qi and Blood Stagnancy

Muscle twinges, chest pain which radiates to the shoulders and back, frequent eructation, unprovoked sighing, a dark purple tongue with ecchymosis, and a submerged, hesitant pulse are often associated with *qi* and blood stagnancy.

Treatment is aimed at the regulation of *qi* and the promotion of blood circulation in order to remove blood stasis and resolve meridional and blood-vessel obstructions. Persica and Achyranthes Combination (*xue fu zhu yu tang*) is effective at achieving these ends.

If the chest pain is acute, add 3 *qian* notoginseng (*san qi*) or 1 bolus of Styrax Formula (*su he xiang wan*).

Accumulation of Turbid Phlegm

Intermittent oppressive chest pain, palpitation, shortness of breath, coughing, viscid sputum, lassitude, drowsiness, a greasy tongue coating and a slippery pulse characterize this conformation.

Treatment attempts to activate *yang*, resolve phlegm and clear obstructions from the meridians and blood vessels. The recommended preparation is Trichosanthes, Bakeri and Pinellia Combination (*gua lou xie bai ban xia tang*), to which has been added 3 *qian* citrus peel (*chen pi*) and 2 *qian* each of cinnamon twig (*gui zhi*) and magnolia bark (*hou pu*).

If the condition is complicated by blood stasis, add 5 *qian* each of salvia (*dan shen*) and red peony (*chi shao*) and 3 *qian* carthamus (*hong hua*).

If the spleen is deficient, add 3 *qian* each of codonopsis (*dang shen*) and white atractylodes (*bai zhu*).

If heat symptoms are present, omit the cinnamon twig (*gui zhi*) and add 3 *qian* each of bamboo shavings (*zhu ru*) and arisaema with bile (*dan nan xing*).

Heart and Kidney *Yang* Deficiency

Palpitation, shortness of breath, lower back pain, listless-ness, an aversion to cold, cold limbs, diarrhea, a white, thin tongue coating, and a submerged and thready or intermittent pulse characterize this conformation.

Treatment attempts to warm and tonify the heart and kid-neys and promote blood circulation in order to remove obstructions from the blood vessels and meridians. The recom-mended preparation is a modification of Ginseng and Aconite Combination (*shen fu tang*), together with Eucommia and Rehmannia Formula (*you gui wan*). The resulting formula is known as Aconite and Cuscuta Combination (*jia jian shen fu you gui yin*).

Aconite and Cuscuta Combination*

Jia Jian Shen Fu You Gui Yin

(Modified Ginseng, Aconite and *You Gui* Decoction)

Codonopsis	*Codonopsitis pilosulae radix*	Dang shen	3.0
Aconite, prepared	*Aconiti carmichaelii praeparata radix*	Zhi fu zi	2.0
Cinnamon twig	*Cinnamomi ramulus*	Gui zhi	2.0
Rehmannia, cooked	*Rehmanniae radix*	Shu di huang	3.0
Lycium fruit	*Lycii fructus*	Gou qi zi	3.0
Epimedium	*Epimedii herba*	Yin yang huo	3.0
Morinda	*Morindae radix*	Ba ji tian	2.0
Eucommia	*Eucommiae cortex*	Du zhong	3.0
Salvia	*Salviae miltiorrhizae radix*	Dan shen	5.0
Carthamus	*Carthami flos*	Hong hua	3.0

*This formula has proved effective in years of clinical practice, though it is not included in most medical texts.

If *qi* deficiency is present, add 3 *qian* astragalus (*huang qi*).

If the patient suffers from spontaneous sweating and has cold limbs, cyanotic lips and nails, and an extremely faint pulse due to *yang* exhaustion, add 1 *qian* red ginseng powder (*hong shen*).

Heart and Kidney *Yin* Deficiency

This conformation is characterized by chest pain, palpitation, dizziness, insomnia, listlessness, lower back pain, tinnitus, a dry mouth, fidgeting, hot flashes, dry stools, a red tongue with a thin coating and a thready, wiry pulse.

Treatment attempts to nourish the heart and kidneys and promote blood circulation in order to remove obstructions from the blood vessels and meridians. The recommended preparation is Generate the Pulse Powder (*sheng mai san*), to which has been added 3 *qian* each of raw rehmannia (*sheng di huang*), fleece-flower root (*shou wu*), lycium fruit (*gou qi zi*) and ligustrum (*nu zhen zi*), as well as 5 *qian* each of salvia (*dan shen*) and hairy holly root (*mao dong qing*).

If the patient suffers from insomnia and palpitation, add 2 *qian* prepared polygala (*yuan zhi*) and 3 *qian* each of hoelen (*fu ling*) and zizyphus (*suan zao ren*).

_Qi_ and _Yin_ Deficiency

This conformation is marked by chest pain; palpitation; shortness of breath; dizziness; listlessness; insomnia; fidgeting; pallor; a red tongue with teeth marks and ecchymosis; and a thready and weak, thready and rapid, or intermittent pulse.

Treatment is aimed at replenishing *qi*, nourishing *yin* and promoting blood circulation in order to remove obstructions from the meridians. The preferred remedy is Ginseng and Longan Combination (*gui pi tang*), to which has been added 3 *qian* each of salvia (*dan shen*), tang-kuei (*dang gui*), carthamus (*hong hua*) and persica (*tao ren*).

If the patient has an intermittent pulse, administer Baked Licorice Combination (*zhi gan cao tang*) in addition to the above modification of Ginseng and Longan Combination.

Acupuncture and Moxibustion Treatment

Common Points

- *zhongwan* (CV 12)
- *zhigou* (TE 6)
- *qimen* (Liv 14)
- *daling* (P 7)
- *neiguan* (P 6)
- *ximen* (P 4)
- *taichong* (Liv 3)

Treatment Method

Three or four of the above points should be used during each treatment session.

Section 6
Stomachache

Stomachaches, termed epigastralgia, are characterized by pain in the epigastric region and are often accompanied by eructation, acid regurgitation and abdominal distention. Stomachaches are frequently observed in patients with acute and chronic gastritis, peptic ulcers and gastroptosis.

Causes of Stomachache

Attack by External Pathogens

Cold evil or excess intake of raw or cold foods will cause cold to accumulate in the middle energizer, thereby obstructing the flow of *qi*, which, in turn, results in a stomachache.

Alternately, excess consumption of spicy foods will cause heat to accumulate in the stomach, and excess consumption of greasy or sweet foods causes heat-dampness to develop. Retention of food in the stomach will prevent stomach *qi* from descending properly, thereby causing a stomachache.

Liver *Qi* Stagnancy

An emotional disorder will prompt the stagnation of liver *qi*, which attacks the stomach and leads to the stagnation of stomach *qi* and, consequently, to a stomachache. If *qi* stagnates and transforms into fire, scorching stomach pain will be induced as well. If *qi* remains stagnant, blood circulation will become obstructed and blood stasis will occur, thereby aggravating the stomachache.

Spleen and Stomach Deficiency

A cold-type stomachache can be caused by one or more of the following conditions: deficient *yang* in the spleen and stomach, dysfunctions of the spleen in transporting and transforming fluids and nutrients, or failure of stomach *qi* to descend. Additionally, stomach *yin* deficiency results in a lack of nourishment for the stomach and, hence, to the *yin*-deficient type of stomachache.

In general, *qi* disorders bring about stomachaches. When *qi* is stagnant, blood stasis develops. Though the stomachache is located in the stomach, it is closely related to the liver and spleen. If the stomachache lingers, meridians and collaterals will become impaired, and hematemesis or hematochezia will occur.

Diagnosis and Herbal Treatment

The most common types of stomachache are deficiency-cold of the spleen and stomach, and disharmony between the liver and stomach. Treatment attempts to warm the middle energizer and regulate liver *qi*. If stomach *yin* is deficient, treatment aims to nourish *yin* and harmonize the stomach. If the pain lingers and is accompanied by blood stasis and bleeding, blood circulation must be activated to remove stasis in the meridians and blood heat must be cooled to stop bleeding.

Deficiency-cold of the Spleen and Stomach

An aversion to cold; dull pain in the stomach region that is relieved by pressure or the intake of food or warm drinks, but aggravated when the stomach is empty; regurgitation of watery fluids; a poor appetite; a sallow complexion; lassitude; cold limbs; loose stools; a pale, swollen tongue with a white, slippery coating; and a thready, weak pulse characterize deficiency-cold of the spleen and stomach.

Treatment is aimed at warming the middle energizer, reinforcing the spleen, regulating *qi* and harmonizing the stomach. Astragalus Combination (*huang qi jian zhong tang*) and Ginseng and Ginger Combination (*ren shen tang*) can be used.

If the stomachache is serious, add 3 *qian* each of cyperus (*xiang fu zi*) and corydalis (*yan hu suo*).

If vomiting is severe, add 3 *qian* pinellia (*ban xia*) and 1 *qian* evodia (*wu zhu yu*).

Astragalus Combination[1]

Huang Qi Jian Zhong Tang
(Astragalus Decoction to Construct the Middle)[2]

Astragalus	*Astragali radix*	*Huang qi*	1.5
Cinnamon twig	*Cinnamomi ramulus*	*Gui zhi*	2.0
Peony	*Paeoniae radix*	*Shao yao*	4.0
Licorice	*Glycyrrhizae radix*	*Gan cao*	2.0
Ginger, fresh	*Zingiberis rhizoma*	*Sheng jiang*	2.0
Jujube	*Zizyphi fructus*	*Da zao*	9.0
Maltose	*Oryza sativa*	*Yi tang*	10.0

Disharmony Between the Liver and Stomach

This conformation is marked by stomach distention, fullness and pain which radiates out to the hypochondrium. The pain moves about and is aggravated by emotional depression. Acid regurgitation, repeated eructation, a thin tongue coating and a wiry pulse are also common characteristics.

Treatment attempts to soothe the liver, regulate *qi*, harmonize the stomach and relieve pain. Bupleurum and Cyperus Combination (*chai hu shu gan tang*) is recommended.

If stagnant *qi* is transformed into fire and is marked by a bitter taste in the mouth and a red tongue with a yellow coating, add 1 *qian* coptis (*huang lian*) and 3 *qian* each of gardenia (*zhi zi*) and scute (*huang qin*).

If the patient complains of gastric discomfort and acid regurgitation, add 5 *qian* each of cuttlebone (*hai piao xiao*) and ark shell (*wa leng zi*).

Bupleurum and Cyperus Combination[1]
Chai Hu Shu Gan Tang
(Bupleurum Powder to Spread the Liver)[2]

Bupleurum	Bupleuri radix	Chai hu	3.0
Peony	Paeoniae radix	Shao yao	2.0
Chih-ko	Citri fructus	Zhi ke	2.0
Cnidium	Cnidii rhizoma	Chuan xiong*	2.0
Cyperus	Cyperi rhizoma	Xiang fu	2.0
Licorice	Glycyrrhizae radix	Gan cao	1.0

*Ligustici rhizoma, also known as chuan xiong, may be substituted for Cnidii rhizoma.

Stomach Yin Deficiency

This conformation is marked by a dull pain in the stomach region; a feeling of fullness in the stomach after eating; a dry mouth and throat; emaciation; dry stools; a dry, red tongue with a thin coating or with no coating; and a thready, wiry pulse.

Treatment focuses on the nourishment of yin, the tonification of the stomach, the regulation of qi and the alleviation of pain. Glehnia and Rehmannia Combination (yi guan jian) can be used.

If qi is also deficient, add 3 qian each of codonopsis (dang shen) and astragalus (huang qi).

If dyspepsia is present, add 3 qian each of crataegus (shan zha), shen-chu (shen qu) and chicken gizzard lining (ji nei jin).

Blood Stasis in the Stomach

This conformation is characterized by a fixed and stabbing pain in the stomach which is aggravated by pressure or by eating. Although stomach distention is also present, the pain is more severe than the distention. Hematemesis, hematochezia (or melena), a dark purple tongue and a submerged pulse or a thready and hesitant pulse are also signs of blood stasis in the stomach.

To treat this conformation, the following should be administered: Pteropus and Bulrush Formula (*shi xiao san*), to which has been added 5 *qian* salvia (*dan shen*), 3 *qian* each of *tang-kuei* (*dang gui*) and corydalis (*yan hu suo*), 1.5 *qian* each of frankincense (*ru xiang*) and myrrh (*mo yao*), and 0.5 *qian* notoginseng (powder of *san qi*).

If hematemesis or hemafecia (melena) is also present, add 3 *qian* each of gelatin (*a jiao*) and bletilla (*bai ji*) and 2 *qian* rhubarb (*da huang*).

Pteropus and Bulrush Formula[1]

Shi Xiao San
(Sudden Smile Powder)[2]

Cattail pollen*	Typhae pollen	Pu huang	9.0
Pteropus	Trogopterorum faeces	Wu ling zhi	9.0

*also known as bulrush

Acupuncture and Moxibustion Treatment

Deficiency-cold of the Spleen and Stomach

- *zhongwan* (CV 12)
- *zhangmen* (Liv 13)
- *neiguan* (P 6)
- *zusanli* (S 36)
- *pishu* (B 20)
- *weishu* (B 21)

Disharmony Between the Liver and Stomach

- *zhongwan* (CV 12)
- *qimen* (Liv 14)
- *neiguan* (P 6)
- *zusanli* (S 36)
- *yanglingquan* (G 34)

Section 7
Hiccuping

A hiccup is a sudden, involuntary intake of breath which is quickly checked by the closure of the glottis and which produces a characteristic sound in the throat due to an adverse rush of *qi*. The sound is short, repeated, frequent and uncontrollable by the patient. Hiccups were first mentioned in TCM literature in *Nei Jing* (Internal Classic), which maintained that hiccuping can be stopped by inducing sneezing or distracting the patient's attention.

Clinically, hiccups, belching and retching result from an ascent of stomach *qi*, though some differences are worth mentioning. In the chapter on hiccups in *Jing Yue Quang Shu* (The Complete Works of Jing-yue Zhang), it is stated: "*Yue* (噦) means hiccup; *gan ou* (乾嘔) means retching or vomiting without vomitus; *ye* (噫) means eructation after a heavy meal, that is, belching." In order to make an accurate diagnosis, it is important to differentiate between retching and eructation.

Hiccups are a common sign of a nervous stomach. This section deals with diseases of the stomach, intestines, peritoneum, mediastinum and esophagus--all of which may induce spasms of the diaphragm, thereby producing hiccups.

Hiccups result from stomach *qi* adversely stimulating the diaphragm. Pathogenic factors cause the reversal of stomach *qi*, thus inducing an accumulation of cold *qi*, an excess of internal heat-dryness, a stagnation of *qi*, a deficiency of vital *qi* or an obstruction of phlegm. Pathogenic factors which invade the lungs or stomach will impede the passage of *qi* through the diaphragm. This will cause stomach *qi* to rush upwards through the throat, thereby producing hiccups.

The severity of the hiccuping can range from mild to severe. A mild case usually occurs occasionally and stops spontaneously, though if the hiccups continue, medicine must be taken. When the hiccups are associated with an acute or chronic disorder, this usually signifies a deterioration of the disease condition, and the patient must be treated accordingly.

Diagnosis and Herbal Treatment

In order to properly treat a case of the hiccups, excess or deficiency and heat or cold must first be differentiated. Treatments vary according to the conformation, and they may eliminate cold, clear heat, relieve stagnancy, resolve phlegm, warm and tonify the spleen and kidneys, or nourish *yin* fluids. Herbs to harmonize the stomach, suppress the adverse flow of stomach *qi* and relieve hiccups should be given. The most commonly prescribed herbs are clove (*ding xiang*) and kaki (*shi di*).

Excess Conformations

1. Cold in the stomach

The sound of the hiccup is dull and slow, and there is discomfort in the diaphragm and epigastrium. The hiccuping is relieved with hot food and drink, but aggravated by cold food and beverages. The patient's appetite is poor and he or she has little desire to drink. The tongue coating is white and moist, and the pulse is slow.

Treatment attempts to eliminate cold and thereby relieve the hiccups. Kaki Combination (*shi di tang*) can be used.

Kaki Combination[1]

Shi Di Tang

(Persimmon Calyx Decoction)[2]

Kaki*	*Kaki calyx*	Shi di	1.5
Clove	*Caryophylli flos*	Ding xiang	1.5
Ginger, fresh	*Zingiberis rhizoma*	Sheng jiang	4.0

*also known as persimmon

If cold symptoms are severe, add 1 *qian* evodia (*wu zhu yu*) and 0.5 *qian* cinnamon bark (*gui pi*) for warming *yang*.

Two *qian* each of *chih-shih* (*zhi shi*), malt (*mai ya*) and citrus peel (*chen pi*) should be added for activating *qi* circulation, resolving phlegm, promoting digestion and relieving dyspepsia.

2. Ascent of stomach fire

The hiccup is loud and sudden, the breath is foul, and the patient is troubled by a severe thirst with a preference for cold drinks. Small amounts of dark yellow urine, constipation, a yellow tongue coating, and a slippery, rapid pulse also characterize this condition.

Treatment is focused on purging heat, softening stools and relieving the hiccups. Minor Rhubarb Combination (*xiao cheng qi tang*), plus 1.5 *qian* kaki (*shi di*), may be used.

If severe heat is present but the patient is not constipated, Bamboo Leaf and Gypsum Combination (*zhu ye shi gao tang*), to which has been added 1.5 *qian* kaki, can be used.

Bamboo Leaf and Gypsum Combination[1]
Zhu Ye Shi Gao Tang
(Bamboo Leaf and Gypsum Decoction)

Bamboo leaf	*Bambusae folium*	Zhu ye	3.0
Gypsum	*Gypsum fibrosum*	Shi gao	10.0
Ginseng	*Ginseng radix*	Ren shen	3.0
Ophiopogon	*Ophiopogonis rhizoma*	Mai men dong	5.0
Pinellia	*Pinellia rhizoma*	Ban xia	3.0
Rice	*Oryzae semen*	Jing mi	5.0
Licorice	*Glycyrrhizae radix*	Gan cao	2.0

3. Adverse flow of *qi* and phlegm accumulation

This condition, which is exacerbated by depression and anger, is characterized by continuous hiccups and distention and fullness of the chest and hypochondrium. Frequent nausea, an inability to eat, dizziness, a thin, greasy tongue coating and a wiry, slippery pulse are also common signs.

Treatment is aimed at promoting the descent of *qi*, resolving phlegm, regulating the stomach and relieving hiccups. Inula and Hematite Combination (*xuan fu hua dai zhe shi tang*) can be used.

Inula and Hematite Combination[1]

*Xuan Fu Hua Dai Zhe Shi Tang**
(Inula and Hematite Decoction)[2]

Inula	*Inulae flos*	*Xuan fu hua*	3.0
Hematite	*Haematitum*	*Dai zhe shi*	3.0
Ginseng	*Ginseng radix*	*Ren shen*	3.0
Pinellia	*Pinellia rhizoma*	*Ban xia*	3.0
Ginger, fresh	*Zingiberis rhizoma*	*Sheng jiang*	3.0
Licorice, baked	*Glycyrrhizae radix*	*Gan cao*	2.0
Jujube	*Zizyphi fructus*	*Da zao*	3.0

*also known as *xuan fu dai zhe tang*

If liver *qi* is stagnant, add 3 *qian* each of melia (*chuan lian zi*) and turmeric (*yu jin*).

If phlegm-dampness is serious, Citrus and Pinellia Combination (*er chen tang*) can also be given.

Deficiency Conformations

1. *Yang* deficiency of the spleen and stomach

This conformation is characterized by a dull, weak hiccuping sound, a weak voice, shortness of breath, a pale complexion, cold limbs, a poor appetite, lassitude, a pale tongue with a white coating, and a thready, weak pulse.

Treatment warms and tonifies the spleen and stomach, regulates the middle energizer and halts the hiccuping. Ginseng and Ginger Combination (*li zhong tang*), to which has been added 2 *qian* evodia (*wu zhu yu*) and 1 *qian* clove (*ding xiang*), can be used.

If kidney *yang* is also deficient, add 1 *qian* prepared aconite (*zhi fu zi*) and 1.5 *qian* cinnamon bark (*gui pi*).

If food is retained in the stomach, add 3 *qian* citrus peel chen pi) and 5 *qian* malt (*mai ya*).

If *qi* is seriously deficient in the middle energizer, Ginseng and Astragalus Combination (*bu zhong yi qi tang*) should be used.

2. Stomach *yin* deficiency

The main clinical manifestations are sporadic hiccuping, a dry mouth and tongue, anxiety, a dry, red tongue with fissures, and a thready, rapid pulse.

Treatment is aimed at promoting the production of body fluids, nourishing the stomach and relieving the hiccups. Glehnia and Ophiopogon Combination (*yi wei tang*), to which has been added 3 *qian* each of eriobotrya (*pi pa ye*), dendrobium (*shi hu*) and jack bean (*dao dou zi*), as well as 1.5 *qian* kaki (*shi di*), can be used for reducing the adverse flow of lung and stomach *qi* and thereby halting the hiccups.

Acupuncture and Moxibustion Treatment

Points of First Choice

- *tiantu* (CV 22)
- *neiguan* (P 6)
- *geshu* (B 17)

Reserved Points

- *zhongwan* (CV 12)
- *tanzhong* (CV 17)
- *zusanli* (S 36)
- *zanzhu* (B 2)

Treatment Method

1. Use the points of first choice first.

2. Add two or three of the reserved points if the desired effect is not achieved.

3. Treat the patient once or twice daily, or if the condition is severe, treat three or four times daily.

Section 8
Vomiting

Vomiting is due to one of two causes: the inability of stomach *qi* to descend or the adverse ascent of turbid *qi*. It occurs in various diseases, such as acute gastritis, peptic ulcer, pyloric spasms or obstruction, pancreatitis, cholecystitis and diseases of the central nervous system. Although its etiology is complex, vomiting can generally be classified into two types-- excess and deficiency.

Excess conformations commonly result from damage due to external pathogens, improper diet or emotional disturbances. All these conditions promote excess liver *qi*. The onset is more rapid and the disease course is shorter than with vomiting due to deficiency conformations. Treatment emphasizes the elimination of pathogens and the extrication of turbid *qi*.

Deficiency, on the other hand, usually results from dysfunctions of the spleen and stomach in the transportation and transformation of food. The onset is insidious and the symptoms linger. Treatment warms the middle energizer, strengthens the stomach and nourishes stomach *yin*.

Diagnosis and Herbal Treatment

Excess Conformations

1. Attack on the stomach by external pathogens

An attack by wind, cold, summer heat or dampness, or fetid turbid *qi* invading the stomach and injuring stomach *qi*, all prevent the descent of *qi* and so cause vomiting.

This condition is characterized by sudden-onset vomiting, chills, fever, headache, pantalgia, an oppressive sensation in the chest, heartburn, pain in the epigastrium, diarrhea, loose stools, a white, greasy tongue coating and a floating pulse.

Treatment is aimed at dispelling the external pathogen, relieving the exterior and eliminating dampness with aromatics. Agastache Formula (*huo xiang zheng qi san*) can be given.

If accompanied by stagnant food, epigastric distention and a sensation of fullness in the chest, add 3 *qian shen-chu* (*shen qu*).

For unabated pathogenic factors attacking the exterior of the body, as well as chills without sweat, add 3 *qian* siler (*fang feng*) and 2 *qian* schizonepeta (*jing jie*).

If the patient is infected with summer heat-dampness evils, with the characteristic symptoms of fever and severe thirst, add 1 *qian* coptis (*huang lian*) and 3 *qian* bamboo shavings (*zhu ru*).

2. Improper digestion

Excess consumption of any type of food or ingestion of raw, cold or greasy foods may cause stomach *qi* to reverse its flow and ascend, thereby causing vomiting. Improper digestion or retention of food is characterized by the vomiting of acid and fetid food, a sensation of fullness in the epigastrium, belching, lack of appetite, loose stools or constipation, a thick, greasy tongue coating and a slippery pulse.

Treatment is aimed at promoting digestion, removing stagnant food and regulating stomach functioning to affect the descent of turbid *qi*. Citrus and Crataegus Formula (*bao he wan*) can be administered.

If there is severe indigestion with constipation, add 3 *qian* each of *chih-shih* (*zhi shi*) and rhubarb (*da huang*).

If the patient has diarrhea due to spleen deficiency, add 3 *qian* white atractylodes (*bai zhu*) and 10 *qian* furnace soil (*zao xin tu*).

3. Phlegm and fluid retention

This condition is characterized by the vomiting of phlegm, saliva and watery fluids; a feeling of oppression in the epigastrium; a loss of appetite; dizziness; palpitation; a white, greasy tongue coating; and a slippery pulse.

Treatment attempts to warm and resolve phlegm, as well as regulate stomach functions, in order to promote the descent of turbid *qi*. Minor Pinellia and Hoelen Combination (*xiao ban xia jia fu ling tang*) can be administered.

If stagnant *qi* transforms into fire and the condition is marked by a bitter-tasting, dry mouth and a red tongue with a yellow coating, add 3 *qian* each of gardenia (*zhi zi*) and scute (*huang qin*).

If the patient is vexed by acid regurgitation, add 1 *qian* Coptis and Evodia Formula (*zuo jin wan*).

If the patient is constipated, has a yellow, greasy tongue coating, and evidences abdominal distention, add 1 *qian* rhubarb (*da huang*) and 3 *qian* *chih-shih* (*zhi shi*).

Minor Pinellia and Hoelen Combination[1]
Xiao Ban Xia Jia Fu Ling Tang
(Pinellia and Hoelen Decoction)

Pinellia	Pinellia rhizoma	Ban xia	4.0
Hoelen	Poria sclerotium	Fu ling	3.0
Ginger, fresh	Zingiberis rhizoma	Sheng jiang	2.0

Coptis and Evodia Formula
Zuo Jin Wan[9]
(Left Metal Pill)[2]

| Coptis | Coptidis rhizoma | Huang lian | 6.0 |
| Evodia | Evodiae fructus | Wu zhu yu | 1.0 |

4. Emotional disturbances

Anxiety and anger result in the failure of the liver to properly control the distribution of *qi*. Liver *qi* then attacks the stomach, which leads to an ascent of stomach *qi* and subsequent vomiting.

Deficiency Conformations

1. Spleen *yang* deficiency

Distention and discomfort in the epigastrium, nausea, vomiting, a pale complexion, an aversion to cold, cold limbs, weakness, fatigue, a dry mouth, loose stools, a pale tongue with a white, greasy coating, and a soft, thready pulse characterize spleen *yang* deficiency.

Treatment is aimed at warming the middle energizer, invigorating the spleen, regulating stomach functioning and promoting the descent of turbid *qi*. Ginseng and Ginger Combination (*ren shen tang*), to which has been added 2 *qian* prepared pinellia (*zhi ban xia*) and 3 *qian* each of citrus peel (*chen pi*) and hoelen (*fu ling*), is the recommended remedy.

If the patient is vomiting watery liquids, add 2 *qian* evodia (*wu zhu yu*) and 10 *qian* furnace soil (*zao xin tu*).

If the patient's limbs are cold, add 1 *qian* cinnamon bark (*gui pi*) and 3 *qian* prepared aconite (*zhi fu zi*).

2. Stomach *yin* deficiency

Recurrent vomiting in small amounts, retching, a dry mouth and pharynx, a red tongue with little saliva, and a thready or rapid pulse characterize this condition.

Treatment focuses on nourishing stomach *yin* and facilitating the descent of turbid *qi* in order to halt vomiting. Ophiopogon Combination (*mai men dong tang*) can be given.

If body fluids are severely depleted and the patient is extremely thirsty, add 3 *qian* polygonatum (*yu zhu*), 4 *qian* trichosanthes root (*gua lou gen*) and 10 *qian* phragmites (*lu gen*).

If the patient's stools are dry, add 3 *qian* each of raw rehmannia (*sheng di huang*), linum (*ma zi ren*) and trichosanthes seed (*gua lou ren*).

Acupuncture and Moxibustion Treatment

Points of First Choice

- *neiguan* (P 6)
- *gongsun* (Sp 4)

Reserved Points

- *zusanli* (S 40)
- *zhongwan* (CV 12)
- *weishu* (B 21)

Treatment Method

1. Use the reducing method in the case of an excess conformation and the reinforcing method or moxibustion for deficiency conformations.

2. Needles should be retained for 15-20 minutes.

3. Treat once daily for 3-10 days.

Section 9
Abdominal Pain

Abdominal pain is a common disorder which involves many of the viscera, as well as the meridians in the abdomen. These viscera and meridians are either attacked by external pathogens or damaged by food stagnancy. *Qi* stagnancy, blood stasis or blood deficiency, or cold of the spleen and stomach can also cause abdominal pain.

The pain must be differentiated into cold or heat and deficiency or excess. *Qi* stagnancy and blood stasis, as manifestations of excess, must also be identified. The following are general guidelines for making these distinctions.

If the pain is sharp, persistent and relieved by heat, it is a cold conformation, while intermittent pain relieved by cold characterizes a heat conformation.

A hunger pain that is not fixed and is lessened when pressure is applied characterizes a deficiency conformation, whereas fixed pain following a meal which is exacerbated when pressure is applied characterizes an excess conformation.

When the abdominal pain is not fixed and the abdomen is distended, the conformation is *qi* stagnancy, but if the pain is fixed and stabbing, or there is an abdominal mass upon palpation, the conformation is blood stasis.

In general, treatment of abdominal pain aims to regulate *qi* functioning, clear the meridians and relieve pain, however, different conformations call for specialized treatments according to an overall analysis of the patient's signs and symptoms.

Diagnosis and Herbal Treatment

Cold Pain

This type of severe abdominal pain is relieved by warmth, but aggravated by cold. Accompanying signs and symptoms may include clear urine, loose stools, a pale tongue with a white, moist coating, a submerged and wiry pulse, and an absence of thirst.

Treatment attempts to warm the middle energizer, dispel cold, regulate the flow of *qi* and alleviate pain through the use of Galanga and Cyperus Formula (*liang fu wan*), to which has been added 3 *qian* corydalis (*yan hu suo*), 2 *qian* prepared aconite (*zhi fu zi*) and 1 *qian* each of zanthoxylum (*chuan jiao*) and dried ginger (*gan jiang*).

If the patient is also vomiting, add 3 *qian* each of pinellia (*ban xia*) and citrus peel (*chen pi*).

If the patient has diarrhea, add 3 *qian* each of white atractylodes (*bai zhu*) and hoelen (*fu ling*).

Galanga and Cyperus Formula

Liang Fu Wan[9]

(Galanga and Cyperus Pill)[2]

Galanga	*Alpiniae officinarum rhizoma*	*Liang jiang*	3.0
Cyperus	*Cyperi rhizoma*	*Xiang fu zi*	3.0

Heat Pain

Severe pain and distention, both of which are exacerbated when pressure is applied; fever; thirst; constipation; oliguria; red urine; a yellow, greasy tongue coating; and a surging, rapid pulse characterize a heat conformation.

Treatment focuses on clearing and purging heat and regulating the flow of *qi* to alleviate pain. Major Rhubarb Combination (*da cheng qi tang*), to which has been added 1 *qian* coptis (*huang lian*) and 3 *qian* gardenia (*zhi zi*), can be given.

If the fever is high and the patient has normal bowel movements, delete the mirabilitum (*mang xiao*) from Major Rhubarb Combination and add 3 *qian* each of lonicera (*jin yin hua*) and forsythia (*lian qiao*).

If the pain is located in the lower right quadrant, delete the mirabilitum and add 10 *qian* each of thlaspi (*bai jiang cao*) and sargentodoxa (*hong teng*). Also apply garlic (*da suan*), mirabilitum and rhubarb (*da huang*) externally.

Deficiency-type Pain

Intermittent pain which is lessened when pressure is applied, aggravated by hunger and fatigue, and relieved after rest or the intake of foods characterizes deficiency pain. Accompanying signs and symptoms may include fatigue, weakness, a lusterless complexion, an aversion to cold, loose stools, a pale tongue with a white coating, and a thready, submerged pulse.

Treatment attempts to reinforce *qi* and warm the middle energizer. Ginseng and Ginger Combination (*ren shen tang*) and Astragalus Combination (*huang qi jian zhong tang*) should be administered.

If the pain is severe, add 3 *qian* each of prepared cyperus (*xiang fu zi*) and corydalis (*yan hu suo*).

Excess-type Pain

1. *Qi* stagnancy

Distention, fullness and pain in the epigastrium characterize this condition. The pain is not fixed and sometimes radiates to the lower abdomen. Belching and flatulence are common signs, as are emotional instability, a thin, greasy tongue coating and a thready, wiry pulse.

Treatment concentrates on soothing the liver and regulating the flow of *qi*. Bupleurum and *Chih-shih* Formula (*si ni san*), to which has been added 3 *qian* each of prepared cyperus (*xiang fu zi*) and melia (*chuan lian zi*), as well as 2 *qian* saussurea (*mu xiang*) and 1 *qian* cluster (*bai dou kou*), is recommended.

If the pain is severe, administer 0.3 *qian* aquilaria powder (*chen xiang*) b.i.d or t.i.d.

2. Blood stasis

Indications of blood stasis include severe, persistent and fixed abdominal pain which is aggravated by pressure; a dark complexion; a purple tongue; and an uneven pulse. The treatment of choice is Cnidium and Bulrush Combination (*shao fu zuo yu tang*), which promotes blood circulation by removing blood stasis.

If the pain is severe and a mass of blood or tissue can be felt upon examination, add 2 *qian* carthamus (*hong hua*) and 3 *qian* each of persica (*tao ren*), sparganium (*san ling*) and zedoaria (*e shu*).

Cnidium and Bulrush Combination
Shao Fu Zuo Yu Tang[8]
(Drive Out Blood Stasis in the Lower Abdomen Decoction)[2]

Tang-kuei	Angelicae radix	Dang gui	3.0
Cnidium	Cnidii rhizoma	Chuan xiong*	3.0
Bulrush	Typhae pollen	Pu huang	3.0
Pteropus	Trogopterorum faeces	Wu ling zhi	3.0
Cinnamon bark	Cinnamomi cortex	Gui pi	1.0
Myrrh	Myrrha	Mo yao	2.0
Corydalis	Corydalis rhizoma	Yan hu suo	3.0
Ginger, dried	Zingiberis siccatum rhizoma	Gan jiang	1.0
Fennel	Foeniculi fructus	Xiao hui xiang	1.0
Peony, red	Paeoniae rubra radix	Chi shao	3.0

Ligustici rhizoma, also known as *chuan xiong*, may be substituted for *Cnidii rhizoma*.

Functions: promotes the flow of *qi* by warming the meridians; removes blood stasis to relieve pain.

Explanation: *Tang-kuei*, cnidium and red peony promote blood circulation and remove blood stasis, while bulrush and pteropus, assisted by myrrh and corydalis, relieve blood stasis and alleviate pain. Cinnamon bark and fennel treat deficiency-cold of the lower energizer, as well as lower abdominal pain due to blood stasis. Dried ginger warms the middle energizer and dispels cold.

3. Food retention

This condition is characterized by abdominal distention; abdominal pain which is aggravated by pressure and relieved by vomiting or diarrhea; fetid eructation; acid regurgitation; nausea; vomiting; constipation or diarrhea; a thick, greasy tongue coating; and a slippery, excess pulse.

The treatment of choice is Citrus and Crataegus Formula (*bao he wan*) for removing undigested food and regulating stomach *qi*.

If the pain is accompanied by abdominal distention and constipation, add 3 *qian* each of rhubarb (*da huang*) and *chih-shih* (*zhi shi*).

Acupuncture and Moxibustion Treatment

Cold Pain

- *zhongwan* (CV 12)
- *shenjue* (CV 8)
- *guanyuan* (CV 4)
- *zusanli* (S 36)
- *gongsun* (Sp 4)

Deficiency-type Pain

- *pishu* (B 20)
- *weishu* (B 21)
- *zhongwan* (CV 12)
- *qihai* (CV 6)
- *zhangmen* (Liv 13)
- *zusanli* (S 36)

Food Stagnancy

- *zhongwan* (CV 12)   • *qihai* (CV 6)
- *zusanli* (S 36)   • *tianshu* (S 25)

Section 10
Diarrhea

Diarrhea refers to loose stools and frequent defecation. The organs involved are the spleen, stomach and colon. Causes include infections due to external pathogens, injury to the internal organs due to improper diet, and a deficiency or dysfunction of one or more of the internal organs, chiefly severe dampness and malfunctioning of the spleen. Alternately, in Western medicine, the causes of diarrhea include acute and chronic colonitis, intestinal tuberculosis, gastrointestinal dysfunctions and dyspepsia.

As regards external causes, the main culprit is dampness invading the spleen and stomach. *Su Wen* (Plain Questions) states: "Excess dampness causes diarrhea."

The most common internal cause is spleen deficiency. The spleen's inability to adequately and properly transport moisture and transform food into refined essence leads to diarrhea, since failure to transport moisture can lead to dampness, which will further injure the spleen and thereby aggravate the deficiency. In general, acute diarrhea is primarily due to excess dampness, while spleen deficiency is chiefly responsible for chronic diarrhea.

Etiology

External Pathogens

Cold, dampness, heat and summer heat can all cause diarrhea. Of these, dampness is the most common cause, since dampness injures spleen *yang*, resulting in impaired transportation and transformation functions and, consequently, diarrhea. Clinically speaking, cold, heat and summer heat are often combined with dampness and can be more correctly termed cold-dampness, heat-dampness and summer heat-dampness, respectively.

Improper Diet

Overeating leads to food stagnancy, while excess consumption of greasy or sweet foods or the eating of raw, cold or contaminated foods injures the spleen and stomach, resulting in the impairment of the transportation and transformation functions of the spleen and, ultimately, diarrhea.

Spleen and Stomach Deficiency

As discussed above, the primary functions of the spleen are the transportation and transformation of food and fluids. When the spleen is functioning properly, spleen *qi* ascends and stomach *qi* descends. Improper food intake, fatigue, internal injury or a lingering illness can lead to a weakness of the spleen and stomach, thereby prompting dysfunctions in the transportation and transformation processes.

Kidney *Yang* Deficiency

Kidney *yang*, also known as fire from the gate of life, controls visceral *yang*, which is closely related to spleen *yang* and, indeed, aids the latter in the transportation of fluids and the transformation of food into refined essence. If kidney *yang* is deficient, food stagnancy and diarrhea will result.

Excess Liver *Qi* Attacking the Stomach

Emotional disturbances may impair spleen functions. For instance, anxiety and anger can impair the normal flow of liver *qi*. This excess liver *qi* then invades the spleen, which leads to transportation and transformation dysfunctions and, eventually, diarrhea.

Diagnosis and Herbal Treatment

Diarrhea can be classified into two types--acute and chronic--based on its onset and course. Furthermore, it is necessary to differentiate between excess and deficiency, and between cold and heat. If the diarrhea is acute at the onset and the abdominal pain is aggravated by pressure, but relieved by defecation, it is an excess conformation. If the disease course is lengthy with persistent abdominal pain which is lessened by pressure and warmth, it is a deficiency conformation. If the stools are watery, odorless and clear with undigested food, it is a cold conformation. If the stools are yellowish brown and fetid, and the anus burns following defecation, it is a heat conformation.

In the treatment of diarrhea, herbs inducing diuresis are often administered. Diuresis can remove dampness through the urine, thus easily curing diarrhea. Generally speaking, treatment for an excess conformation focuses on the elimination of the pathogenic factor, while the strengthening of the body's natural resistance is stressed in the case of a deficiency conformation.

Acute Diarrhea

1. Infection by external pathogens

    a. cold-dampness

An abrupt onset, loose or watery stools, abdominal pain with borborygmus or abdominal pain accompanied by chills, fever, headache, general body aches, a thin, white or white greasy tongue coating, and a soft, floating pulse characterize diarrhea caused by cold-dampness.

The treatment of choice is Agastache Formula (*huo xiang zheng qi san*), which relieves exterior symptoms, dispels cold and eliminates dampness.

If exterior symptoms, such as chills and arthralgia, are present, add 3 *qian* each of schizonepeta (*jing jie*) and siler (*fang feng*).

If watery diarrhea and borborygmus are present, add 3 *qian* atractylodes (*cang zhu*) and 4 *qian* plantago (*che qian zi*).

b. heat-dampness

The following signs and symptoms indicate diarrhea induced by heat-dampness: abdominal pain while defecating; diarrhea; brownish yellow, fetid stools; a burning sensation in the anus; frequent micturition of dark urine; fidgeting; thirst; fever; headache; general body aches; a greasy, yellow tongue coating; and a rapid, soft or rapid, slippery pulse.

The treatment of choice is Pueraria, Coptis and Scute Combination (*ge gen huang lian huang qin tang*), which clears heat and promotes diuresis.

If dampness is severe and if the patient has a thick, greasy tongue coating, add 3 *qian* each of atractylodes (*cang zhu*) and perilla leaf (*zi su ye*) and 2 *qian* magnolia bark (*huo pu*).

If the patient has a high fever, a yellow tongue coating and a bitter taste in his mouth, add 3 *qian* each of lonicera (*jin yin hua*), forsythia (*lian qiao*) and gardenia (*zhi zi*).

If the pain is severe, add 5 *qian* peony (*shao yao*) and 3 *qian* saussurea (*mu xiang*).

If the patient experiences nausea and vomiting, add 3 *qian* prepared pinellia (*zhi ban xia*) and 2 *qian* each of bamboo shavings (*zhu ru*) and fresh ginger (*sheng jiang*).

y

stools having the stench of rotten eggs, ~~lomi~~dominal pain with distention which is relieved fetid eructation, acid regurgitation, a dirty, greasy tongue coating and a slippery, wiry pulse characterize diarrhea provoked by food stagnancy.

Citrus and Crataegus Formula (*bao he wan*) is the treatment of choice for removing food stagnancy.

If the indigestion, abdominal pain and distention are severe, and if defecation is uncomfortable and the stools are odorless, add 3 *qian* each of rhubarb (*da huang*), areca seed (*bing lang*) and *chih-shih* (*zhi shi*).

Chronic Diarrhea

1. Spleen and stomach deficiency

This conformation is marked by recurrent episodes of diarrhea, the stools of which are sometimes loose and sometimes watery. The patient has a poor appetite, a sallow complexion, a pale tongue with a white coating and a thready, weak pulse. Other indications include an uncomfortable sensation of fullness after eating, an increase in defecation after eating small amounts of greasy foods, lassitude and undigested food in the stools.

Treatment attempts to strengthen the spleen and stomach, regulate the middle energizer and eliminate dampness. Ginseng and Atractylodes Formula (*shen ling bai zhu san*) can be used.

If there is incessant diarrhea with undigested food, add 3 *qian* each of terminalia (*ke zi*) and myristica (*rou dou kou*) and 10 *qian* furnace soil (*zao xin tu*).

If the diarrhea persists and the rectum is prolapsed, add 3 *qian* astragalus (*huang qi*), 5 *qian* pueraria (*ge gen*) and 1 *qian* cimicifuga (*sheng ma*).

2. Spleen and kidney *yang* deficiency

Periumbilical pain, diarrhea and borborygmus shortly before dawn; abdominal pain which is intensified by cold compresses, but relieved with hot compresses; cold extremities; lower back pain; weak knees; a pale tongue with a white coating and a submerged, thready and weak pulse characterize spleen and kidney *yang* deficiency.

Treatment attempts to warm the kidneys and strengthen the spleen. The remedy of choice is Psoralea and Myristica Formula (*si shen wan*), to which has been added 3 *qian* each of codonopsis (*dang shen*), white atractylodes (*bai zhu*), terminalia (*ke zi*) and saussurea (*mu xiang*) and 1 *qian* cinnamon bark (*gui pi*).

If there is a *qi* deficiency or an adverse descent of *qi*, as is often seen in the elderly, add 3 *qian* astragalus (*huang qi*) and 1 *qian* baked ginger (*pao jiang*).

Psoralea and Myristica Formula
Si Shen Wan[8]
(Four Miracle Pill)[2]

Psoralea	*Psoraleae semen*	*Bu gu zhi*	120.0
Schizandra	*Schizandrae fructus*	*Wu wei zi*	60.0
Myristica	*Myristicae semen*	*Rou dou kou*	60.0
Evodia	*Evodiae fructus*	*Wu zhu yu*	30.0

These four herbs are ground into a powder. A decoction is then made which consists of 250 *qian* fresh ginger (*sheng jiang*) and 180 *qian* jujube. The pieces of ginger are discarded, as are the jujube kernels and outer skins. The meat of the jujube is made into a paste and added to the powderized

Psoralea and Myristica Formula. The juice from the decoction is gradually added to the powder to form a paste, being careful not to add too much juice. Pills which are 2-3 *qian* apiece are made from the paste. If the paste does not stay together to form pills, wheat flour may be added as a binder. One pill should be taken two or three times daily with warm water on an empty stomach.

Functions: warms and reinforces the spleen and kidneys; relieves diarrhea.

Explanation: Psoralea warms and reinforces kidney *yang*. This imperial herb is assisted by schizandra, which warms the middle energizer and dispels cold, and by myristica and evodia, which astringe the intestines to correct the diarrhea. Jujube and ginger regulate the functioning of the spleen and stomach. Together the herbs warm and reinforce the spleen and kidneys, though they primarily work on the kidneys.

3. Excess liver *qi* invading the spleen

Abdominal pain and borborygmus before defecation, a sensation of fullness and oppression in the chest and hypochondrium, belching and poor appetite are induced by emotional stress or nervousness, both of which cause excess liver *qi* to invade the spleen. A thin tongue coating and a wiry pulse may also be observed.

Treatment focuses on soothing the liver and strengthening the spleen. The following is recommended: Siler and Atractylodes Formula (*tong xie yao fang*), to which has been added 3 *qian* each of saussurea (*mu xiang*), turmeric (*yu jin*) and cyperus (*xiang fu*).

If the patient's appetite is especially poor, add 3 *qian* each of *shen-chu* (*shen qu*), chicken gizzard lining (*ji nei jin*), germinated rice (*gu ya*) and malt (*mai ya*).

Siler and Atractylodes Formula
Tong Xie Yao Fang[11]
(Important Formula for Painful Diarrhea)[2]

Atractylodes, white	*Atractylodis rhizoma*	*Bai zhu*	3.0
Peony	*Paeoniae radix*	*Shao yao*	3.0
Citrus peel	*Citri pericarpium*	*Chen pi*	2.0
Siler	*Ledebouriellae radix*	*Fang feng*	2.0

Functions: nourishes the liver to relieve pain; strengthens the spleen to stop diarrhea.

Explanation: White atractylodes strengthens the spleen and tonifies the middle energizer, while peony nourishes the liver to relieve pain. Citrus peel regulates the flow of *qi* and strengthens the spleen. Siler, with its ascending and dispelling nature, aids in halting diarrhea. Together the four herbs restore proper functioning to the liver and spleen.

Acupuncture and Moxibustion Treatment

Acute Diarrhea

- *zhongwan* (CV 12)
- *zusanli* (S 36)
- *tianshu* (S 25)
- *yinlingquan* (Sp 9)

Chronic Diarrhea

- *pishu* (B 20)
- *zhangmen* (Liv 13)
- *zusanli* (S 36)
- *zhongwan* (CV 12)
- *tianshu* (S 25)

Spleen and Kidney *Yang* Deficiency

- *mingmen* (GV 4)
- *guanyuan* (CV 4)

Section 11
Dysentery

The common symptoms of dysentery are abdominal pain, tenesmus and diarrhea with bloody and mucous stools. Dysentery is usually seen in summer and autumn, and is generally caused by both external and internal pathogenic factors.

Etiology

Attack by External Evils

Summer dampness and external pathogens invade the gastrointestinal tract, causing heat-dampness to accumulate in the body, thereby obstructing the circulation of *qi* and blood, eventually creating *qi* stagnancy and blood stasis. The stagnant *qi* and blood, combined with dampness and external pathogens, result in bloody, pus-containing stools.

Improper Diet or the Consumption of Contaminated Foods

Either factor can cause intestinal *qi* and heat-dampness to accumulate, leading to *qi* stagnancy and blood stasis. Cold-dampness may also accumulate, thereby damaging the stomach and intestines, blocking the *qi* of the large intestine and ultimately leading to functional disturbances of *yin* and blood. *Qi* and blood stagnancy, combined with impure *qi* in the intestines, will result in the formation of bloody, pus-containing stools and the development of cold-conformation dysentery.

If dampness surpasses heat, the evil will damage *qi* and the stools will contain white, mucous pus. This is known as white dysentery. If heat surpasses dampness, the evil will damage the blood, resulting in bloody stools. This is known as red dysentery. If both dampness and heat are in excess, both *qi* and blood will be damaged. In this case, the stools will contain both pus and blood. This is known as red-white dysentery.

If the evil does not recede, spleen *qi* will become weak, resulting in chronic or repeated attacks of dysentery. Damage to the spleen, stomach and kidneys will result, leading to spleen and kidney deficiency.

Diagnosis and Herbal Treatment

Dysentery initially is classified as an excess-heat conformation, which is treated by clearing heat, resolving dampness, detoxifying evils, regulating *qi* and activating blood circulation.

If the disease persists for several weeks, months or even years, it transforms into a deficiency-cold conformation. At this stage, treatment is focused on warming the middle energizer and dispersing cold. Sometimes deficiencies are complicated by excess conformations and the treatment should include both purging and tonifying herbs. If the dysentery is chronic and without remission, astringent herbs should be used to stop the diarrhea.

Heat-dampness Dysentery

Characterized by bloody, mucoid stools, abdominal pain, fever, tenesmus, a burning sensation in the anus, small quantities of dark urine, a red tongue with a yellow, greasy coating, and a slippery, rapid pulse, heat-dampness dysentery is treated by clearing and detoxifying heat, regulating *qi* and promoting blood circulation. Peony Combination (*shao yao tang*) can be used.

Peony Combination[1]

Shao Yao Tang

(Peony Decoction)[2]

Peony	*Paeoniae radix*	*Shao yao*	4.0
Coptis	*Coptidis rhizoma*	*Huang lian*	2.0
Scute	*Scutellariae radix*	*Huang qin*	2.0
Rhubarb	*Rhei rhizoma*	*Da huang*	1.0
Tang-kuei	*Angelicae radix*	*Dang gui*	2.0
Cinnamon bark	*Cinnamomi cortex*	*Gui pi*	1.0
Saussurea	*Saussureae radix*	*Mu xiang*	1.0
Areca seed	*Arecae semen*	*Bing lang*	1.0
Licorice	*Glycyrrhizae radix*	*Gan cao*	1.0

If dampness is more of a problem than heat or if stools contain more white mucus than they do blood, 3 *qian* atractylodes (*cang zhu*), 2 *qian* magnolia bark (*hou pu*) and 5 *qian* coix (*yi yi ren*) may be added to Peony Combination.

If heat is more egregious than dampness, if stools contain more blood than they do white mucous or if stools sometimes contain only blood and no mucous, Anemone Combination (*bai tou weng tang*) can be used instead of Peony Combination.

If the patient has a headache, an aversion to cold and general body aches from the outset, add 3 *qian* pueraria (*ge gen*) and 2 *qian* each of schizonepeta (*jing jie*) and siler (*fang feng*) to Peony Combination.

If food stagnation lingers and is accompanied by tenesmus and abdominal pain which is aggravated by pressure to the point that the patient resists palpation, *Chih-shih* and Rhubarb Formula (*zhi shi dao zhi wan*) may be used instead of Peony Combination.

Chih-shih and Rhubarb Formula
Zhi Shi Dao Zhi Wan[19]
(Immature Bitter Orange Pill to Guide Out Stagnation)[2]

Rhubarb	Rhei rhizoma	Da huang	30.0
Chih-shih	*Citri fructus immaturus*	*Zhi shi*	15.0
Shen-chu	*Massa medicata fermentata*	*Shen qu*	15.0
Hoelen	*Poria sclerotium*	*Fu ling*	9.0
Scute	*Scutellariae radix*	*Huang qin*	9.0
Coptis	*Coptidis rhizoma*	*Huang lian*	9.0
Atractylodes, white	*Atractylodis rhizoma*	*Bai zhu*	9.0
Alisma	*Alismatis rhizoma*	*Ze xie*	6.0

Functions: promotes digestion; alleviates laxation; clears heat; eliminates dampness.

Explanation: Rhubarb and *chih-shih* relieve fullness and distention, expel retained food, and clear heat-dampness to stop diarrhea. *Shen-chu* is an adjuvant herb for promoting digestion and regulating the middle energizer. Hoelen, white atractylodes and alisma invigorate the spleen to dispel dampness, while scute and coptis aid in the elimination of heat-dampness.

Cold-dampness Dysentery

Signs and symptoms characterizing this condition include the following: stools which contain more mucous than blood; abdominal pain; tenesmus; a poor appetite; epigastric distention; a heavy feeling in the head and body; lassitude; a pale, thick tongue with a white, greasy coating; and a slow pulse.

Treatment aims to eliminate cold-dampness with warming herbs. The following should be employed to achieve this end: Magnolia and Hoelen Combination (*wei ling tang*), plus 3 *qian* tang-kuei (*dang gui*), 2 *qian* saussurea (*mu xiang*) and 1 *qian* each of coptis (*huang lian*), roasted ginger (*pao jiang*) and cinnamon bark (*gui pi*).

If cold is severe, 1.5 *qian* prepared aconite (*zhi fu zi*) should be added to the above formula.

Deficiency-cold Dysentery

Signs and symptoms of this type of dysentery include: incontinence of feces or watery stools with white mucous, a poor appetite, lassitude, cold limbs, lower back pain, an aversion to cold, emaciation, a pale tongue with a white coating, and a thready, weak pulse.

Treatment attempts to invigorate the spleen, warm the kidneys and strengthen the intestines with astringents to stop diarrhea. Peony and Poppy Combination (*zhen ren yang zang tang*), together with Kaolin and Oryza Combination (*tao hua tang*), can be used.

Peony and Poppy Combination
Zhen Ren Yang Zang Tang[20]
(True Man's Decoction for Nourishing the Organs)[2]

Atractylodes, white	*Atractylodis rhizoma*	Bai zhu	3.0
Codonopsis	*Codonopsitis pilosulae radix*	Dang shen	3.0
Myristica	*Myristicae semen*	Rou dou kou	3.0
Poppy capsule	*Papaveris pericarpium*	Ying su ke	3.0
Peony	*Paeoniae radix*	Shao yao	3.0
Tang-kuei	*Angelicae radix*	Dang gui	2.0
Cinnamon bark	*Cinnamomi cortex*	Gui pi	1.0
Saussurea	*Saussureae radix*	Mu xiang	1.5
Licorice	*Glycyrrhizae radix*	Gan cao	2.0
Terminalia	*Chebulae fructus*	Ke zi	2.0

Functions: warms the middle energizer; tonifies deficiency; strengthens the intestines with astringents to stop diarrhea.

Explanation: Atractylodes, codonopsis and licorice tonify *qi* and invigorate the spleen, while myristica and cinnamon bark warm the middle energizer to reduce diarrhea. Poppy capsule and terminalia are astringent herbs for the alleviation of diarrhea. Peony and *tang-kuei* regulate blood circulation to reduce pain, and saussurea promotes *qi* functioning.

Kaolin and Oryza Combination[1]
Tao Hua Tang
(Peach Blossom Decoction)[2]*

Kaolin	Halloysitum rubrum	Chi shi zhi	4.0
Ginger, dried	Zingiberis siccatum rhizoma	Gan jiang	1.5
Rice	Oryzae semen	Jing mi	8.0

*The chief ingredient, kaolin, is the color of peach blossoms, hence the name.

Acupuncture and Moxibustion Treatment

Points of First Choice

- *tianshu* (S 25)
- *shangjuxu* (S 37)
- *qihai* (CV 6)

If heat is severe, add *quchi* (LI 11) and *hegu* (LI 4).

Reserved Points

- *guanyuan* (CV 4)
- *zusanli* (S 36)
- *weizhong* (B 40, prick to induce bleeding)

Treatment Method

1. Retain the needle for 30 minutes.

2. Treat once or twice daily.

3. In the case of heat-dampness dysentery, the reducing method should be used.

4. In the case of cold-dampness or deficiency-cold dysentery, the reinforcing method should be employed.

Section 12
Dampness Retention

Dampness retention means that the dampness evil has stagnated in the spleen and stomach. The common symptoms are lassitude, chest fullness, abdominal distention, a loss of the sensation of taste, a poor appetite, and a greasy tongue coating. This disease is usually seen in the rainy season.

Dampness evil is the chief pathogenic factor and its invasion of the body is associated with a damp environment, frequent standing in water or being caught in the rain.

Interior dampness is related to the excess consumption of raw, cold foods, especially melons and other fruits, or of greasy or sweet foods, all of which can impair the digestion and transportation functions of the spleen and stomach. Such impairments can develop into cold-dampness or heat-dampness syndromes. If the patient has a pre-existing cold deficiency of both the spleen and stomach, the dampness evil is liable to cause symptoms of cold-dampness. However, if the patient has pre-existing heat accumulation in the stomach and intestines or a *yin* deficiency with excess fire, dampness evil will cause symptoms of heat-dampness.

Dampness evil transformed into cold easily damages spleen *yang*; transformed into heat, it consumes stomach *yin*. Dampness is a *yin* evil and thus is characterized as being "sticky." If the dampness is excessive, *yang* will be suppressed, resulting in the transformation of dampness into cold evil. In general, the disease is caused by dampness evil. Thus, in clinical practice, cold-dampness is seen more often than heat-dampness.

Diagnosis and Herbal Treatment

This disease has an insidious onset and, at times, a prolonged course, since dampness, by nature, is sticky and difficult to resolve. The primary symptoms of dampness retention are lassitude, soreness and a heavy sensation of the limbs, chest fullness, abdominal distention, a diminished sense of taste, a greasy tongue coating and a soft, floating pulse.

Dampness Stagnancy in the Spleen and Stomach

Symptoms include fatigue, weak limbs, a heavy feeling in the head as if it were tightly bandaged, a feeling of oppression in the chest, abdominal distention, a loss of the sense of taste or a sweet taste in the mouth, a sticky mouth, a white, greasy tongue coating and a soft, floating and slippery pulse.

Treatment seeks to eliminate dampness evil with aromatic herbs. Agastache Formula (*huo xiang zheng qi san*) can be given.

If the patient retains food, add 5 *qian* crataegus (*shan zha*) and 3 *qian* each of *shen-chu* (*shen qu*) and chicken gizzard lining (*ji nei jin*).

If there is chest and abdominal fullness and distention, as well as loose stools and a white, thick, greasy tongue coating, use Magnolia and Ginger Formula (*ping wei san*).

Heat-dampness Accumulation in the Middle Energizer

Symptoms and signs include a bitter taste in the mouth; a sticky, greasy mouth; loss of appetite; chest fullness; abdominal distention; a dry mouth with little desire to drink; red urine; a low-grade fever; a yellow, greasy tongue coating; and a soft, floating and rapid pulse.

Treatment aims to clear heat and resolve dampness. Coptis and Acorus Combination (*lian pu yin*) may be selected.

Coptis and Acorus Combination
Lian Pu Yin[9*]
(Coptis and Magnolia Bark Decoction)

Coptis	*Coptidis rhizoma*	*Huang lian*	1.0
Acorus	*Acori rhizoma*	*Chang pu*	1.0
Magnolia bark	*Magnoliae officinalis cortex*	*Hou pu*	2.0
Pinellia	*Pinellia rhizoma*	*Ban xia*	1.0
Soja	*Sojae semen praeparatum*	*Dan dou chi*	3.0
Gardenia	*Gardeniae fructus*	*Zhi zi*	3.0
Phragmites	*Phragmitis rhizoma*	*Lu gen*	2.0

*also spelled *lian po yin*

Functions: clears heat; eliminates dampness; regulates the flow of *qi*; harmonizes the middle energizer.

Explanation: Bitter-tasting coptis and gardenia help eliminate heat-dampness. Magnolia bark, pinellia and soja eliminate dampness for the relief of chest and abdominal distention. Acorus and phragmites harmonize the middle energizer and eliminate heat. This prescription can be used to treat a severe heat-dampness conformation.

If this condition occurs in summer, a piece of fresh lotus leaf (*xian he ye*) may be added.

Spleen Deficiency with Dampness Accumulation

This condition is characterized by a sallow complexion; lassitude; heavy, weak limbs; epigastric discomfort; a poor appetite; an aversion to oily foods; loose stools or watery diarrhea; a thin, greasy tongue coating or a thick, pale tongue; and a soft, floating and slow pulse.

Treatment is aimed at reinforcing the spleen and resolving dampness. Saussurea and Cardamom Combination (*xiang sha liu jun zi tang*) can be used.

Saussurea and Cardamom Combination[1]

Xiang Sha Liu Jun Zi Tang

(Six-gentleman Decoction with Aucklandia and Amomum)[2]

Saussurea	Saussureae radix*	Mu xiang	1.5
Cardamom	Amoni semen	Sha ren	1.5
Atractylodes, white	Atractylodis radix	Bai zhu	3.0
Ginseng	Ginseng radix	Ren shen	3.0
Hoelen	Poria sclerotium	Fu ling	4.0
Citrus peel	Citri pericarpium	Chen pi	3.0
Pinellia	Pinellia rhizoma	Ban xia	3.0
Licorice, baked	Glycyrrhizae radix	Zhi gan cao	1.5

Aucklandiae lappae radix may be substituted.

If the patient is troubled by diarrhea and borborygmus, add 3 *qian* each pueraria (*ge gen*) and agastache (*huo xiang*).

If edema of the face and extremities is present, add 3 *qian* each astragalus (*huang qi*), dolichos (*bai bian dou*) and coix (*yi yi ren*).

Dampness transformed into cold can damage spleen *yang*, thus, warm or hot herbs should be used to reinforce *yang* and thereby dry dampness. Besides these bitter-tasting herbs, other warm-natured herbs which strengthen the functioning of spleen *yang* can also be added--herbs such as dried ginger (*gan jiang*) and prepared aconite (*zhi fu zi*).

If dampness transforms into heat and damages stomach *yin*, herbs to nourish *yin* and eliminate dampness should be used. Treatment centers on clearing heat and eliminating dampness without damaging *yin*, as well as promoting the production of body fluids and nourishing *yin* without increasing dampness.

To these ends, the following herbs are recommended: glehnia (*sha shen*), dendrobium (*shi hu*), fresh lotus leaf (*xian he ye*), phragmites (*lu gen*), talc (*hua shi*), agastache (*huo xiang*) and coix (*yi yi ren*).

Acupuncture and Moxibustion Treatment

- *zhongwan* (CV 12)
- *zusanli* (S 36)
- *fenlong* (S 40)
- *gongsun* (Sp 4)
- *shanyinjiao* (Sp 6)
- *yinlingquan* (Sp 9)

Section 13
Jaundice

Jaundice is clinically characterized by dark yellow urine and yellow pigmentation of the sclera and skin. It is frequently seen in acute and chronic hepatitis, liver cirrhosis, liver cancer, cholecystitis, cholelithiasis and pancreatic cancer.

Etiology

Attack by External Pathogens

Attack by pestilent toxins or heat evil can result in heat stagnancy, which then combines with dampness and accumulates in the spleen and stomach. The liver and gallbladder are adversely affected by this heat-dampness, which causes bile to stray from its normal pathway and extravasate into the skin and sclera, thereby manifesting as jaundice.

Excess Consumption of Food and Drink

Excessive consumption of alcoholic beverages or irregular eating habits (sometimes overeating and then skipping meals for days) may damage the spleen and stomach, impairing their normal transportation functions. In this way, dampness will collect in the body and be transformed into heat. Heat will then adversely affect the liver and gallbladder, impairing the liver's function to extravasate bile. Bile will then be deposited in the muscles and skin and flow downward into the urinary bladder, creating the yellow color of the eyes, face and urine.

Spleen *Yang* Deficiency

Constitutional *yang* deficiency or damage to spleen *yang* following an illness will result in dampness, which will transform into cold. Cold-dampness then stagnates in the middle energizer, interfering with the dispersion and discharge functions of the liver and gallbladder. Thus, bile accumulates in the muscles and skin, flows to the urinary bladder and causes dark yellow jaundice.

Qi and Blood Stagnancy

A prolonged disease course may result in a deficiency of both the spleen and kidneys. Dampness turbidity will linger, and the icterus will appear dark and dingy. This is known as jaundice with blood stasis.

Diagnosis and Herbal Treatment

In order to make an accurate diagnosis, a differentiation between *yang* jaundice and *yin* jaundice must be made. The former has a short disease course, is characterized by a bright yellow color and is associated with an excess-heat conformation. The latter has a prolonged course, is characterized by a dark yellow color and is associated with a deficiency-cold conformation.

In some cases, *yang* jaundice can transform into *yin* jaundice and vice versa. If *yang* jaundice is not treated properly, the course of illness is prolonged, and, consequently, spleen *yang* is weakened. Cold will turn into dampness, and then *yang* jaundice may change into *yin* jaundice. If *yin* jaundice is severely affected by external heat-dampness, bile will extravasate to the muscles and skin. Thus *yin* jaundice will transform into *yang* jaundice. The clinical features of this type of *yang* jaundice, however, are more complex, as a deficiency conformation is mixed with an excess conformation.

Yang Jaundice

Signs and symptoms include bright orange-yellow skin and sclera, fever, thirst, chest fullness, abdominal distention, constipation, small quantities of red urine, a greasy, yellow tongue coating and a slippery, rapid pulse.

1. More heat than dampness

Both the skin and sclera are bright orange-yellow. The patient has a fever, abdominal distention, a feeling of oppression in the chest, nausea, constipation, a greasy, yellow tongue coating and a wiry, rapid pulse. In addition, the patient is thirsty, though only small amounts of red urine are passed.

Treatment aims at clearing heat and promoting diuresis in order to eliminate dampness. Capillaris Combination (*yin chen hao tang*) can be used.

Capillaris Combination[1]
Yin Chen Hao Tang
(Artemisia *Yinchenhao* Decoction)[2]

Capillaris	*Artemisiae capillaris herba*	*Yin chen hao*	4.0
Gardenia	*Gardeniae fructus*	*Zhi zi*	3.0
Rhubarb	*Rhei rhizoma*	*Da huang*	1.0

2. More dampness than heat

The skin and sclera are yellow, though not as bright yellow as they are in jaundice with excess heat. There is a low-grade, lingering fever. The patient may be tired and complain of heavy-headedness. The patient also has a distended feeling in the chest and epigastrium, a loss of appetite, abdominal distention, loose stools, a dry mouth, a thick, greasy and slightly yellow tongue coating and a soft, floating and slow pulse.

Treatment is centered on the promotion of diuresis in order to eliminate dampness turbidity, clear heat and reduce jaundice. Capillaris and Hoelen Five Formula (*yin chen wu ling san*) is recommended.

Capillaris and Hoelen Five Formula[1]

Yin Chen Wu Ling San

(Artemisia *Yinchenhao* and Five Ingredient Powder with Poria)[2]

Capillaris	*Artemisiae capillaris herba*	*Yin chen hao*	3.0
Hoelen	*Poria sclerotium*	*Fu ling*	4.0
Alisma	*Alismatis rhizoma*	*Ze xie*	4.0
Atractylodes, white	*Atractylodis rhizoma*	*Bai zhu*	4.0
Cinnamon twig	*Cinnamomi ramulus*	*Gui zhi*	2.0
Polyporus	*Polyporus sclerotium*	*Zhu ling*	4.0

For an exterior conformation in the early stage of jaundice, 1 *qian* ma-huang (*ma huang*), 3 *qian* forsythia (*lian qiao*) and 5 *qian* phaseolus (*chi xiao dou*) may be added to relieve exterior symptoms, eliminate heat and remove dampness through diuresis.

Yin Jaundice

The skin and sclera are a dark, dingy yellow. There is a feeling of fullness in the chest and abdomen, and the stools are loose. Cold-dampness due to spleen deficiency is usually manifested as *yin* jaundice.

1. Cold-dampness due to spleen deficiency

The clinical manifestations are dark yellow jaundice, a poor appetite, loose stools, lassitude, an aversion to cold, a pale tongue with a white, greasy coating and a soft, floating and slow pulse.

Treatment focuses on warming *yang*, reinforcing the spleen, dissolving dampness and eliminating jaundice. Capillaris, Atractylodes and Aconite Combination (*yin chen zhu fu tang*) can be used.

Capillaris, Atractylodes and Aconite Combination
Yin Chen Zhu Fu Tang [10]
(Capillaris, Atractylodes and Aconite Decoction)

Capillaris	*Artemisiae capillaris herba*	*Yin chen hao*	5.0-10.0*
Atractylodes, white**	*Atractylodis rhizoma*	*Bai zhu*	3.0
Aconite, prepared	*Aconiti carmichaelii praeparata radix*	*Zhi fu zi*	2.0

* If the jaundice is mild, select a dose near the low end of the range, whereas if the jaundice is serious, select a dose near the high end of the range.
** Atractylodes (*cang zhu*) may be substituted for white atractylodes.

Functions: warms *yang*; reinforces the spleen; removes dampness; eliminates jaundice.

Explanation: Capillaris eliminates heat-dampness and reduces jaundice, while prepared aconite is an auxiliary herb which warms *yang* and removes dampness. Either form of atractylodes strengthens the spleen and dispels dampness.

2. Jaundice due to blood stasis

The clinical features are dark yellow skin and sclera, emaciation, abdominal distention or an abdomen with a palpable mass, stabbing pain in the chest and hypochondrium, keratinized skin, spider telangiectasia, liver pains and, in severe cases, epistaxis and bleeding gums. The tongue substance is purplish red and may have ecchymosis, and the pulse is thready and wiry.

Treatment is aimed at activating blood circulation and relieving stasis. Persica and Carthamus Combination (*ge xia zhu yu tang*) may be used.

Persica and Carthamus Combination

Ge Xia Zhu Yu Tang[8]

(Drive Out Blood Stasis Below the Diaphragm Decoction)[2]

Tang-kuei	Angelicae radix	Dang gui	3.0
Cnidium	Cnidii rhizoma	Chuan xiong*	2.0
Persica	Persicae semen	Tao ren	3.0
Pteropus	Trogopterorum faeces	Wu ling zhi	3.0
Moutan	Moutan radicis cortex	Mu dan pi	3.0
Peony, red	Paeoniae rubra radix	Chi shao	3.0
Lindera	Linderae radix	Wu yao	3.0
Cyperus	Cyperi rhizoma	Xiang fu zi	3.0
Carthamus	Carthami flos	Hong hua	3.0
Chih-ko	Citri fructus	Zhi ke	3.0
Corydalis	Corydalis rhizoma	Yan hu suo	3.0
Licorice	Glycyrrhizae radix	Gan cao	1.0

Ligustici rhizoma, also known as *chuan xiong*, may be substituted for *Cnidii rhizoma*.

Functions: activates blood circulation; relieves blood stasis; dissolves the abdominal mass; stops pain.

Explanation: *Tang-kuei*, cnidium, persica and carthamus activate blood to dispel stasis, while pteropus and corydalis also alleviate pain. Moutan and peony cool blood heat and dissipate blood stasis. Lindera, cyperus and *chih-ko* regulate *qi* by activating blood circulation, and licorice harmonizes the actions of the other herbs.

If pain in the hypochondriac region is severe, 3 *qian* each of melia (*chuan lian zi*) and turmeric (*yu jin*) may be added to the above formula.

If the patient has ascites and oliguria, add 3 *qian* alisma (*ze xie*), 10 *qian* bottle gourd peel (*chen hu lu*) and 4 *qian* plantago (*che qian zi*).

If the abdominal mass is quite prominent, but the patient is otherwise in good condition, 3 *qian* each of pangolin scale (*chuan shan jia*), sparganium (*san ling*) and zedoaria (*e zhu*) may be added.

If the patient's abdomen in distended, add 3 *qian* each of areca peel (*da fu pi*) and chih-shih (*zhi shi*).

Acupuncture and Moxibustion Treatment

Yang Jaundice

- *danshu* (B 19)
- *yanglingquan* (G 34)
- *yinlingquan* (Sp 9)
- *neiting* (S 44)
- *taicong* (Liv 3)

Yin Jaundice

- *zhiyang* (GV 9)
- *pishu* (B 20)
- *dashu* (B 11)
- *zhongwan* (CV 12)
- *zusanli* (S 36)
- *weishu* (B 21)
- *sanyinjiao* (Sp 6)

Section 14
Hypochondriac Pain

Hypochondriac or subcostal pain is a common symptom which, as far back as the writing of *Nei Jing* (Internal Classic), has been attributed to hepatobiliary pathology: "If the evil is in the liver, there also is hypochondriac pain."

The liver is located under the hypochondrium, and the liver's meridians and vessels distribute *qi* and blood to both hypochondriac regions. The gallbladder attaches to the liver, and its meridians run along the hypochondrium, thus hypochondriac pain is mainly caused by hepatobiliary diseases.

The liver has the functions of smoothing and regulating the flow of *qi* and blood, and when this flow is interrupted, hypochondriac pain occurs. Any of the following will impair the functions of the liver and create a disturbance in *qi* and blood flow, leaving the meridians and vessels without the proper nourishment: emotional upsets, heat-dampness accumulation following a prolonged illness, external trauma or a deficiency of *yin* or blood.

Diagnosis and Herbal Treatment

Differential diagnosis of hypochondriac pain is primarily based on changes in *qi* and blood. Generally speaking, distending pain which is migratory in character indicates a *qi* stagnancy; fixed, stabbing pain indicates blood stasis; and a dull, lingering ache is associated with blood deficiency. Severe hypochondriac pain, which is usually accompanied by a bitter taste in the mouth and a yellow tongue coating, is the result of heat-dampness in the liver and gallbladder.

Liver *Qi* Stagnancy

This type of hypochondriac pain is usually migratory in character and accompanied by distention. The pain changes in intensity according to fluctuations in the patient's emotional disposition. In addition, the patient experiences chest fullness, a lack of appetite and frequent belching. A thin tongue coating and a wiry pulse may also be seen.

Treatment attempts to soothe the liver and regulate *qi*. Bupleurum and Cyperus Combination (*chai hu shu gan tang*) can be given.

If the pain is severe, add 3 *qian* each of immature citrus peel (*qing pi*) and brassica (*bai jie zi*).

If the pain is accompanied by nausea and vomiting, also use Inula and Hematite Combination (*xuan fu dai zhe tang*).

Blood Stasis

The hypochondriac pain is stabbing and fixed, increasing in severity at night. There may be a mass in the subcostal region, the tongue is dark purple, and the pulse is submerged and hesitant.

Treatment is aimed at the removal of blood stasis, including obstructions from the meridians and collaterals. *Tang-kuei* and Persica Combination (*fu yuan huo xue tang*) is recommended.

Tang-kuei and Persica Combination[1]
Fu Yuan Huo Xue Tang
(Revive Health by Invigorating the Blood Decoction)[2]

Tang-kuei	Angelicae radix	Dang gui	3.0
Persica	Persicae semen	Tao ren	4.0
Carthamus	Carthami flos	Hong hua	2.0
Rhubarb	Rhei rhizoma	Da huang	3.0
Pangolin scale	Manitis squama	Chuan shan jia	3.0
Trichosanthes root	Trichosanthis radix	Gua lou gen	3.0
Bupleurum	Bupleuri radix	Chai hu	4.0
Licorice	Glycyrrhizae radix	Gan cao	2.0

Heat-dampness of the Liver and Gallbladder

The hypochondriac pain is accompanied by a bitter taste in the mouth, chest fullness, loss of appetite, nausea and vomiting. The eyes are congested or icteric, the skin is generally yellow, and the urine is dark yellow. The tongue coating is yellow and greasy, and pulse is wiry and rapid.

Treatment is aimed at clearing heat and removing dampness. Gentian Combination (*long dan xie gan tang*) may be used.

For severe jaundice, add 10 *qian* capillaris (*yin chen hao*) and 3 *qian* phellodendron (*huang bo*).

If heat-dampness prompts the formation of small, sand-like gallstones, the hypochondriac pain may radiate to the shoulders and back. In this case, add 10 *qian* desmodium (*jin qian cao*), 5 *qian* lygodium (*hai jin sa*) and 3 *qian* turmeric (*yu jin*).

If heat-dryness in the gastrointestinal tract causes constipation, add 2 *qian* each of rhubarb (*da huang*) and mirabilitum (*mang xiao*).

Liver *Yin* Deficiency

The hypochondriac pain is dull, lingering and accompanied by a dry mouth and pharynx, a red tongue with a thin coating, a rapid and wiry pulse, fidgeting and dizziness.

Treatment is aimed at nourishing *yin* and soothing the liver. Glehnia and Rehmannia Combination (*yi guan jian*), plus 3 *qian* albizzia (*he huan pi*), 2 *qian* rose bud (*mei gui hua*) and 3 *qian* tribulus (*ji li*), is recommended.

If the patient is restless, add 3 *qian* zizyphus (*suan zao ren*) and 5 *qian* salvia (*dan shen*).

If the patient suffers from dizzy spells, add 3 *qian* each of mulberry seed (*sang shen zi*) and ligustrum (*nu zhen zi*).

Acupuncture and Moxibustion Treatment

Liver *Qi* Stagnancy

- *neiguan* (P 6)
- *zhigou* (TE 6)
- *yanglingquan* (G 34)

Blood Stasis

- *zhangmen* (Liv 13)   • *zhigou* (TE 6)
- *yanglingquan* (G 34)

Liver *Yin* Deficiency

- *zhangmen* (Liv 13)   • *zhigou* (TE 6)
- *neiguan* (P 6)

Section 15
Palpitation

According to TCM theory, palpitation is classified into two types: (1) mild palpitation which is temporarily induced by fear and (2) chronic and continuous palpitation when the patient feels an "uneasiness of the heart." According to Western medicine, palpitation occurs when a vegetative nervous dysfunction develops, such as anemia, arrhythmia or similar heart problems; whereas TCM attributes palpitation to anxiety, a deficiency of heart blood, a weakness of heart *yang*, a deficiency of kidney *yin* or a deficiency of kidney *yang*.

Fear and other emotional disturbances create an uneasiness of the mind and, so, palpitation. So do a severe blood loss or a deficiency of both *qi* and blood. Old age and a heart *qi* or heart *yang* deficiency also induce palpitation. Deficiency of kidney *yin* due to consumption, lingering diseases and sexual indulgence all create abnormal flare-ups of heart fire, which, in turn, induce palpitation and an uneasiness of the mind. Furthermore, kidney deficiency, which is characterized by fluid retention, can manifest itself in palpitation when these excess fluids invade the heart.

In clinical differentiation, deficiency should be distinguished from excess, however, there are more deficiency conformations than there are excess conformations. At times a patient will show both deficiency and excess conformations simultaneously. Since excess conformations include both those associated with blood stasis and those related to phlegm retention, a practitioner must differentiate between the primary and secondary causes. All conformations are either caused by or aggravated by emotional instability, and so tranquilizing herbs may be added to the recommended formulas.

Diagnosis and Herbal Treatment

Emotional Instability

Palpitation, susceptibility to fear, nightmares, fidgeting, a normal tongue coating and a somewhat rapid pulse are associated with emotional instability. The mind can be calmed and the heart nourished with Licorice and Jujube Combination (*gan mai da zao tang*), to which has been added 3 *qian* each of hoelen (*fu ling*) and polygala (*yuan zhi*), 2 *qian* acorus (*chang pu*) and 6 *qian* dragon bone (*long gu*).

If there is heat-phlegm and a yellow, greasy tongue coating, add 1 *qian* coptis (*huang lian*) and 3 *qian* each of bamboo shavings (*zhu ru*) and trichosanthes fruit (*gua lou*).

If there is a feeling of oppression in the chest, fidgeting, cyanosed lips and a purple tongue due to blood stasis, add 3 *qian* tang-kuei (*dang gui*), 2 *qian* cnidium (*chuan xiong*) and 4 *qian* salvia (*dan shen*).

Heart *Qi* and Heart Blood Deficiencies

These deficiencies are manifested by palpitation; dizziness; lassitude; a pale complexion, lips and tongue; and a thready, weak pulse.

Treatment focuses on replenishing *qi* and blood, nourishing the heart and tranquilizing the mind with Ginseng and Longan Combination (*gui pi tang*).

If the blood is severely deficient, add 3 *qian* gardenia (*zhi zi*) and 4 *qian* each of raw rehmannia (*sheng di huang*) and cooked rehmannia (*shu di huang*).

Excess Fire Due to *Yin* Deficiency

This condition is characterized by palpitation, fidgeting, a feeling of uneasiness while sleeping, dizziness, lower back pain, tinnitus, hectic fever, night sweats, feverish sensation in the palms and soles, a red tongue with no coating, and a thready, rapid pulse.

Treatment attempts to nourish *yin* in order to clear fire and reinforce the heart in an effort to tranquilize the mind with Ginseng and Zizyphus Formula (*tian wang bu xin dan*).

If there is a feverish sensation in the heart region or in the palms and soles, as well as a dry mouth with a bitter taste, add 1 *qian* coptis (*huang lian*) and 3 *qian* dioscorea (*shan yao*).

If the patient is troubled by hectic fever and night sweats, add 3 *qian* each of anemarrhena (*zhi mu*) and *ching-hao* (*qing hao*), as well as 5 *qian* each of dragon bone (*long gu*) and oyster shell (*mu li*).

Heart *Yang* Deficiency

Heart *yang* deficiency is characterized by palpitation; shortness of breath; chills; cold limbs; a feeling of oppression in the chest and heart region; spontaneous perspiration; a pale complexion; a pale, thick and tender tongue with a thin, white coating; and a thready, weak pulse.

Treatment consists in warming *yang* to arrest palpitation. Cinnamon and Dragon Bone Combination (*gui zhi long gu mu li tang*) should be used.

If heart *yang* deficiency is aggravated by *yang* deficiency, resulting in excess fluid retention, palpitation, dizziness, edema and loose stools, 3 *qian* of each of the following should be added: codonopsis (*dang shen*), white atractylodes (*bai zhu*) and dioscorea (*shan yao*).

Should retained fluids invade the heart, add 3 *qian* each of prepared aconite (*zhi fu zi*) and dried ginger (*gan jiang*).

Cinnamon and Dragon Bone Combination[1]

Gui Zhi Long Gu Mu Li Tang

(Cinnamon Twig, Dragon Bone and Oyster Shell Decoction)

Cinnamon twig	Cinnamomi ramulus	Gui zhi	4.0
Peony	Paeoniae radix	Shao yao	4.0
Ginger, fresh	Zingiberis rhizoma	Sheng jiang	4.0
Dragon bone	Draconis os	Long gu	3.0
Oyster shell	Ostreae testa	Mu li	3.0
Licorice	Glycyrrhizae radix	Gan cao	2.0
Jujube	Zizyphi fructus	Da zao	12.0

Acupuncture and Moxibustion Treatment

Common Points

- *neiguan* (P 6)
- *shenmen* (H 7)
- *tanzhong* (CV 17)
- *xinshu* (B 15)
- *shaohai* (H 3)
- *yinxi* (H 6)
- *ximen* (P 4)
- *tongli* (H 5)

Treatment Method

Three or four points should be used daily for 10 days.

Section 16
Sweat Conformation

A sweat conformation results from an imbalance of *yin* and *yang*, a disharmony between *ying* (nutrients) and *wei* (the body's defense mechanisms) or a malfunctioning of the sweat pores. According to its clinical manifestations, sweat conformation is classified as either spontaneous sweating or night sweats. The former is frequent sweating which is not provoked by exercise, while the latter occurs during sleep.

A functional disturbance of the autonomic nervous system, such as shock, hypoglycemia (insulin shock) or illnesses such as tuberculosis, hyperthyroidism and the full range of febrile diseases can be differentiated and treated according to sweat conformation.

Perspiration is the body's means of eliminating excess heat and pathogenic factors. According to traditional Chinese medicine, sweat is the fluid of the heart and is formed from essence and *qi*. The loss of too much sweat, therefore, also results in a loss of vital essence and *qi*. Perspiration due to hot weather, the wearing of too much clothing, the drinking of hot beverages, labor, strenuous exercise or the use of diaphoretics is considered normal when the quantity of sweat expelled is relatively small. Excess perspiration, on the other hand, is usually caused by a dysfunction of *wei qi* (defensive *qi*), a deficiency of *yang qi* or hyperactivity of fire due to *yin* deficiency.

Diagnosis and Herbal Treatment

Clinically, sweat conformations should be classified as deficiency or excess and cold or heat. In spontaneous sweating, all of the above conformations can be observed; however, in night sweats, only deficiency-heat is common.

Spontaneous Sweating

1. Disharmony between *ying* and *wei*

This condition is marked by excess perspiration and accompanied by an aversion to wind, general body aches, alternating sensations of heat and cold, a thin, white tongue coating and a moderately slow pulse. In the case of insomnia accompanied by anxiety, the perspiration may be either spontaneous or aggravated, as is also the case with a deficiency associated with an exterior conformation when the patient is subjected to wind.

Disharmony between *ying* and *wei* is treated by harmonizing the two with Cinnamon Combination (*gui zhi tang*).

If the patient is experiencing palpitation and insomnia, add 5 *qian* dragon bone (*long gu*) and 10 *qian* oyster shell (*mu li*).

If there is a deficiency associated with an exterior conformation with profuse sweating, add 3 *qian* astragalus (*huang qi*).

2. Lung *qi* deficiency

Profuse sweating when exercising, an aversion to cold, lingering illness, a weak constitution, weak resistance to wind and cold, susceptibility to the common cold, a pale complexion, a thready, weak pulse and a thin, white tongue coating are all characteristic of lung *qi* deficiency.

Treatment replenishes *qi* and consolidates superficial resistance with Siler and Astragalus Formula (*yu ping feng san*).

Siler and Astragalus Formula

Yu Ping Feng San

(Jade Windscreen Powder)[2]

Astragalus	Astragali radix	Huang qi	10.0
Atractylodes (white)	Atractylodis rhizoma	Bai zhu	20.0
Siler	Ledebouriellae radix	Fang feng	10.0

3. Excess heat in the interior

Unprovoked or excessive sweating, thirst with a preference for cold beverages, a flushed, warm face, fidgeting, fever, constipation, a red tongue with a yellow coating, and a large, surging pulse characterize excess heat in the interior.

This conformation is treated by clearing heat with Gypsum Combination (*bai hu tang*).

Should there be profuse sweating and severe thirst, add 10 *qian* phragmites (*lu gen*) and 5 *qian* each of trichosanthes root (*gua lou gen*) and dendrobium (*shi hu*).

If the patient is also constipated, add 2 *qian* rhubarb (*da huang*).

If the sweating is accompanied by fidgeting, add 1 *qian* coptis (*huang lian*) and 3 *qian* each of gardenia (*zhi zi*) and lophatherum (*dan zhu ye*).

Night Sweats
1. Heart blood deficiency

A deficiency of heart blood is characterized by night sweats, a sallow complexion, shortness of breath, listlessness, a pale tongue with a thin coating, and a weak pulse.

Treatment is concerned with nourishing the heart, tonifying the blood and arresting the sweat with Ginseng and Longan Combination (*gui pi tang*).

If the sweating is profuse, also administer Dragon Bone and Oyster Shell Combination (*long gu mu li tang*).

2. Hyperactivity of fire due to *yin* deficiency

This condition is characterized by hectic fever; night sweats; fidgeting; insomnia; dysphoria with a feverish sensation in the heart area, palms and soles; a thin physique; irregular menstruation in women or nocturnal emission in men; a red tongue with no coating; and a wiry, thready and rapid pulse.

Treatment consists of nourishing *yin* and removing fire with *Tang-kuei* and Six Yellow Combination (*dang gui liu huang tang*).

Tang-kuei and Six Yellow Combination
Dang Gui Liu Huang Tang[21]
(*Tang-kuei* and Six Yellow Decoction)[2]

Tang-kuei	Angelicae radix	Dang gui	3.0
Rehmannia, raw	Rehmanniae radix	Sheng di huang	3.0
Rehmannia, cooked	Rehmanniae radix	Shu di huang	3.0
Scute	Scutellariae radix	Huang qin	3.0
Phellodendron	Phellodendri cortex	Huang bo	3.0
Coptis	Coptidis rhizoma	Huang lian	1.0
Astragalus	Astragali radix	Huang qi	5.0

Functions: nourishes *yin*; removes fire; consolidates superficial resistance; inhibits perspiration.

Explanation: *Tang-kuei* and both forms of rehmannia nourish *yin* and blood to remove internal fire. Scute, phellodendron and coptis remove fire to relieve fidgeting, as well as clear heat to preserve *yin*. Astragalus replenishes *qi* and consolidates superficial resistance to stop perspiration.

If the illness lingers and is accompanied by kidney *yin* deficiency, treat the patient with Rehmannia and Schizandra Formula (*qi wei du qi wan*).

If the hectic fever is serious, add 3 *qian* each of anemarrhena (*zhi mu*) and lycium bark (*di gu pi*), as well as 2 *qian* each of tortoise shell (*gui pan*) and turtle shell (*bie jia*).

Acupuncture and Moxibustion Treatment

Common Points

- *fuliu* (K 7)
- *qihai* (CV 6)
- *shenshu* (B 23)
- *houxi* (SI 3)
- *hegu* (LI 4)

Treatment Method

Three points may be selected for each treatment.

Section 17
Insomnia

Difficulties in falling or staying asleep must be differentiated into several categories, including the inability to fall asleep quickly, awakening shortly after falling asleep and being unable to resume sleeping, the inability to sleep soundly or the inability to sleep at all. Insomnia is often accompanied by dizziness, a feeling of fullness in the head, palpitation and poor memory. It can be observed in patients with neurosis, emotional instability, high fever and menopausal disorders.

Etiology

Injury Due to Emotional Excesses

Some violent emotions impair liver *qi*, which stagnates, transforms into fire, invades heart *shen* and causes mental derangement and insomnia.

Improper Diet

Excess consumption of greasy or sweet foods can result in the retention of fluids and phlegm in the stomach, causing stomach *qi* malfunctioning and, eventually, insomnia.

Senility or Blood *Qi* Deficiency of the Heart

Palpitation and insomnia are the result of exhaustion of liver and kidney essence. If vital essence is prevented from replenishing the heart, the breakdown of the normal physiological coordination between the heart and the kidneys will occur. These conditions may also result in excess heart fire or blood *qi* deficiency in the heart and gallbladder. Any one of these scenarios can manifest as fear and timidity on the part of the patient.

Diagnosis and Herbal Treatment

A differentiation between deficiency and excess conformations must be made to assure proper treatment. The former is generally due to blood and *yin* deficiencies of the heart, spleen, liver and kidneys, while the latter is usually caused by stagnant liver *qi* transformed into fire or by the retention of food and turbid phlegm, which results in stomach disorders. Treatment of deficiency conformations consists of reinforcing *qi* replenishing blood and nourishing *yin* to eliminate deficient fire, while excess conformations are treated by clearing the liver, purging fire, removing the retained food and phlegm, harmonizing the stomach and tranquilizing the mind.

Stagnant Liver *Qi* Transformed Into Fire

Fidgeting, irritability, insomnia, a dry mouth with a bitter taste, a bitter taste, headache, conjunctiva congestion, dark yellow urine, constipation, a red tongue with a yellow coating, and a wiry, rapid pulse characterize stagnant liver *qi* transformed into fire.

Treatment attempts to purge liver fire, while simultaneously tranquilizing the mind. Administer Gentian Combination (*long dan xie gan tang*), to which has been added 4 *qian* dragon teeth (*long chi*) and 5 *qian* magnetite (*ci shi*). Dragon bone (*long gu*) may be substituted for dragon teeth if the latter is unavailable.

Should the patient complain of a feeling of oppression in the chest and should distention in the hypochondriac region be observed, add 3 *qian* each of turmeric (*yu jin*) and *chih-ko* (*zhi ke*).

If the patient is constipated, add 2 *qian* raw rhubarb (*sheng da huang*).

Heat-phlegm Invading the Heart

This condition is characterized by insomnia, dizziness, a feeling of oppression in the chest, a bitter taste in the mouth, fidgeting, acid regurgitation, nausea, a yellow, greasy tongue coating and a slippery, rapid pulse.

Treatment aims at clearing heat, resolving phlegm, harmonizing the stomach and tranquilizing the mind. Hoelen and Bamboo Combination (*wen dan tang*), along with 1 *qian* coptis (*huang lian*), can be given.

If the insomnia is caused by food retention due to stomach disharmony, add 3 *qian* pinellia (*ban xia*) and 10 *qian* husked sorghum (*shu mi*).

Timidity Due to Deficiencies of *Qi* and Heart Blood

Insomnia, absent-mindedness, the propensity to daydream, frequent awakenings from sleep which are due to fright, timidity, palpitation, a pale tongue with a thin, white coating, and a thready pulse are all associated with deficiencies of *qi* and heart blood.

Treatment replenishes *qi* and tranquilizes the mind. Hoelen and Acorus Formula (*an shen ding zhi wan*) is recommended.

If the insomnia is due to anxiety, use Zizyphus Combination (*suan zao ren tang*) instead.

Hoelen and Acorus Formula

An Shen Ding Zhi Wan[22]

(Bolus for Tranquilizing the Mind and Calming the Spirit)[22]

Hoelen	Poria sclerotium	Fu ling	30.0
Fu-shen	Poria cor	Fu shen	30.0
Ginseng	Ginseng radix	Ren shen	30.0
Acorus	Acori rhizoma	Chang pu	15.0
Dragon teeth	Mastodi dentis fossilia	Long chi	15.0

These herbs are made into honeyed, two-*qian* boluses. One bolus is taken three times daily.

Functions: relieves fright and sleeplessness.

Explanation: Hoelen and *fu-shen* tranquilize the mind. Ginseng replenishes *qi*, acorus calms the mind and relieves fright, and sedation is affected with dragon teeth.

Zizyphus Combination[1]

Suan Zao Ren Tang

(Sour Jujube Decoction)[2]

Zizyphus*	Zizyphi spinosi semen	Suan zao ren	10.0
Hoelen	Poria sclerotium	Fu ling	5.0
Cnidium	Cnidii rhizoma	Chuan xiong**	6.0
Anemarrhena	Anemarrhenae rhizoma	Zhi mu	3.0
Licorice	Glycyrrhizae radix	Gan cao	1.0

*also known as sour jujube

**Ligustici rhizoma*, also known as *chuan xiong*, may be substituted for *Cnidii rhizoma*.

Heart and Spleen Deficiency

Palpitation, a poor memory, drowsiness, the propensity to be easily awakened at night, dizziness, lassitude, a loss of the sensation of taste, pallor, a pale tongue with a thin, white coating, and a thready, weak pulse characterize heart and spleen deficiency.

Treatment is directed at tonifying the heart and spleen. Ginseng and Longan Combination (*gui pi tang*) can be given.

If the patient's appetite is poor and his or her abdomen is distended, delete the astragalus (*huang qi*) and add 4 *qian shen-chu* (*shen qu*).

In case of a serious blood deficiency, add 4 *qian* cooked rehmannia (*shu di huang*) and 3 *qian* lycium fruit (*gou qi zi*), or use Ginseng and Longan Combination (*gui pi tang*) in combination with Astragalus and Zizyphus Combination (*yang xin tang*).

Hyperactivity of Fire Due to *Yin* Deficiency

Fidgeting, insomnia, dizziness, tinnitus, a dry mouth and throat, a burning sensation in the palms and soles, lower back pain, a red tongue and a thready, rapid pulse signal hyperactivity of fire due to *yin* deficiency.

Treatment consists of nourishing *yin* and removing fire. Coptis and Gelatin Combination (*huang lian a jiao tang*) can be used.

If insomnia is due to anxiety or other emotional instability and if excess fire is not severe, Ginseng and Zizyphus Formula (*tian wang bu xin dan*) can be given instead.

Acupuncture and Moxibustion Treatment

Basic Points for Any Type of Insomnia

- *shenmen* (H 7)
- *sanyinjiao* (Sp 6)

Additional Points for Heart and Spleen Deficiency

- *xinshu* (B 15)
- *jueyinshu* (B 14)
- *pishu* (B 20)

Additional Points for Kidney Deficiency

- *xinshu* (B 15)
- *shenshu* (B 23)
- *taixi* (K 3)

Additional Points for Heart and Gallbladder *Qi* Deficiency

- *xinshu* (B 15)
- *danshu* (B 10)
- *daling* (P 7)
- *qiuxu* (G 40)

Additional Points for Excess Liver *Yang*

- *ganshu* (B 18)
- *jianshi* (P 5)
- *taichong* (Liv 3)

Additional Points for Spleen and Stomach Disharmony

- *weishu* (B 21)
- *zusanli* (S 36)

Section 18
Dizziness

Dizziness is a common symptom of many diseases, including hypertension, anemia, auditory vertigo and neurosis. During episodes of dizziness, the patient feels as if he were on a rocking boat. In mild cases in which the dizziness is often associated with blurry or otherwise abnormal vision, the condition can usually be relieved by closing one's eyes and allowing them to rest. In severe cases, nausea, vomiting, sweating and fainting may also occur.

The most common etiology, from a TCM viewpoint, is stagnant liver *qi* which transforms into fire. This fire injures liver *yin*, creating excess liver *yang* which ascends to the head and causes dizziness. Dizziness can also occur when kidney *yin* deficiency results in inadequate nourishment of the liver, causing excess liver *yang* to invade the head, or when malfunctions in the spleen's transformation and transportation functions cause phlegm-dampness to accumulate and thereby prevent the ascension of *yang* and the descent of turbid *yin*.

Dizziness due to a deficiency is commonly caused by *qi* and blood deficiencies and the resulting failure of the brain to be nourished with adequate supplies of *qi* and blood. Because the kidneys store essence, which nourishes the marrow, deficiency of kidney essence results in malnourishment of the marrow, thus creating a deficiency in both the lower and upper parts of the body and, ultimately, dizziness.

Diagnosis and Herbal Treatment

Excess Liver *Yang*

Dizziness; tinnitus; distention and pain in the head which are aggravated by fidgeting, fatigue and violent emotions;

irritability; insomnia; drowsiness; a flushed face; a bitter taste in the mouth; a red tongue with a thin, yellow coating; and a wiry pulse characterize an excess of liver *yang*.

Treatment is aimed at calming the liver and suppressing liver *yang*, for which Gastrodia and Uncaria Combination (*tian ma gou teng yin*) can be given.

If the dizziness is severe, add 0.1 *qian* antelope horn (*ling yang jiao*).

Kidney Essence Deficiency

Kidney essence deficiency is marked by dizziness, lassitude, memory loss, soreness and weakness of the lower back and knees, tinnitus, and seminal emission in men. If *yang* deficiency is also present and acute, symptoms of cold limbs, a pale tongue and a submerged, thready pulse may also appear. If *yin* deficiency is present and acute, a burning sensation in the palms, soles and heart region, as well as a red tongue and a wiry, thready pulse, may also be seen.

Treatment of *yang* deficiency concentrates on tonifying the kidneys and strengthening *yang*. Eucommia and Rehmannia Formula (*you gui wan*) is recommended.

Tonification of the kidneys and nourishment of *yin* are the aims of *yin* deficiency treatment. To achieve these ends, the following should be given: Rehmannia Six Formula (*liu wei di huang wan*), plus 5 *qian* tortoise shell (*gui ban*), 3 *qian* lycium fruit (*gou qi zi*) and 4 *qian* ligustrum (*nu zhen zi*).

Accumulation of Turbid Phlegm

This condition is marked by dizziness, heavy-headedness, distention and fullness in the chest and upper abdomen, nausea, poor appetite, drowsiness, a white, greasy tongue coating and a soft, floating and slippery pulse.

Treatment is aimed at removing dampness, resolving phlegm, tonifying the spleen and harmonizing the stomach. Pinellia and Gastrodia Combination (*ban xia bai zhu tian ma tang*) can be given.

If there is severe dizziness and frequent vomiting, add 5 *qian* hematite (*dai zhe shi*).

If turbid phlegm is transformed into fire and accompanied by a bitter taste in the mouth, fidgeting, and distention and pain in the head and eyes, add 1 *qian* coptis (*huang lian*) and 3 *qian* each of bamboo shavings (*zhu ru*) and *chih-ko* (*zhi ke*). Alternately, Alisma Combination (*ze xie tang*) may be taken in addition to Pinellia and Gastrodia Combination.

Pinellia and Gastrodia Combination[1]
Ban Xia Bai Zhu Tian Ma Tang
(Pinellia, White Atractylodes Macrocephala and Gastrodia Decoction)[2]

Pinellia	*Pinellia rhizoma*	*Ban xia*	3.0
Atractylodes, white	*Atractylodis rhizoma*	*Bai zhu*	3.0
Gastrodia	*Gastrodiae rhizoma*	*Tian ma*	2.0
Hoelen	*Poria sclerotium*	*Fu ling*	3.0
Citrus peel	*Citri pericarpium*	*Chen pi*	3.0
Ginger, fresh	*Zingiberis rhizoma*	*Sheng jiang*	2.0

Alisma Combination[1]
Ze Xie Tang
(Alisma Decoction)

Alisma	*Alismatis rhizoma*	*Ze xie*	5.0
Atractylodes, white	*Atractylodis rhizoma*	*Bai zhu*	2.0

Qi and Blood Deficiency

Dizziness, blurred or otherwise abnormal vision, pallor, pale lips and nails, lassitude, poor appetite, shortness of breath, lack of strength to speak, palpitation, a pale tongue and a thready, weak pulse characterize *qi* and blood deficiency.

Treatment aims to replenish *qi* and blood with Ginseng and Longan Combination (*gui pi tang*).

If palpitation is serious, add 5 *qian* each of dragon bone (*long gu*) and oyster shell (*mu li*) and 10 *qian* mother of pearl (*zhen zhu mu*).

In the case of serious insomnia, add 3 *qian* zizyphus (*suan zao ren*) and 5 *qian* polygonum stem (*ye jiao teng*).

If there is a severe blood deficiency, add 3 *qian* gelatin (*a jiao*).

If *qi* of the middle energizer is deficient, use Ginseng and Astragalus Combination (*bu zhong yi qi tang*).

After the dizziness is relieved, Lycium, Chrysanthemum and Rehmannia Formula (*qi ju di huang wan*) can be used to improve deficiencies of both *qi* and blood and so prevent dizziness from occurring in the future.

Acupuncture and Moxibustion Points

Excess Liver *Yang*

- *fengchi* (G 20)
- *hegu* (LI 4)
- *ganshu* (B 18)

Kidney Essence Deficiency

- *fengchi* (G 20)
- *shangxing* (GV 23)
- *baihui* (GV 20)

Accumulation of Turbid Phlegm

- *shangxing* (GV 23)
- *fenglong* (S 40)
- *taiyang* (EX-HN5)
- *hegu* (LI 4)

Blood *Qi* Deficiency

- *shangxing* (GV 23)
- *hegu* (LI 4)
- *baihui* (GV 20)
- *zusanli* (S 36, apply moxibustion)

Section 19
Headache

The head is the point where the three *yang* meridians of the hands and feet, the *dumai* (GV) and the *qi* of the internal organs meet. Therefore, it is said in Chinese medicine: "The head is the gathering place of the various *yang*." And: "The head is the repository of lucid *yang*."

In Western medicine, a headache may commonly be observed in infectious diseases, hypertension, intracranial tumors, trigeminal neuralgia and neurosis.

Diagnosis and Herbal Treatment

According to TCM theory, a headache is either induced by external pathogens or internal injury. Generally speaking, the onset of a headache due to external pathogens is rapid, and the headache itself is very painful. It is excess in nature and should be treated by dispelling the external pathogens. On the other hand, the onset of a headache due to an internal injury is usually slow. The pain is slight, though the condition is chronic and often accompanied by some symptoms in the internal organs. This type of headache is deficient in nature and should be treated through tonification. A headache due to turbid phlegm or blood stasis, in turn, is due to a deficiency complicated by an excess, or a deficiency in origin, but an excess in superficiality.

Headache Due to External Pathogens

This type of headache is induced by external wind, cold, dampness or heat, or combinations thereof. Wind is the most common of these external pathogens, though it is generally accompanied by one or more of the other factors.

1. Wind-cold

At the onset, the patient experiences only chills and a tightness and aching in the head. These symptoms, which are aggravated by exposure to wind and cold, gradually spread to the neck and back. An absence of thirst, a thin, white tongue coating and a floating, tense pulse may also be observed.

Treatment is aimed at dispelling wind-cold, for which Schizonepeta and Siler Formula (*jing fang bai du san*) or Cnidium and Tea Formula (*chuan xiong cha tiao san*) can be used.

Cnidium and Tea Formula[1]

Chuan Xiong Cha Tiao San

(Ligusticum *Chuanxiong* Powder to be Taken with Green Tea)[2]

Cnidium	Cnidii rhizoma	Chuan xiong*	3.0
Chiang-huo	Notopterygii rhizoma	Qiang huo	2.0
Angelica	Angelicae dahuricae radix	Bai zhi	2.0
Asarum	Asari herba cum radice	Xi xin	1.0
Schizonepeta	Schizonepetae herba	Jing jie	2.0
Siler	Ledebouriellae radix	Fang feng	2.0
Mentha	Menthae herba	Bo he	1.0
Licorice	Glycyrrhizae radix	Gan cao	1.5
Green tea leaf	Camelliae folium	Cha ye	1.5

Ligustici rhizoma, also known as *chuan xiong*, may be substituted for *Cnidii rhizoma*.

2. Wind-heat

A splitting headache, an aversion to wind, fever, a flushed face, conjunctiva congestion, thirst, constipation, dark yellow urine, a yellow tongue coating and a floating, rapid pulse are induced by wind-heat.

Treatment attempts to dispel wind and clear heat with Morus and Chrysanthemum Combination (*sang ju yin*).

If the patient is fidgety and irritable, and has a bitter taste in his or her mouth and a yellow, greasy tongue coating, add 3 *qian* gentian (*long dan cao*).

If the tongue is red and dry, add 3 *qian* each of dendrobium (*shi hu*) and trichosanthes root (*gua lou gen*).

If the patient is constipated, add 3 *qian* rhubarb (*da huang*).

3. Wind-dampness

A headache with a tight and heavy feeling, dizziness, lassitude, a sensation of oppression in the chest, poor appetite, a white, greasy tongue coating and a soft, floating pulse are associated with wind-dampness.

Treatment concentrates on dispelling wind and removing dampness, for which *Chiang-huo* and Vitex Combination (*qiang huo sheng shi tang*) is recommended.

If dampness is prominently marked by a sensation of severe oppression in the chest, poor appetite and a white, thick, greasy tongue coating, add 3 *qian* each of atractylodes (*cang zhu*) and magnolia bark (*hou pu*).

In the case of nausea and vomiting, add 3 *qian* pinellia (*ban xia*).

Chiang-huo and Vitex Combination

Qiang Huo Sheng Shi Tang[19]

(Notopterygium Decoction to Overcome Dampness)[2]

Chiang-huo	Notopterygii rhizoma	Qiang huo	2.0
Tu-huo	Angelicae tuhuo radix	Du huo	2.0
Kao-pen	Ligustici sinensis rhizoma et radix	Gao ben	3.0
Siler	Ledebouriellae radix	Fang feng	1.5
Cnidium	Cnidii rhizoma	Chuan xiong*	2.0
Vitex	Viticis fructus	Man jing zi	3.0
Licorice	Glycyrrhizae radix	Gan cao	1.0

Ligustici rhizoma, also known as *chuan xiong*, may be substituted for *Cnidii rhizoma*.

Functions: dispels wind-heat; relieves headache.

Explanation: *Chiang-huo* and *tu-huo* dispel general wind-heat symptoms, ease joint movement and alleviate headache, while siler dispels wind to relieve pain. Cnidium promotes *qi* and blood circulation, while *kao-pen* and vitex treat heaviness and pain in the head. Licorice coordinates the actions of the other herbs.

Headache Due to Internal Injury

This type of headache is often attributed to disorders of the liver, spleen or kidneys, or to disharmony of *qi* and blood.

1. Headache due to excess liver *yang*

Emotional instability causes liver *qi* to stagnate and transform into fire. This fire invades the head, exhausts *yin* and so causes *yin* deficiency of the liver and kidneys, as well as excess liver *yang*. These conditions result in a headache which is located in both temples and is accompanied by dizziness, fidgeting, irritability, insomnia, a bitter taste in the mouth, pain in the hypochondrium, a wiry pulse and a thin, yellow tongue coating or a red tongue with scant coating.

Treatment is designed to calm the liver and suppress excess liver *yang*. Gastrodia and Uncaria Combination (*tian ma gou teng yin*) is recommended.

If liver *qi* is stagnant, add 3 *qian* each of turmeric (*yu jin*) and bupleurum (*chai hu*).

If excess liver fire is present, add 3 *qian* each of moutan (*mu dan pi*) and gentian (*long dan cao*).

If *yin* is severely deficient, add 3 *qian* raw rehmannia (*sheng di huang*) and 4 *qian* lycium fruit (*gou qi zi*).

2. Headache due to turbid phlegm

Fatigue or a weak constitution following an illness are usually responsible for spleen disorders. The impaired spleen is unable to generate and transform enough *qi* and blood to nourish the brain and marrow, thus inducing a headache. Furthermore, the spleen fails to transform and transport fluids, and so turbid phlegm develops and accumulates. This phlegm invades and obstructs *yang*, thus exacerbating the headache, which is generally accompanied by heavy-headedness, fullness and distention in the chest and upper abdomen, nausea, vomiting of sputum, a white, greasy tongue coating and a slippery pulse.

Treatment seeks to tonify the spleen to resolve phlegm with Pinellia and Gastrodia Combination (*ban xia bai zhu tian ma tang*).

3. Headache due to kidney deficiency

Inherent kidney defects, kidney *yang* deficiency, kidney infections and diseases associated with sexual promiscuity tend to deplete kidney essence, which then is not present in sufficient amounts to adequately nourish the brain and marrow, thus causing a headache.

A dull, numbing headache which the patient describes as feeling as if his head were empty is characteristic of kidney deficiency. The headache is often accompanied by dizziness, tinnitus, soreness and weakness in the lower back and knees, seminal emission in men and profuse leukorrhea in women.

A patient with kidney *yin* deficiency will also exhibit fidgeting, a feverish sensation in the palms, soles and heart region, a red tongue with scant coating and a thready, rapid pulse; while a patient with kidney *yang* deficiency will have chills, cold limbs, a pale, thick tongue and a submerged, thready and weak pulse.

Kidney *yin* deficiency is treated with Achyranthes and Rehmannia Formula (*zuo gui wan*) to nourish kidney *yin*, while Eucommia and Rehmannia Formula (*you gui wan*) is recommended for strengthening kidney *yang*.

4. Headache due to *qi* and blood deficiency

A mild, chronic headache which is accompanied by dizziness and aggravated by fatigue is a sign of *qi* and blood deficiency. Lassitude, palpitation, shortness of breath, a pale tongue and a thready, weak pulse may also be observed.

Treatment replenishes *qi* and blood through the use of *Tang-kuei* and Ginseng Eight Combination (*ba zhen tang*).

5. Headache due to blood stasis

A fixed, stabbing and chronic headache induced by a traumatic head injury are generally associated with blood stasis. A dark purple tongue with ecchymosis or petechiae and a hesitant pulse may also be observed.

Treatment stimulates blood circulation to remove blood stasis. The following remedy is recommended: *Tang-kuei* Four

Combination (*si wu tang*), plus 3 *qian* each of persica (*tao ren*), achyranthes (*niu xi*), angelica (*bai zhi*) and earthworm (*di long*), as well as 2 *qian* carthamus (*hong hua*) and 1 *qian* asarum (*xi xin*).

If the headache is severe, add 1 *qian* scorpion (*quan xie*) and 2 pieces centipede (*wu gong*).

Acupuncture and Moxibustion Treatment

Headache at the Back of the Head
- *fengfu* (GV 16)
- *houxi* (SI 3)
- *fengchi* (G 20)

Headache on the Side(s) of the Head
- *zulinqi* (G 41)
- *waiguan* (TE 5)
- *xuanzhong* (G 39)

Headache in the Forehead
- *yintang* (EX-HN3)
- *tou wei* (S 8)
- *hegu* (LI 4)

Headache at the Top of the Head
- *taicong* (Liv 3)
- *xingjian* (Liv 2)
- *fengfu* (GV 16)

Headache Due to Wind-cold
- *fengfu* (GV 16)
- *fengchi* (G 20, apply moxibustion)
- *dazhui* (GV 14)
- *hegu* (LI 4)

Headache Due to Wind-heat
- *taiyang* (EX-HN5)
- *shaoshang* (L 11)
- *dazhui* (GV 14)
- *lieque* (L 7)

Headache Due to Excess Liver *Yang*
- *taicong* (Liv 3)
- *tongziliao* (G 1)
- *ganshu* (B 18)
- *fengchi* (G 20)
- *taixi* (K 3)

Headache Due to Blood and *Qi* Deficiency

- *baihui* (GV 20)
- *qihai* (CV 6)
- *ganshu* (B 18)
- *pishu* (B 20)
- *shenshu* (B 23)
- *hegu* (LI 4)
- *zusanli* (S 36)

Headache Due to the Accumulation of Turbid Phlegm

- *baihui* (GV 20)
- *shangxing* (GV 23)
- *taiyang* (EX-HN5)
- *zusanli* (S 36)
- *hegu* (LI 4)

Section 20
Apoplexy (Stroke)

"*Zhong feng*" is Chinese for "cerebrovascular accident," and "*zu zhong*" is the TCM term for stroke. Together they are the TCM equivalent for apoplexy. This group of diseases is characterized by a sudden deviation of the eyes and mouth, dysphasia, hemiplegia, an inability to remain standing, loss of consciousness and even coma. Cerebral hemorrhaging, cerebral thrombosis or peripheral facial paralysis may also be observed.

Apoplexy is generally caused by a disharmony of *qi* and blood. In addition, emotional upsets, improper diet, inadequate sleep, worry, anger and heart fire can damage liver and kidney *yin*, which then will be unable to control *yang*. The latter condition results in an excess of liver *yang*, the accumulation of blood in the upper body and, consequently, apoplexy.

Alternately, improper diet and fatigue may injure the spleen, thereby prompting a failure in its ability to transport and convert nutritional essence and dampness. The latter then accumulates and produces phlegm, which stagnates and transforms into heat or, occasionally, into internal wind. Wind then carries phlegm upwards to block the orifice and the meridians, causing sudden coma, hemiplegia and deviation of the eyes and mouth.

In general, wind (chiefly liver wind), fire (usually heart or liver fire), phlegm (phlegm-dampness or wind-phlegm), *qi* (either *qi* deficiency or an adverse flow of *qi*), blood (deficiency or stasis), *yin* deficiency and *yang* excess may influence each other and so induce apoplexy.

A less frequently seen scenario involves a deficiency of *qi* and blood, which enables wind evil to invade the meridians. Furthermore, some patients have a constitution of *yin* deficiency complicated by excesses of *yang*, phlegm and dampness. If such a patient is affected by external wind evil, the latter will prompt interior wind to induce apoplexy.

Apoplexy is deficient in nature, but appears as an exterior excess. The deficiency is usually manifested in the blood, *qi*, liver or kidneys; while the exterior excess refers to the accumulation of wind, fire, phlegm and dampness, as well as the adverse flow of *qi* and blood.

Patient conditions vary greatly as regards the severity of the disease course. Usually, apoplexy can be divided into two types: that involving the meridians and collaterals, and that involving the internal organs. The former is milder and does not affect mental functioning, while the latter is usually severe and entails a loss of consciousness.

Diagnosis and Herbal Treatment

Apoplexy Involving the Meridians and Collaterals

When the patient exhibits dizziness, headache, tinnitus, vertigo, insomnia and drowsiness, he may suddenly suffer from dysphasia, stiffness of the tongue, deviation of the mouth and eyes, hemiplegia, a red tongue with a greasy, yellow coating, and a wiry and slippery or wiry, thready and rapid pulse.

Treatment nourishes *yin*, suppresses excess *yang* and tranquilizes liver wind. Dragon Bone and Two Shells Combination (*zhen gan xi feng tang*), plus 3 *qian* raw rehmannia (*sheng di huang*) and 4 *qian* uncaria (*gou teng*), can be used.

Dragon Bone and Two Shells Combination
Zhen Gan Xi Feng Tang[23]
(Sedate the Liver and Extinguish the Wind Decoction)[2]

Achyranthes	*Achyranthis radix*	Niu xi	10.0
Hematite	*Haematitum*	Dai zhe shi	10.0
Dragon bone	*Draconis os*	Long gu	5.0
Oyster shell	*Ostreae testa*	Mu li	5.0
Tortoise shell	*Testudinis plastrum*	Gui ban	5.0
Peony	*Paeoniae radix*	Shao yao	5.0
Scrophularia	*Scrophulariae radix*	Xuan shen	5.0
Asparagus	*Asparagi radix*	Tian men dong	5.0
Melia	*Meliae toosendan fructus*	Chuan lian zi	2.0
Ching-hao	*Artemisiae ching hao herba*	Qing hao	2.0
Malt	*Hordei germinatus fructus*	Mai ya	2.0
Licorice	*Glycyrrhizae radix*	Gan cao	1.5

Functions: regulates the liver; calms wind.

Explanation: Achyranthes is the principal herb for stimulating the flow of blood to the lower body. Oyster shell, hematite, dragon bone, tortoise shell, scrophularia and asparagus nourish *yin* and suppress *yang*. Peony soothes the liver, while melia and malt promote the flow of *qi* and alleviate pain. *Ching-hao* helps stop pain, and licorice harmonizes the actions of the other herbs.

If there is profuse sputum, add 3 *qian* arisaema with bile (*dan nan xing*) and 10 *qian* bamboo juice (*zhu li*).

In the case of a severe headache, add 10 *qian* haliotis (*shi jue ming*) and 3 *qian* prunella (*xia ku cao*).

If the patient is plagued by fidgeting, add 3 *qian* each of scute (*huang qin*) and gardenia (*zhi zi*).

If the patient has a thick, greasy tongue coating due to phlegm-dampness, the dosage of Dragon Bone and Two Shells Combination should be reduced.

Apoplexy Involving the Solid and Hollow Organs

The primary feature of this type of apoplexy is a sudden loss of consciousness. In order to further differentiate this condition, two subtypes are identified: the stroke of excess and the stroke of prostration. The former involves pathogenic evils inside the body, while the latter often involves the collapse of *yang qi.*

1. Stroke of excess (closed conformation)

This type of stroke is characterized by spasms of the limbs, a closed mouth, lock jaw, clenched fists, anuria, a sudden loss of consciousness, cessation of bowel movement, and coma. Depending on the presence or absence of heat, the stroke of excess may be further divided into *yang* closed stroke and *yin* closed stroke.

a. *yang* closed stroke

In addition to the symptoms mentioned above, the patient is listless and has a flushed face, fever, foul-smelling breath, a yellow, greasy tongue coating and a wiry, slippery and rapid pulse.

Treatment is aimed at inducing resuscitation and tranquilizing liver wind with cold, pungent herbs. Antelope Horn and

Uncaria Combination (*ling jiao gou teng tang*) and one bolus of Rhinoceros and Amber Formula (*zhi bao dan*) can be given.

If there is profuse phlegm, add 10 *qian* bamboo juice (*zhu li*) and 2 *qian* arisaema with bile (*dan nan xing*).

Rhinoceros and Amber Formula
Zhi Bao Dan[20]
(Greatest-treasure Special Pill)[2]

Rhinoceros horn	Rhinocerotis cornu	Xi jiao	3.2
Cinnabar	Cinnabaris	Zhu sha	3.2
Realgar	Realgar	Xiong huang	3.2
Hawksbill shell	Eretmochelytis carapax	Dai mao	3.2
Amber	Succinum	Hu pu	3.2
Musk	Moschus	She xiang	0.4
Borneol	Borneolum	Bing pian	0.4
Cow gallstone	Bovis bezoar	Niu huang	1.6
Benzoin	Benzoinum	An xi xiang	4.8
Gold foil	Aurum	Jin bo	5 pieces
Silver foil	Argentum	Yin bo	5 pieces

Functions: clears heat; induces resuscitation; resolves phlegm; detoxifies.

Explanation: Rhinoceros horn, cow gallstone and hawksbill shell clear excess heat and detoxify, while musk, borneol and benzoin resolve phlegm and induce resuscitation. Cinnabar, hawksbill shell and amber tranquilize the mind and treat mental disturbances due to turbid phlegm. Gold and silver foil, as well as cinnabar and realgar, may be omitted if costs prohibit their use, and buffalo horn (*shui niu jiao*) may be substituted for the rhinoceros horn, which is banned from sale in the United States.

b. *yin* closed stroke

In addition to the general symptoms noted above for closed-conformation strokes, the following may also be observed: a pale complexion, cyanosis of the lips, profuse phlegm and saliva, cold limbs, lying supine without movement, a white, greasy tongue coating and a slow, slippery pulse.

Treatment induces resuscitation, resolves phlegm and subdues wind with warm, pungent herbs. Arisaema and Acorus Combination (*die tan tang*) and one pill of Styrax Formula (*su he xiang wan*), dissolved in warm water, may be used.

Arisaema and Acorus Combination
Die Tan Tang[9]
(Expectorate Phlegm Decoction)

Pinellia	Pinellia rhizoma	Ban xia	2.0
Citrus peel	Citri pericarpium	Chen pi	2.0
Hoelen	Poria sclerotium	Fu ling	3.0
Licorice	Glycyrrhizae radix	Gan cao	1.0
Chih-shih	Citri fructus immaturus	Zhi shi	2.0
Arisaema	Arisaematis rhizoma	Tian nan xiang	2.0
Bamboo shavings	Bambusae caulis in taeniis	Zhu ru	3.0
Acorus	Acori rhizoma	Chang pu	3.0
Ginseng	Ginseng radix	Ren shen	1.0
Jujube	Zizyphi fructus	Da zao	5.0

Function: expectorates phlegm.

Explanation: This formula is a modification of Citrus and Pinellia Combination (*er chen tang*), which is used to resolve phlegm by drying interior dampness. *Chih-shih*, bamboo shavings and arisaema have been added to expel wind, clear heat and dispel phlegm. Acorus, a warm, pungent herb, opens the nasal passages and throat, while ginseng tonifies *qi* in order to induce resuscitation.

2. Stroke of prostration

This condition is characterized by a sudden collapse into coma, closed eyes, an open mouth, a dry nose, shallow breathing, hands lying beside the body with fingers unclenched, cold limbs, profuse sweating, incontinence of urine and feces, quadriplegia, paralysis of the tongue and a weak pulse.

Dragon Bone, Oyster Shell, Ginseng and Aconite Combination (*shen fu long mu tang*) may be used.

If profuse sweating cannot be controlled, add 5 *qian* astragalus (*huang qi*), 1 *qian* schizandra (*wu wei zi*) and 4 *qian* glutinous rice root (*nuo dao gen*).

Sequelae

1. Hemiplegia

In TCM, this is called *pian ku* or one-sided atrophy. It is due to wind-phlegm flowing into the meridians and collaterals, thereby causing *qi* stagnancy and blood stasis, which prevent the proper movement of *qi* and the unimpeded circulation of blood to nourish the body. Consequently, the limbs will atrophy and become disabled.

Treatment strengthens *qi*, stimulates blood circulation, resolves phlegm and removes obstructions from the meridians. Astragalus and Peony Combination (*bu yang huan wu tang*) is recommended.

Astragalus and Peony Combination
Bu Yang Huan Wu Tang[8]
(Reinforce *Yang* and Restore the Normal Functioning
of the Five Viscera Decoction)

Astragalus	*Astragali radix*	*Huang qi*	10.0
Tang-kuei	*Angelicae radix*	*Dang gui*	3.0
Cnidium	*Cnidii rhizoma*	*Chuan xiong**	2.0
Peony, red	*Paeoniae rubra radix*	*Chi shao*	3.0
Earthworm	*Lumbricus*	*Di long*	3.0
Persica	*Persicae semen*	*Tao ren*	3.0
Carthamus	*Carthami flos*	*Hong hua*	3.0

Ligustici rhizoma, also known as *chuan xiong*, may be substituted for
Cnidii rhizoma.

Functions: invigorates *qi*; stimulates blood circulation;
removes obstructions in the meridians; promotes movement of
the limbs.

Explanation: Astragalus reinforces vital energy, while *tang-kuei*, cnidium, red peony, persica and carthamus are associate
herbs used to activate blood circulation and remove blood
stasis. Earthworm dredges the meridional passages. This formula is commonly prescribed for the treatment of hemiplegia
and paraplegia.

If the patient has a deviation of the mouth and/or eyes, add
3 *qian* silkworm (*bai jiang can*), 1 *qian* giant typhonium tuber
(*bai fu zi*) and 2 *qian* scorpion (*quan xie*).

In case of weakness in the legs, add 3 *qian* each of dipsacus
(*xu duan*), loranthus (*sang ji sheng*) and achyranthes (*niu xi*).

If the patient is constipated, add 5 *qian* linum (*ma zi ren*)
and 3 *qian* apricot seed (*xing ren*).

Should the hemiplegia linger and be accompanied by a
weak pulse, the dose of astragalus may be increased. In an

acute case, however, the astragalus should be reduced to 3 qian, provided the patient's vital energy is not weak.

2. Dysphasia

This is the result of wind-phlegm ascending and so obstructing the meridians and collaterals.

Treatment expels wind evil and eliminates phlegm through the removal of obstructions from the meridians and the opening of the orifices. Typhonium and Acorus Formula (jie yu dan) is the preferred remedy.

Typhonium and Acorus Formula
Jie Yu Dan[22]
(Relieve Dysphasia Powder)

Giant typhonium tuber	*Typhonii rhizoma*	Bai fu zi	3.0
Acorus	*Acori rhizoma*	Chang pu	1.0
Polygala	*Polygalae radix*	Yuan zhi	2.0
Gastrodia	*Gastrodiae rhizoma*	Tian ma	1.0
Scorpion	*Scorpio*	Quan xie	1.0
Chiang-huo	*Notopterygii rhizoma*	Qiang huo	1.0
Arisaema	*Arisaematis rhizoma*	Tian nan xing	3.0
Saussurea	*Saussureae radix*	Mu xiang	1.0
Licorice	*Glycyrrhizae radix*	Gan cao	1.0

Functions: dispels wind; resolves phlegm; opens orifices; restores the ability to speak.

Explanation: Giant typhonium tuber, scorpion and *chiang-huo* dispel wind-phlegm, while acorus, polygala, gastrodia and arisaema resolve phlegm and open the throat and nasal passages. Saussurea activates the flow of *qi*, and licorice invigorates vital energy. Together these herbs restore proper functioning to the tongue, thereby enabling the patient to speak.

In addition to herbal medicine, the use of acupuncture, moxibustion and massage are essential to complete the treatment of apoplexy. Furthermore, it is also very important to encourage the patient to exercise his paralyzed side or members.

Common Acupuncture and Moxibustion Points

Apoplexy Involving the Meridians and Collaterals

1. Headache and dizziness
    a. points of first choice
        - *baihui* (GV 20)
        - *taichong* (Liv 3)

    b. reserved points
        - *sishencong* (EX-HN1)
        - *fengchi* (G 20)
        - *taiyang* (EX-HN5)

2. Dysphasia and numbness of the tongue
        - *yameng* (GV 15)
        - *lianquan* (CV 23)

3. Facial paralysis
    a. points of first choice
        - *xiaguan* (S 7)
        - *dicang* (S 4)
        - *jiache* (S 6)

    b. reserved points
        - *yinxiang* (LI 20)
        - *chengjiang* (CV 24)

4. Paralysis of the upper limbs
    a. points of first choice
        (1) - *tianding* (LI 17)
             - *chuchi* (LI 11)

        (2) - *xiaoluo* (TE 12)
             - *sidu* (TE 9)

        (3) Alternately employ the points of the (1) or (2) group.

        Augment with electric stimulation (electro-acupuncture) for 15-20 minutes.

b. reserved points
- *jianyu* (LI 15)
- *hegu* (LI 4)
- *shousanli* (LI 10)

5. Paralysis of the lower limbs
a. points of first choice
(1) • *huantiao* (G 30) • *weiyang* (B 39)

(2) • *chongmen* (Sp 12) • *piguan* (S 31)

(3) • *zusanli* (S 36) • *yanglingquan* (G 34)

(4) Alternately employ points from the (1), (2) or (3)
group. Augment with electric stimulation for 15-20 minutes.

b. reserved points
- *futu* (S 32)
- *xuanzhong* (G 39)

Apoplexy Involving the Internal Organs

1. Stroke of excess
a. points of first choice
- *shuigou* (GV 26)
- *neiguan* (P 6)
- the 12 well (*jing*) points

b. reserved points
- *fengchi* (G 20)
- *hegu* (LI 4)
- *laogong* (P 8)
- *taichong* (Liv 3)

2. Stroke of prostration
a. points of first choice
- *baihui* (GV 20)
- *zusanli* (S 36)
- *shuigou* (GV 26)

b. reserved points
- *neiguan* (P 6)
- *shenque* (CV 8) (moxibustion)
- *hegu* (LI 14)
- *guanyuan* (CV 4) (moxibustion)

Section 21
Syncope

Syncope, commonly known as fainting, is a transient loss of consciousness, which, according to Western medicine, is due to an inadequate supply of blood to the brain. Usually the patient gradually regains consciousness and there are no subsequent episodes of hemiplegia, aphasia, abnormal focusing of the eyes or "drooping" of the mouth.

According to a Western medical viewpoint, this conformation includes hemorrhagic shock, physical collapse or exhaustion, short-term coma, sunstroke, hypoglycemia, hypertensive crisis, cerebrovascular spasm and hysteria.

Traditional Chinese medicine (TCM) points to the following as causes of syncope: internal injury by excesses of the seven emotions; the six external evils; phlegm retention; and improper diet. The latter two can disrupt the crucial balance between *yin* and *yang*. This imbalance results in disharmonies between *qi*, *yin* and *yang*, which in turn cause syncope.

Before administering first aid, a differentiation must be made between deficiency and excess types. Acupuncture and moxibustion may be given, or the patient can be treated with an integration of Western and TCM therapies. After consciousness is restored, a diagnosis must be made as to whether the syncope was the result of a disorder of *qi*, blood or phlegm, or of improper diet or summer heat.

Diagnosis and Herbal Treatment

Syncope Resulting From a *Qi* Disorder

1. Excess conformation

This conformation is generally induced by emotional irritations which lead to an adverse flow of *qi*. The patient faints, with jaw and fists clenched, limbs cold, tongue coating thin and white, and pulse weak or submerged and wiry.

Treatment consists in restoring the normal flow of *qi* and relieving *qi* stagnancy with Bupleurum and *Chih-shih* Formula (*si ni san*), to which has been added 3 *qian* each of areca seed (*bing lang zi*) and saussurea (*mu xiang*), as well as 0.3 *qian* aquilaria (powder of *chen xiang*). This formula should be taken with warm water.

If there is an excess of liver *yang*, with dizziness, headache and a flushed face, add 10 *qian* each of haliotis (*shi jue ming*) and oyster shell (*mu li*), as well as 3 *qian* uncaria (*gou teng*).

If there is profuse phlegm and tachypnea with the sound of phlegm in the throat, add 10 *qian* bamboo juice (*zhu li*) and 3 *qian* each of arisaema with bile (*dan nan xiang*) and fritillaria (*bei mu*). This concoction is to be taken with warm water.

The patient may also take *Tang-kuei* and Bupleurum Formula (*xiao yao san*) in order to regulate the flow of *qi*, alleviate mental depression and prevent stress-induced relapses.

2 Deficiency conformation

A patient suffering from deficiency-conformation syncope ordinarily is feeble and has relapses which are fright- or fatigue-induced. Manifestations include dizziness, fainting, a pale complexion, perspiration, cold limbs, shallow breathing, a thin tongue coating and a submerged, weak pulse.

Treatment consists in tonifying *qi* and restoring *yang* with Ginseng and Aconite Combination (*shen fu tang*) and Dragon Bone and Oyster Shell Combination (*long gu mu li tang*).

Ginseng and Aconite Combination[1]
Shen Fu Tang
(Ginseng and Prepared Aconite Decoction)[2]

Ginseng	*Ginseng radix*	*Ren shen*	3.0
Aconite, prepared	*Aconiti carmichaelii praeparata radix*	*Zhi fu zi*	2.0

Dragon Bone and Oyster Shell Combination[1]
Long Gu Mu Li Tang
(Dragon Bone and Oyster Shell Decoction)

Dragon bone	*Draconis os*	*Long gu*	5.0
Oyster shell	*Ostreae testa*	*Mu li*	5.0

If *qi* deficiency is serious, add 5 *qian* astragalus (*huang qi*).

If the patient is palpitating, add 3 *qian* each of polygala (*yuan zhi*) and zizyphus (*suan zao ren*).

Syncope Due to Blood Disorders

1. Excess conformation

The patient suddenly loses consciousness and has a clenched jaw, a flushed face, cyanosed lips, a red tongue and a submerged, hesitant pulse.

Treatment promotes blood circulation and the normal flow of *qi* with Persica and Cnidium Combination (*tong qiao huo xue tang*).

Persica and Cnidium Combination
Tong Qiao Huo Xue Tang[8]
(Unblock the Orifices and Invigorate the Blood Decoction)[2]

Peony, red	Paeoniae rubra radix	Chi shao	1.0
Cnidium	Cnidii rhizoma	Chuan xiong*	1.0
Persica	Persicae semen	Tao ren	3.0
Carthamus	Carthami flos	Hong hua	3.0
Allium	Allii fistulosi bulbus	Cong bai	3 pieces
Jujube	Zizyphi fructus	Da zao	5 pieces
Ginger, fresh	Zingiberis rhizoma	Sheng jiang	3.0
Musk	Moschus	She xiang	0.05

*Ligustici rhizoma, also known as chuan xiong, may be substituted for Cnidii rhizoma.

The above ingredients are decocted in water and taken with wine.

Functions: promotes blood circulation; induces resuscitation.

Explanation: Red peony, cnidium, persica and carthamus promote blood circulation and remove blood stasis. Aromatic allium also stimulates blood circulation. Ginger and jujube harmonize ying (nutrients) and wei (defensive mechanism), while musk aids in restoring consciousness. The formula is good for treating blood stasis in the upper body.

2. Deficiency conformation

This type of syncope is due to an excessive loss of blood. The patient suddenly loses consciousness, with such manifestations as a pale complexion, pale lips, slack jaw, tremors in the limbs, spontaneous perspiration, feeble breathing, a pale tongue and a thready, weak pulse or thready, rapid and weak pulse.

Treatment consists of invigorating *qi* and nourishing blood with Ginseng Nutritive Combination (*ren shen yang rong tang*).

Ginseng Nutritive Combination[1]
Ren Shen Yang Rong Tang*
(Ginseng Decoction to Nourish the Nutritive *Qi*)[2]

Ginseng	Ginseng radix	Ren shen	3.0
Rehmannia, cooked	Rehmanniae radix	Shu di huang	4.0
Atractylodes, white	Atractylodis rhizoma	Bai zhu	4.0
Tang-kuei	Angelicae radix	Dang gui	4.0
Peony	Paeoniae radix	Shao yao	4.0
Hoelen	Poria sclerotium	Fu ling	4.0
Astragalus	Astragali radix	Huang qi	2.5
Cinnamon bark	Cinnamomi cortex	Gui pi	2.5
Schizandra	Schizandrae fructus	Wu wei zi	1.5
Polygala	Polygalae radix	Yuan zhi	1.5
Citrus peel	Citri pericarpium	Chen pi	2.5
Licorice	Glycyrrhizae radix	Gan cao	1.5

*also known as *ren shen yang ying tang*

Syncope Due to Phlegm

The patient suddenly becomes unconscious with sounds of phlegm in the throat or the vomiting of foamy saliva. Tachypnea, a white, greasy tongue coating and a submerged, slippery pulse may also be observed.

The condition is treated by promoting *qi* circulation and eliminating phlegm with Hoelen and Bamboo Combination (*wen dan tang*), to which has been added 1 *qian* brassica (*bai jie zi*) and 3 *qian* each of perilla seed (*zi su zi*) and raphanus (*lai fu zi*).

Syncope Due to Crapulence

The patient goes into a coma after crapulence with asphyxia. Abdominal distention, a thick, greasy tongue coating and a slippery, rapid pulse may also be observed.

Treatment involves removing the retained food, promoting digestion and regulating the stomach with Citrus and Crataegus Formula (*bao he wan*), to which has been added 1.5 *qian* coptis (*huang lian*) and 3 *qian* each of *chih-shih* (*zhi shi*), magnolia bark (*hou pu*) and scute (*huang qin*).

If the patient is experiencing constipation and abdominal distention, add 3 *qian* rhubarb (*da huang*). Decoct the rhubarb and administer it after the above remedy has been given. In this way, the rhubarb will more effectively remove retained food and pass it through the bowels.

Syncope Due to Summer Heat

In hot weather, people are susceptible to heat stroke, which is characterized by fainting. The patient feels a sudden sensation of oppression in the chest and also manifests a fever, dizziness, headache, a flushed face, a dry mouth, a red, dry tongue and an excess, surging and rapid pulse.

The condition is treated by clearing summer heat and inducing resuscitation with Gypsum Combination (*bai hu tang*), to which has been added 1.5 *qian* coptis (*huang lian*) and 3 *qian* each of gardenia (*zhi zi*), turmeric (*yu jin*), lophatherum (*dan zhu ye*) and forsythia (*lian qiao*), as well as a half piece of fresh lotus leaf (*lian ye*).

The unconscious patient should be taken to a cool, well-ventilated place. In order to remove the heat from the heart and thereby affect resuscitation, a bolus of Bovis Bezoar and Coptis Formula (*niu huang qing xin wan*) should be given.

Bovis Bezoar and Coptis Formula
Niu Huang Qing Xin Wan[24]
(Cattle Gallstone Pill to Clear the Heart)[2]

Scute	Scutellariae radix	Huang qin	30.0
Coptis	Coptidis rhizoma	Huang lian	30.0
Gardenia	Gardeniae fructus	Zhi zi	30.0
Turmeric	Curcumae rhizoma	Yu jin	30.0
Cow gallstone	Bovis bezoar	Niu huang	10.0

The above herbs are ground into a fine powder and made into 1-*qian* boluses by mixing the powder with honey and coating the mixture with cinnabar (*zhu sha*). One or two boluses are taken daily.

Functions: clears heat; detoxifies; induces resuscitation; acts as a tranquilizer.

Explanation: Scute, coptis and gardenia clear heat and purge fire. Turmeric removes heat and alleviates depression, while cow gallstone clears *ying fen*, removes heat from the blood and detoxifies. The bolus should be taken with cool water.

If the patient suffering from syncope due to summer heat is thirsty and has a dry mouth and a red tongue, add 3 *qian* American ginseng root (*xi yang shen*), which have been decocted separately.

In order to replenish *qi* and promote the production of body fluids, 3 *qian* ophiopogon (*mai men dong*) and 10 *qian* fresh dendrobium (*xian shi hu*) should be added.

When profuse sweating results in *qi* exhaustion, dizziness, palpitation, a pale complexion, cold limbs and a thready, rapid pulse, Dragon Bone and Oyster Shell Combination (*long gu mu li tang*) should be administered, adding 3 *qian* ginseng (*ren shen*), decocted separately, and 3 *qian* prepared aconite (*zhi fu zi*).

If summer-heat pathogens impair *yin*, causing the ascent of liver wind, dizziness, nausea, convulsions of the limbs and a wiry, rapid pulse may be observed. To clear heat, calm the liver, nourish *yin* and tranquilize interior wind, administer Antelope Horn and Uncaria Combination (*ling jiao gou teng tang*).

Acupuncture and Moxibustion Treatment

Excess Conformation

- *renzhong* (GV 26)
- *zhongchong* (P 9)
- *taichong* (Liv 3)
- *hegu* (LI 4)
- *laogong* (P 8)
- *shaoze* (SI 1)

Deficiency Conformation

- *baihui* (GV 20)
- *qihai* (CV 6)
- *guanyuan* (CV 4)
- *neiguan* (P 6)
- *zusanli* (S 36)
- *mingmen* (GV 4)

Section 22
Bleeding Problems

Bleeding is a clinical sign of a great many diseases. Externally, blood can escape from the mouth, nose or skin, or be eliminated through the stools or urine, while internal bleeding includes hemoptysis, hematemesis, epistaxis, hematochezia, hematuria and purpura.

Bleeding problems may be divided into excess or deficiency conformations. The former is associated with hemorrhaging in acute diseases and usually is induced by fire, while the latter is associated with hemorrhaging in chronic diseases and is usually induced by a *qi* deficiency or fire due to *yin* deficiency, though, in a few cases, the hemorrhaging may be related to a deficiency-cold conformation. The causes of hemorrhages are many, though they may be roughly categorized as hemorrhages due to interior factors, those due to external evils and those which result from other exterior factors.

Etiology

Interior Factors

Fatigue, internal injury or extremes of any of the seven emotions can impair the liver and spleen. Hemorrhages develop after an illness or as a result of overwork or a spleen or *qi* deficiency. A deficient spleen cannot properly regulate the blood, thereby causing it to escape from the vessels. Blood escaping from the upper body is termed hemoptysis, whereas that escaping from the lower body is hematuria, and that released from the skin is called purpura. Specifically, anxiety and unresolved or repressed anger can impair the liver, prompting liver fire to invade the lungs and stomach, thereby damaging the collaterals and causing hemoptysis or hematemesis.

Following a lingering illness or as a result of a febrile disease, *yin* essence becomes deficient. Consequently, fire flares up, impairs the lung collaterals and leads to hemoptysis. In the case of a *yin* deficiency of the liver or kidneys, heat forces the blood to descend, resulting in hematuria. Furthermore, should heart fire flare up, heat will invade the urinary bladder and hematuria may occur.

External Evils

When the patient is affected by the evils of wind, heat and dryness, the latter stagnates in the lungs and transforms into fire. Fire and a reversed flow of *qi* will burn the lung collaterals and thereby cause hemoptysis and epistaxis.

Other Exterior Factors

Excess consumption of alcoholic beverages or hot or acrid foods causes heat-dampness to accumulate in the stomach and intestines. This accumulation damages the stomach collaterals and results in hematemesis. Heat-dampness may also descend to the intestines and burn the collaterals, causing the formation of bloody stools.

Diagnosis and Herbal Treatment

Although blood problems can be classified into several categories, such as hemostasis, hematemesis, hematochezia and hematuria, their etiology and pathology have some things in common. Generally speaking, hemorrhaging is associated with fire, heat-dampness, spleen deficiency or kidney deficiency. In the case of loss of blood accompanied by a thready, normal pulse, treatment is relatively easy; however, if the pulse is rapid, large and wiry, treatment is more difficult.

Hemoptysis

In the case of hemoptysis, blood is coughed up from the lungs and phlegm is mixed with blood or bright red blood is coughed up. Hemoptysis may also be manifested as the spontaneous eructation of blood clots. The condition has many causes, the primary ones being respiratory diseases of the lungs and bronchi.

Heart disease can also result in hemoptysis. Clinically, hemoptysis is often induced by tuberculosis, bronchiectasis or pulmonary carcinoma.

1. Wind-heat impairment of the lungs

A cough due to an itchy throat, sputum with blood, a dry mouth and nose, fever, a red tongue with a thin, yellow coating, and a floating, rapid pulse characterize wind-heat impairment of the lungs.

This condition is treated by ventilating the lungs and clearing heat with Morus and Lycium Formula (*xie bai san*), to which has been added 3 *qian* each of apricot seed (*xing ren*), fritillaria (*bei mu*) and soja (*dan dou chi*).

2. Liver fire invading the lungs

Paroxysmal cough, phlegm with blood or the coughing up of blood without phlegm, pain in the chest and hypochondrium during coughing fits, fidgeting, irritability, dry stools, a red tongue with a thin, yellow coating, and a wiry, rapid pulse characterize invasion of the lungs by liver fire.

This disease is treated by removing heat from the lungs, calming the liver and harmonizing the collaterals with 3 *qian* Indigo and Concha Formula (*dai ge san*), to which is added 1 *qian* licorice (*gan cao*) and 3 *qian* each of morus bark (*sang bai pi*) and scute (*huang qin*).

3. *Yin* deficiency inducing fire

A flushed face, fidgeting, a dry throat, a cough due to a scratchy throat, phlegm with blood or repeated hemoptysis, a red tongue with scanty coating, and a thready, rapid pulse characterize a *yin* deficiency which induces fire.

This condition is treated by nourishing *yin*, clearing fire and moistening the lungs with Lily Combination (*bai he gu jin tang*), to which has been added 3 *qian* each of madder (*qian cao gen*), lotus node (*ou jie*) and bletilla (*bai ji*).

Hematemesis

Blood from the stomach is vomited through the mouth. In a serious case of hematemesis, the excessive amounts of dark purple, expectorated blood contain undigested food. Heat accumulated in the stomach, fire transformed from stagnant liver *qi*, stagnation of the stomach collaterals and impairment of blood collaterals can all induce hematemesis. Clinically speaking, hemorrhages due to portal cirrhosis, gastroduodenal ulcers and carcinoma of the stomach are common.

1. Accumulation of stomach heat

This condition is characterized by the following signs and symptoms: distention, fullness and/or pain in the stomach and abdomen; the spitting up of dark purple or bright red blood, or of blood containing food residue; constipation; melena; a red tongue with greasy, yellow coating; and a slippery, rapid pulse.

Treatment clears stomach heat, purges fire, removes heat from the blood and affects hemostasis with Coptis and Rhubarb Combination (*san huang xie xin tang*), to which has been added 3 *qian* each of Japanese thistle (*da ji*), field thistle (*xiao ji*), biota top (*ce bo ye*) and imperata (*bai mao gen*).

2. Liver fire invading the stomach

The spitting up of bright red or purple blood, a bitter taste in the mouth, pain in hypochondrium, irritability, headache, conjunctival congestion, fidgeting, drowsiness, insomnia, a red tongue and a wiry, rapid pulse characterize liver fire invading the stomach.

This condition is treated by purging liver fire, clearing stomach heat and nourishing *yin* fluid with Gentian Combination (*long dan xie gan tang*).

3. Spleen *qi* deficiency

The spitting up of dark or reddish blood, palpitation, shortness of breath, a pale complexion, loss of appetite, cold limbs, melena, a pale tongue and a thready, weak pulse characterize spleen *qi* deficiency.

Treatment strengthens the spleen, replenishes *qi*, tonifies blood and nourishes the heart with Ginseng and Longan Combination (*gui pi tang*).

Apostaxis

Apostaxis involves bleeding of the gums, tongue, ears and skin which is not induced by trauma. Depending on its location, apostaxis is known by various names, two of which are discussed here, namely, epistaxis and bleeding of the gums.

1. Epistaxis

The blood escapes from the nasal cavities and its color is usually bright red. Epistaxis may be associated with one of the following: lung heat, stomach heat or deficiency of *qi* and blood.

a. lung heat

Nasal dryness, cough, absence of sputum, fever, a red tongue with a thin, yellow coating, and a rapid pulse characterize lung heat.

It is treated by clearing lung heat and removing heat from the blood with Morus and Chrysanthemum Combination (*sang ju yin*).

256

b. stomach heat

A nosebleed of bright red blood, thirst, halitosis, constipation, a red tongue with a yellow coating, and a rapid pulse are associated with stomach heat.

Treatment consists in removing heat from the blood with Rehmannia and Gypsum Combination (*yu nu jian*).

Rehmannia and Gypsum Combination
Yu Nu Jian[26]
(Jade Woman Decoction)[2]

Gypsum	Gypsum fibrosum	Shi gao	6.0
Rehmannia, raw	Rehmanniae radix	Sheng di huang	6.0
Ophiopogon	Ophiopogonis rhizoma	Mai men dong	2.0
Anemarrhena	Anemarrhenae rhizoma	Zhi mu	3.0
Achyranthes	Achyranthis radix	Niu xi	3.0

c. deficiency of *qi* and blood

Epistaxis or skin ecchymosis, a pale complexion, listlessness, dizziness, palpitation, sleeplessness, a pinkish tongue and a thready, weak pulse characterize a deficiency of *qi* and blood.

The condition is treated by invigorating *qi* and nourishing blood with *Tang-kuei* and Ginseng Eight Combination (*ba zhen tang*).

2. Bleeding gums

This may be further distinguished as either bleeding gums due to excess stomach heat or bleeding gums associated with fire due to *yin* deficiency.

a. excess stomach heat

Red, swollen and painful gums, the extravasation of bright red blood, headache, halitosis, constipation, a yellow tongue coating and a surging, rapid pulse are associated with excess stomach heat.

The condition is treated by clearing stomach fire with Gypsum Combination (*bai hu tang*), to which has been added 2 *qian* rhubarb (*da huang*) and 10 *qian* imperata (*bai mao gen*).

b. fire due to *yin* deficiency

Pinkish blood, slightly painful and swollen gums, loose teeth, dizziness, lower back pain, a flushed face, a red tongue and a thready, rapid pulse characterize fire due to *yin* deficiency.

The condition is treated by moistening *yin* and removing fire and heat from the blood with Anemarrhena, Phellodendron and Rehmannia Formula (*zhi bo ba wei wan*).

Hematochezia

In the case of hematochezia, the blood hemorrhaged from the lower region of the intestines is bright red and occurs after defecation, whereas dark blood hemorrhaged before defecation is due to bleeding from the upper gastrointestinal tract. The former condition is associated with an excess heat conformation, while the latter is attributable to deficiency of the spleen and stomach.

1. Internal cold and deficiency of the spleen and stomach

Purple or dark, bloody stools or melena or hemorrhaging after defecation, dull pain in the abdomen, a sallow complexion, lassitude, no desire to speak, a pale tongue and a thready pulse characterize internal cold and deficiency of the spleen and stomach.

This condition is treated by replenishing *qi*, nourishing the blood, warming the spleen and controlling the bleeding with *Fu Lung Kan* Combination (*huang tu tang*).

Fu Lung Kan Combination*

Huang Tu Tang
(Decoction of Yellow Earth)[17]

Furnace soil**	*Terra flava usta*	*Fu long gan*	7.0
Atractylodes, white	*Atractylodis rhizoma*	*Bai zhu*	3.0
Aconite, prepared	*Aconiti carmichaelii praeparata radix*	*Zhi fu zi*	1.0
Rehmannia, cooked	*Rehmanniae radix*	*Shu di huang*	3.0
Licorice, baked	*Glycyrrhizae radix*	*Zhi gan cao*	2.0
Gelatin	*Asini gelatinum*	*A jiao*	3.0
Scute	*Scutellariae radix*	*Huang qin*	3.0

* also known as Yellow Earth Combination
**Furnace soil is first decocted with water and then the resulting liquid replaces water for the decocting of the remaining ingredients.

Functions: warms *yang*; strengthens the spleen; arrests bleeding.

Explanation: Furnace soil warms the middle energizer, strengthens the spleen, harmonizes the stomach and halts vomiting, diarrhea and bleeding. White atractylodes and prepared aconite warm *yang* and strengthen the spleen, while cooked rehmannia and gelatin moisten *yin* and nourish the blood. Baked licorice is a sweet herb which harmonizes the middle energizer, whereas bitter, cold-natured scute counteracts hot, dry-natured aconite. When spleen *yang* is deficient and results in hematochezia, the above prescription is especially appropriate.

2. Descent of heat-dampness

Hematochezia of a bright red color or bleeding before defecation, constipation, a yellow, greasy tongue coating and a soft, rapid or slippery, rapid pulse are associated with a descent of heat-dampness.

This condition is treated by clearing heat from the blood and dissolving dampness with Sophora Formula (*huai hua sen*).

Sophora Formula
Huai Hua San[24]
(Sophora Flower Powder)

Sophora	Sophorae flos	Huai hua	3.0
Biota top	Thujae orientalis folium et ramulus	Ce bo ye	3.0
Chih-ko	Citri fructus	Zhi ke	3.0
Schizonepeta, processed	Schizonepetae herba	Jing jie tan	3.0

Functions: clears the large intestine; affects hemostasis.

Explanation: Sophora clears heat-dampness from the large intestine, while biota top clears heat from the blood and stops bleeding. *Chih-ko* regulates intestinal *qi*, prevents heat-dampness stagnancy during hemostasis and halts bleeding caused by hemorrhoids, while schizonepeta expels wind and corrects blood disorders.

If the hemorrhoids are due to occupations or activities involving prolonged standing or walking over the course of many years, Cimicifuga Combination (*yi zi tang*) should be given instead.

Cimicifuga Combination[1]
Yi Zi Tang[1]
(Hemorrhoid Decoction)

Bupleurum	Bupleuri radix	Chai hu	5.0
Cimicifuga	Cimicifugae rhizoma	Sheng ma	1.5
Tang-kuei	Angelicae radix	Dang gui	6.0
Licorice	Glycyrrhizae radix	Gan cao	2.0
Scute	Scutellariae radix	Huang qin	3.0
Rhubarb	Rhei rhizoma	Da huang	1.0

Functions: clears heat; relieves hemorrhoids; promotes bowel movement.

Explanation: Bupleurum and cimicifuga promote the ascent of spleen *qi,* while *tang-kuei* stimulates blood circulation in the large intestine and aids in the recovery of a prolapsed intestine or the alleviation of hemorrhoids. *Tang-kuei* in combination with rhubarb moistens the intestine and promotes bowel movement. Licorice relieves pain and tonifies *qi.* Scute and rhubarb clear intestinal heat and stop bleeding.

Hematuria

Blood or blood clots in the urine are known as hematuria. Unlike strangury, urination for the patient afflicted with hematuria is usually not painful. This condition is commonly associated with renal tuberculosis, kidney or ureter stones, renal carcinoma or bladder carcinoma.

1. Excess heat in the lower energizer

Hot or dark yellow, bloody urine, thirst, a red tongue with a yellow coating, and a rapid pulse are characteristic of excess heat in the lower energizer.

Treatment consists of clearing heat from the blood with Cephalanoplos Combination (*xiao ji yin zi*).

Cephalanoplos Combination

Xiao Ji Yin Zi[13]
(Cephalanoplos Decoction)[2]

Rehmannia, raw	Rehmanniae radix	Sheng di huang	10.0
Field thistle	Cephalanoplos herba	Xiao ji	10.0
Talc	Talcum	Hua shi	5.0
Akebia	Akebiae caulis	Mu tong	1.5
Cattail pollen*	Typhae pollen	Pu huang	3.0
Lophatherum	Lophatheri herba	Dan zhu ye	3.0
Lotus node	Loti rhizomatis nodus	Ou jie	5.0
Tang-kuei	Angelicae radix	Dang gui	3.0
Gardenia	Gardeniae fructus	Zhi zi	3.0
Licorice	Glycyrrhizae radix	Gan cao	1.0

*also known as bulrush

Functions: removes heat from the blood; affects hemostasis.

Explanation: Raw rehmannia, field thistle, lotus node and cattail pollen remove heat from the blood and affect hemostasis. Talc, akebia, lophatherum and gardenia clear heat and treat strangury. *Tang-kuei* and licorice nourish the blood and regulate the stomach. Cephalanoplos Combination is a commonly prescribed remedy for treating hematuria and strangury complicated by hematuria.

2. Fire due to *yin* deficiency

Small amounts of dark yellow, blood-tinged urine, tinnitus, dizziness, lower back pain, weak legs, a red tongue and a thready, rapid pulse characterize fire due to *yin* deficiency.

Treatment nourishes *yin*, removes fire, clears blood heat and affects hemostasis with Anemarrhena, Phellodendron and Rehmannia Formula (*zhi bai ba wei wan*).

3. *Qi* deficiency in the middle energizer

Frequent urination with reddish blood, poor appetite, a sallow complexion, listlessness, shortness of breath, lack of energy to speak, lower back pain, a pale tongue and a weak pulse characterize *qi* deficiency in the middle energizer.

Treatment aims at strengthening the spleen and replenishing *qi* with Ginseng and Astragalus Combination (*bu zhong yi qi tang*).

Section 23
Edema

Edema is fluid accumulation in the connective tissues which appears as swelling in the face or on the eyelids, abdomen or back, or at times all over the body. If severe, it is accompanied by hydrothorax or ascites. Edema often occurs in acute or chronic nephritis, congestive heart failure, cirrhosis of the liver and dystrophy.

A common cause of edema is the invasion of wind evil and the subsequent obstruction of lung *qi*. The lungs regulate the body surface and so are linked to the skin and hair. If wind evil invades the body surface, obstruction of lung *qi* occurs and bladder functions cannot be properly regulated, resulting in edema of the muscles and skin. Specifically, spleen and kidney dysfunctions or deficiencies can cause edema.

Residing in a damp climate or exposure to rainy weather for a prolonged time can result in dampness invading the interior and subsequent damage to the spleen. Such impairment prompts transportation and transformation dysfunctioning, which allows dampness to penetrate the muscles and skin of the lower limbs, thus inducing edema.

Yang deficiency of the spleen and/or kidneys causes fluid retention, while kidney *qi* deficiency disrupts normal bladder functions so that urine cannot be properly voided, resulting in interstitial edema.

Lingering edema induced by external factors can prompt the occurrence of interior factors, such as *yang* deficiency of the spleen and kidneys. This, in turn, will further prolong the disease course. On the other hand, if the edema is induced by interior factors which obstruct lung *qi*, exterior factors invading the interior will abruptly resolve the edema.

Generally speaking, edema caused by external pathogens is considered *yang* edema, whereas *yin* edema is caused by internal injury. Clinically speaking, dampness easily impairs *yang*, causing *yang* deficiency. Furthermore, accumulated dampness may transform into *yin* deficiency or heat.

Edema caused by internal injury or external pathogens is associated with the lungs, spleen and kidneys. As regards pathogenesis, these three organs are interrelated and so influence each other. As the ancient TCM practitioner Jin-yue Zhang said: "All kinds of edema are diseases involving the lungs, spleen and kidneys in which water is transformed into *qi*. Therefore, exterior is in the lungs, but since water is controlled by the earth, it is the spleen which must bring the water under control."

Diagnosis and Herbal Treatment

The treatment of edema consists of six basic methods: (1) diaphoresis, (2) diuresis, (3) dampness removal, (4) dissipation of water retention with warm-natured herbs, (5) *qi* regulation and (6) the use of hydragogues. Depending on the patient's constitution, one method may be used alone, or two or three methods may be combined. *Yang* edema is treated by ventilating and removing the obstruction, whereas *yin* edema is treated with warming and tonifying methods. After the edema subsides, the therapeutic effect can be enhanced through the use of herbs to replenish *qi* and strengthen the spleen.

In general, all patients with edema should attempt to eliminate salt from their diets or strictly limit its use. Shellfish, raw and cold foods, and alcoholic beverages should also be avoided.

Yang Edema

Characterized by a rapid onset, *yang* edema begins in the face and spreads to the chest, abdomen and limbs. It is predominantly located above the waist. Sunken dimples appear on the skin when pressed, though these readily disappear when the pressure is relieved and the skin is quickly restored to its former state. This disease is often accompanied by some symptoms of heat-dampness.

1. Wind edema

Before the edema occurs, the patient usually has a wind-evil conformation, which is characterized by fever, an aversion to wind and cold, headache, aching pain in the extremities, cough, dyspnea, a red, swollen and sore throat, a thin, white tongue coating and a floating pulse. Generally, edema of the face is observed first, then it spreads to the entire body and difficulty in urination occurs. The illness breaks abruptly.

Wind edema is treated by ventilating the lungs and draining fluids with Atractylodes Combination (*yue bi jia zhu tang*).

Atractylodes Combination[1]
Yue Bi Jia Zhu Tang
(Maidservant from the *Yue* Decoction plus Atractylodes)[2]

Atractylodes, white	Atractylodis rhizoma	Bai zhu	4.0
Ma-huang	Ephedrae herba	Ma huang	3.0
Gypsum	Gypsum fibrosum	Shi gao	8.0
Ginger, fresh	Zingiberis rhizoma	Sheng jiang	3.0
Licorice	Glycyrrhizae radix	Gan cao	2.0
Jujube	Zizyphi fructus	Da zao	15.0

To treat a bad cough, add 2 *qian* platycodon (*jie geng*) and 3 *qian* each of peucedanum (*qian hu*) and arctium (*niu bang zi*).

If there is a red, swollen and sore throat, add 3 *qian* lonicera (*jin yin hua*), 5 *qian* dandelion (*pu gong ying*) and 1 *qian* cicada (*chan tui*).

If there is a cough with a great deal of phlegm, add 3 *qian* each of lepidium (*ting li zi*) and inula (*xuan fu hua*).

If the edema is serious, add 4 *qian* plantago (*che qian zi*) and 5 *qian* alisma (*ze xie*).

If the patient's constitution is delicate, with such symptoms as perspiration, an aversion to wind, heaviness in the limbs, lingering edema and *wei yang* deficiency, treat with Stephania and Astragalus Combination (*fang ji huang qi tang*).

Stephania and Astragalus Combination[1]

Fang Ji Huang Qi Tang

(Stephania and Astragalus Decoction)[2]

Astragalus	Astragali radix	Huang qi	5.0
Stephania	Aristolochiae fangchi radix	Fang ji	5.0
Atractylodes, white	Atractylodis rhizoma	Bai zhu	3.0
Ginger, fresh	Zingiberis rhizoma	Sheng jiang	3.0
Licorice, baked	Glycyrrhizae radix	Zhi gan cao	1.5
Jujube	Zizyphi fructus	Da zao	5.0

2. Inundation of dampness

Generalized edema occurs mainly in the abdomen and lower limbs. It is accompanied by oliguria, heaviness in the torso and limbs, lassitude, poor appetite, a feeling of oppression in the chest, nausea, a greasy tongue coating and a soft pulse. Its onset is slow and its course long.

Treatment activates *yang* and promotes diuresis with Hoelen Five Herb Formula (*wu ling san*) and Hoelen and Areca Combination (*wu pi yin*).

Hoelen Five Herb Formula[1]

Wu Ling San

(Five-ingredient Powder with Poria)[2]

Alisma	Alismatis rhizoma	Ze xie	6.0
Atractylodes, white	Atractylodis rhizoma	Bai zhu	4.5
Cinnamon twig	Cinnamomi ramulus	Gui zhi	1.5
Hoelen	Poria sclerotium	Fu ling	4.5
Polyporus	Polyporus sclerotium	Zhu ling	4.5

Hoelen and Areca Combination[1]
Wu Pi Yin
(Five Peel Decoction)[2]

Hoelen peel	*Poria cocos sclerotium*	*Fu ling pi*	3.0
Morus bark	*Mori radicis cortex*	*Sang bai pi*	3.0
Ginger peel, fresh	*Zingiberis pericarpium*	*Sheng jiang pi*	2.0
Areca peel	*Arecae pericarpium*	*Da fu pi*	3.0
Citrus peel	*Citri pericarpium*	*Chen pi*	2.0

If the edema occurs above the waist, add 2 *qian ma-huang* (*ma huang*) and 3 *qian* apricot seed (*xing ren*).

If the edema occurs below the waist, add 2 *qian* pepper (*shan jiao*), 3 *qian* stephania (*fang ji*) and 4 *qian* plantago (*che qian zi*).

If the patient has an aversion to cold, cold limbs and a submerged, slow pulse, add 2 *qian* each of prepared aconite (*zhi fu zi*) and dried ginger (*gan jiang*).

3. Accumulation of heat-dampness

Generalized edema, thin skin, a feeling of oppression in the chest, abdominal distention, fidgeting, thirst, small amounts of dark yellow urine, constipation, a greasy, yellow tongue coating and a submerged, rapid pulse are characteristic of an accumulation of heat-dampness.

This form of edema is treated by clearing heat and removing dampness with Alisma and Areca Combination (*shu zuo yin zi*).

Alisma and Areca Combination

Shu Zuo Yin Zi

(Decoction for Diuresis)[12]

Alisma	*Alismatis rhizoma*	*Ze xie*	4.0
Small red bean	*Phaseoli semen*	*Chi xiao dou*	5.0
Chiang-huo	*Notopterygii rhizoma*	*Qiang huo*	3.0
Poke root	*Phytolaccae radix*	*Shang lu*	5.0
Areca peel	*Arecae pericarpium*	*Da fu pi*	5.0
Zanthoxylum	*Zanthoxyli fructus*	*Shan jiao*	3.0
Akebia	*Akebiae caulis*	*Mu tong*	4.0
Chin-chiu	*Gentianae macrophyllae radix*	*Qin jiao*	3.0
Hoelen peel	*Poria pericarpium*	*Fu ling pi*	10.0
Ginger, fresh	*Zingiberis rhizoma*	*Sheng jiang*	3.0

Functions: clears heat; removes dampness; stimulates urination; eliminates edema.

Explanation: Alisma, small red bean, zanthoxylum and hoelen peel promote urination and so remove dampness. *Chiang-huo*, *chin-chiu* and fresh ginger expel wind, remove dampness and promote urination. Poke root removes water retention by stimulating urination. Areca peel promotes *qi* circulation to induce diuresis. This formula is recommended for edema with a short disease course which is due to either exterior or interior causes.

If excess heat is present, add 4 *qian* forsythia (*lian qiao*) and 2 *qian* lophatherum (*dan zhu ye*).

If the patient is only able to expel small quantities of urine, add 4 *qian* benincasa peel (*dong gua pi*) and 5 *qian* imperata (*bai mao gen*) to the basic formula.

If there is a severe shortness of breath, add 3 *qian* lepidium (*ting li zi*).

If the abdominal distention is not alleviated and the patient becomes constipated, 2 *qian* each of rhubarb (*da huang*) and *chih-shih* (*zhi shi*) can be added.

Yin Edema

Its onset is slow, and its course is prolonged and subject to recurring episodes. The edema begins in the legs, then moves to the abdomen, chest, upper limbs and face, though it continues to be more pronounced below the waist. Deep dimples appear when the skin is pressed, and it is difficult to restore the skin to its state before dimpling. The disease is often accompanied by symptoms of *yang* deficiency of the spleen and kidneys.

1. Spleen *yang* deficiency

The edema is most severe in the legs. There is abdominal and stomach fullness and distention. Other manifestations may include a poor appetite, loose stools, a sallow complexion, lassitude, cold limbs, decreased urination, a pale tongue with a white, slippery coating, and a slow pulse.

Treatment warms the middle energizer, strengthens the spleen and promotes *qi* to induce diuresis with Magnolia and Atractylodes Combination (*shi pi yin*).

If the edema is severe, add 3 *qian* each of cinnamon twig (*gui zhi*), polyporus (*zhu ling*) and alisma (*ze xie*).

If there are symptoms of *qi* deficiency, add 3 *qian* each of codonopsis (*dang shen*) and astragalus (*huang qi*).

2. Kidney *yang* deficiency

Generalized severe edema, especially below the waist, with pain and heaviness in the lower back is characteristic of kidney *yang* deficiency. In addition, the patient is only able to expel small quantities of urine. Cold limbs, an aversion to cold, lassitude, a gray or pale complexion, a thick, pale tongue with a white coating, and a submerged, thready pulse may also be observed.

Treatment warms the kidneys with Vitality Combination (*zhen wu tang*) to induce diuresis.

If deficiency-cold is serious with soreness and weakness in the lower back and knees, an aversion to cold and cold limbs, add 1 *qian* cinnamon bark (*gui pi*) and 3 *qian* each of fenugreek (*hu lu pa*) and morinda (*ba ji tian*).

If there is a shortness of breath, spontaneous perspiration and difficulty in lying supine, add 3 *qian* codonopsis (*dang shen*), 2 *qian* schizandra (*wu wei zi*) and 10 *qian* calcined oyster shell (*duan mu li*).

Common Acupuncture and Moxibustion Points

Yang Edema

1. Points of first choice
   - *fengchi* (G 20)
   - *hegu* (LI 4)
   - *fengmen* (B 12)
   - *shuifen* (CV 9)

2. Reserved points
   - *feishu* (B 13)
   - *taiyuan* (L 9)
   - *zhongfu* (L 1)
   - *huizong* (S 7)

Yin Edema

1. Points of first choice
   - *zusanli* (S 36)
   - *pishu* (B 20, moxibustion)
   - *shenshu* (B 23, moxibustion)
   - *mingmen* (D 4, moxibustion)

2. Reserved points
   - *zhangmen* (Liv 13)
   - *taibai* (Sp 3)
   - *taixi* (K 3)
   - *jingmen* (G 25)
   - *fenglong* (S 40)

Section 24
Strangury

The conformation of strangury is characterized by frequent, painful, scanty, interrupted urination which is expelled in drops rather than in a stream. In addition, vesical tenesmus, cramps in the lower abdomen or pain radiating out from the lower back or abdomen may also be observed.

Ancient TCM physicians classified strangury into five types:
1. *qi lin*, strangury caused by a *qi* disorder
2. *xue lin*, strangury complicated by hematuria
3. *gao lin*, strangury marked by chyluria
4. *shi lin*, strangury due to the passage of urinary stones
5. *lao lin*, strangury due to strain on the body

Descriptions of the symptoms which accompany these types are similar to those given in Western medicine for urinary calculus, chyluria, bladder tumor, prostatic hyperplasia, urinary tract infections and tuberculosis of the urinary system.

From a TCM standpoint, the principal cause of strangury is the accumulation of heat-dampness in the lower energizer. After a prolonged disease course, strangury can transform from an excess condition to one of deficiency, or become a combination of excess and deficiency.

Etiology
Accumulation of Heat-dampness

The main cause of strangury is the accumulation of heat-dampness in the lower energizer. Heat-dampness can arise from external pathogenic factors or can be induced by excess consumption of wine or greasy, spicy or sweet foods, which prompt the formation of heat-dampness in the middle energizer and its subsequent descent to the bladder. Prolonged accumulation of heat-dampness results in *shi lin*, strangury due to the passage of urinary stones. Heat-dampness burns blood collaterals, forcing the blood to circulate abnormally, thus causing *xue lin*. Accumulation of heat-dampness in the lower energizer results in disturbances in *qi* transformation. Consequently, lymphatic fluids are no longer properly regulated. The passing of chyloid urine characterizes *gao lin*.

Liver *Qi* Stagnancy

Liver *qi* disorders result in the accumulation of liver *qi* and its subsequent transformation into fire. From the liver, fire descends to the lower energizer and disrupts the normal functioning of bladder *qi*. The patient thus experiences difficulty and pain in micturition of urine which is expelled in dribbles rather than in streams. This is known as *qi lin*.

Spleen and Kidney Deficiency

Prolonged strangury, exhaustion and impairment of vital *qi* by heat-dampness, senility, weakness due to a protracted illness, fatigue, anxiety, sexual intemperance or the descent of *qi* can all lead to a deficiency of both the spleen and kidneys.

Difficulty and pain in urination owing to overwork or strain on the body is known as *lao lin*, whereas strangury due to weakness following a prolonged illness or to a deficiency and descent of *qi* in the middle energizer is a *qi lin* dysfunction in the storage of essence. This dysfunction is related to kidney deficiency and the descent of lymphatic fluids, which result in the formation of chyloid *lin*. Disturbances of *yin* and blood due to the fire of kidney *yin* deficiency may also induce *xue lin*.

Diagnosis and Herbal Treatment

Although strangury can be classified into five types, clinically, it is divided into two: excess or deficiency. The former is due to heat-dampness in the bladder and liver *qi* stagnancy. It is treated by clearing heat, dispelling dampness and regulating the flow of *qi*. Deficiency strangury is caused by a spleen and kidney deficiency. It is treated by strengthening the spleen, reinforcing the kidneys and tonifying *qi*.

Prolonged strangury causes difficulty in differentiating between deficiency and excess. Therefore, the original cause of the disease should be differentiated by the symptoms. Furthermore, acute and chronic strangury must be distinguished in order to properly treat the patient.

Qi Lin: Strangury Caused by a *Qi* Disorder

The symptoms of the excess conformation are difficulty in urination, abdominal pain, a thin, white tongue coating and a submerged, wiry pulse. If there is weakness due to a prolonged illness and a descent of *qi* of the middle energizer, distention and a bearing-down sensation in the lower abdomen may develop. Should this occur, other symptoms which may be observed include a pale complexion and tongue, and a thready, weak pulse.

Treatment regulates *qi* with Aquilaria Formula (*chen xiang san*).

Aquilaria Formula
Chen Xiang San[27]
(Aquilaria Powder)

Aquilaria	*Aquilariae lignum*	*Chen xiang*	0.3
Pyrrosia	*Pyrrosiae folium*	*Shi wei*	5.0
Talc	*Talcum*	*Hua shi*	3.0
Tang-kuei	*Angelicae radix*	*Dang gui*	3.0
Vaccaria	*Vaccariae semen*	*Wang bu liu xing*	3.0
Dianthus	*Dianthi herba*	*Qu mai*	3.0
Abutilon	*Abutili semen*	*Dong kui zi*	3.0
Peony, red	*Paeoniae rubra radix*	*Chi shao*	3.0
Atractylodes, white	*Atractylodis rhizoma*	*Bai zhu*	3.0
Licorice, baked	*Glycyrrhizae radix*	*Zhi gan cao*	2.0

Function: regulates *qi* in order to treat strangury.

Explanation: Aquilaria promotes the descent of abnormally ascending *qi* and regulates the middle energizer. Pyrrosia, talc, vaccaria, dianthus and abutilon expel urine. *Tang-kuei* and red peony promote blood circulation and abate pain, while white atractylodes strengthens the spleen and reinforces *qi*. Licorice harmonizes the actions of the other herbs.

Deficiency *qi lin*, on the other hand, is treated by tonifying the middle energizer and reinforcing *qi* with Ginseng and Astragalus Combination (*bu zhong yi qi tang*).

Xue Lin: Strangury Complicated by Hematuria

Purplish urine or urine with blood streaks or clots, difficulty in urination, a stabbing pain and a burning sensation during urination, a yellow tongue coating and a rapid, weak pulse characterize *xue lin*. If the illness is prolonged, the urine is pinkish and the patient is listless.

Excess-type *xue lin* is treated by clearing heat, dispelling dampness and affecting hemostasis with Dianthus Formula (*ba zheng san*) and Cephalanoplos Combination (*xiao ji yin zi*).

The deficiency type is treated by nourishing *yin*, clearing heat and controlling blood flow with Anemarrhena, Phellodendron and Rehmannia Formula (*zhi bo ba wei wan*).

Gao Lin: Strangury Marked by Chyluria

The excess type is marked by a red tongue with a greasy coating and burning, difficult and painful micturition of cloudy, milk-like or greasy urine.

Treatment is aimed at clearing heat, removing dampness and separating turbid and clear urine with Tokoro Combination (*bi xie fen qing yin*).

Tokoro Combination[1]

Bi Xie Fen Qing Yin
(Tokoro Decoction)

Tokoro	Dioscoreae sativa rhizoma	Bi xie	4.0
Alpinia fruit	Alpinia oxyphyllae fructus	Yi zhi ren	4.0
Acorus	Acori rhizoma	Chang pu	4.0
Lindera	Linderae radix	Wu yao	4.0

As regards deficiency-type *gao lin*, should the disease persist over a long period of time and should the patient lose weight, or should the strangury be due to fatigue, a deficiency of both the spleen and kidneys is involved. The following manifestations will be seen: greasy urine, difficult and painful urination, dizziness, weakness in the lower back and knees, lassitude and a thready, weak pulse.

The deficiency type is treated by strengthening the kidneys with Rehmannia Six Formula (*liu wei di huang wan*), to which is added 3 *qian* cherokee rose (*jin yin zi*) and 5 *qian* each of dragon bone (*long gu*) and oyster shell (*mu li*).

Should *qi* deficiency occur in the middle energizer, use Ginseng and Astragalus Combination (*bu zhong yi qi tang*) instead.

Shi Lin: Strangury Due to the Passage of Urinary Stones

Gritty substances in the urine; difficulty, discontinuity or pain in micturition; a cramping sensation in the lower abdomen with pain radiating to the umbilicus or pain in the lower back and abdomen; hematuria; a normal tongue with a thin, white or greasy, yellow coating; and a wiry, tense pulse characterize *shi lin*.

This type of strangury is treated by clearing heat, dispelling dampness and removing urinary calculus with Dianthus Formula (*ba zheng san*) and Gardenia and Hoelen Formula (*wu lin san*).

Lao Lin: Strangury Due to Strain on the Body

Dribbling urination, lassitude in the lower back and knees, listlessness, general weakness which is exacerbated by fatigue, a prolonged disease course and a feeble pulse characterize *lao lin.*

Treatment seeks to tonify the kidneys and reinforce the spleen with Ginseng and Astragalus Combination (*bu zhong yi qi tang*) and Rehmannia Eight Formula (*ba wei di huang wan*).

If kidney *yin* is deficient, Anemarrhena, Phellodendron and Rehmannia Formula (*zhi bo ba wei wan*) can be used.

Common Acupuncture and Moxibustion Points

Basic Points for All Types of Strangury

- *zhongji* (CV 3)
- *pangguangshu* (B 28)
- *yinlingquan* (Sp 9)
- *sanyinjiao* (Sp 6)

Additional Point for *Qi Lin*

- *xingjian* (Liv 2)

Additional Points for *Xue Lin*

- *xuehai* (Sp 10)
- *pishu* (B 20)

Additional Points for *Gao Lin*

- *shenshu* (B 23)
- *zhaohai* (K 6)

Additional Points for *Shi Lin*

- *weiyang* (B 39)
- *zhaohai* (K 6)

Additional Points for *Lao Lin*

- *zusanli* (S 36)
- *guanyuan* (CV 4)
- *baihui* (GV 20)

Section 25
Uroschesis

Uroschesis is the retention or suppression of urine with symptoms such as difficulty in urination and obstruction of the urinary passage. According to Western medicine, it can be categorized into bradyuria, oliguria, dysuria and anuria.

A TCM understanding of uroschesis associates its onset with disturbances to *qi* transformation in the urinary bladder, since the functional activity of bladder *qi* is closely connected to that of the triple energizer, especially the lower energizer. Specifically, there are four reasons for such a *qi* imbalance:

1. An obstruction of lung *qi* in the upper energizer, which is due to an accumulation of lung heat, prevents the normal regulation of water.

2. A spleen *yang* and/or spleen *qi* deficiency results in the failure of the middle energizer to affect the descent of turbid *yin*.

3. Heat-dampness accumulation and kidney *yang* deficiency result in the body's inability to promote water circulation in the lower energizer and so induce diuresis.

4. An obstruction in the urethra or trauma may also cause uroschesis.

Diagnosis and Herbal Treatment

The manifestations of the disease are primarily slow, dribbling micturition or an inability to void. Onset can be sudden or gradual. Though uroschesis and strangury are, in some ways, symptomatically similar, the former involves the voiding of abnormally small amounts of urine or none at all, while the latter involves the voiding of normal amounts of urine.

The herbal treatments discussed below can be combined with acupuncture, moxibustion and massage. The following formulas are used to correct a retention of urine, but are ineffective against true anuria.

Accumulation of Heat-dampness

Anuria or the micturition of only small quantities of dark urine, accompanied by a burning sensation; distention and fullness in the lower abdomen; a dry, sticky mouth; constipation; a red tongue with a greasy, yellow coating; and a submerged, rapid pulse characterize an accumulation of heat-dampness.

The condition is treated by eliminating dampness, clearing heat and inducing diuresis with Dianthus Formula (*ba zheng san*).

If the patient has a thick, yellow tongue coating, add 3 *qian* each of atractylodes (*cang zhu*) and phellodendron (*huang bo*).

If the patient is restless, suffers from insomnia or has an ulcer on the tongue or elsewhere in the mouth, use Rehmannia and Akebia Formula (*dao chi san*) instead.

Obstruction of Lung *Qi*

Difficulty in urination or anuria, a dry throat, extreme thirst, shortness of breath or a cough, a thin, yellow tongue coating and a rapid pulse characterize an obstruction of lung *qi*.

Treatment consists in clearing lung heat and facilitating the passage of water with Platycodon and Fritillaria Combination (*qing fei tang*).

If the patient has a red tongue tip, add 1 *qian* coptis (*huang lian*) and 3 *qian* lophatherum (*dan zhu ye*).

If the patient has a red tongue, lung *yin* deficiency and an absence of saliva, add 3 *qian* each of glehnia (*bei sha shen*) and lily (*bai he*).

Should the patient be constipated, add 1 *qian* rhubarb (*da huang*) and 3 *qian* apricot seed (*xing ren*) in order to ventilate the lungs and stimulate bowel movement.

Descent of Middle Energizer *Qi*

A bearing-down sensation, distention of the lower abdomen, vesicle tenesmus, listlessness, a poor appetite, shortness of breath with a low, feeble voice, a pale tongue with a thin coating, and a submerged, weak pulse are common manifestations of a descent of middle energizer *qi.*

Treatment attempts to affect the ascent of *qi* and the concurrent descent of turbid water with Ginseng and Astragalus Combination (*bu zhong yi qi tang*), to which is added 0.5 *qian* cinnamon bark (*gui pi*), 1 *qian* tetrapanax (*tong cao*) and 3 *qian* plantago (*che qian zi*).

Liver *Qi* Stagnancy

Melancholia, restlessness, irritability, an obstruction to the passage of urine or bradyuria, fullness in the hypochondrium and abdomen, a thin, yellow tongue coating or a red tongue, and a wiry pulse are common manifestations of liver *qi* stagnancy.

This condition is treated by promoting the functional activities of *qi* to affect diuresis with Bupleurum and Peony Formula (*jia wei xiao yao san*), to which is added 1 *qian* aquilaria (*chen xiang*) and 3 *qian* each of citrus peel (*chen pi*), pyrrosia leaf (*shi wei*), abutilon (*dong kui zi*), talc (*hua shi*), cyperus (*xiang fu zi*) and lindera (*wu yao*).

Kidney *Qi* Deficiency

An obstruction to the passage of urine, dribbling urination or the absence of urine; a pale complexion; lassitude; cold, aching, weak lower back and knees; a pale tongue; a submerged, thready pulse; and a weak cubit pulse can be observed in a patient suffering from kidney *yin* deficiency.

The conformation is treated by warming *yang*, reinforcing *qi*, tonifying the kidneys and promoting diuresis with Achyranthes and Plantago Formula (*niu che shen qi wan*).

If the patient is senile and primordial *qi* is seriously deficient, add 2 *qian* red ginseng (*hong shen*) and 3 *qian* each of antler (*lu jiao*), curculigo (*xian mao*) and epimedium (*yin yang huo*).

If kidney *qi* deficiency is accompanied by exterior cold, use *Ma-huang* and Asarum Combination (*ma huang fu zi xi xin tang*) instead of Achyranthes and Plantago Formula. Supplement the former with 3 *qian* each of achyranthes (*niu xi*) and plantago (*che qian zi*).

Achyranthes and Plantago Formula[1]
Niu Che Shen Qi Wan
(Tonify Kidney *Qi* with Achyranthes and Plantago Pill)

Rehmannia, cooked	*Rehmanniae radix*	Shu di huang	3.0
Dioscorea	*Dioscorea batatis rhizoma*	Shan yao	3.0
Cornus	*Corni fructus*	Shan zhu yu	3.0
Hoelen	*Poria sclerotium*	Fu ling	3.0
Moutan	*Moutan radicis cortex*	Mu dan pi	3.0
Alisma	*Alismatis rhizoma*	Ze xie	3.0
Achyranthes	*Achyranthis radix*	Niu xi	3.0
Plantago	*Plantaginis semen*	Che qian zi	3.0
Aconite, prepared	*Aconiti carmichaelii praeparata radix*	Zhi fu zi	0.5
Cinnamon twig	*Cinnamomi ramulus*	Gui zhi	1.0

Ma-huang and Asarum Combination[1]

Ma Huang Fu Zi Xi Xin Tang

(Ephedra, Asarum and Prepared Aconite Decoction)[2]

Ma-huang	Ephedrae herba	Ma huang	3.0
Aconite, prepared	Aconiti carmichaelii praeparata radix	Zhi fu zi	1.0
Asarum	Asari herba cum radice	Xi xin	1.0

Obstruction of the Urethra

The passing of urine is at times impossible or is but a mere dribbling. Other manifestations are fullness and pain in the lower abdomen, a dark purple tongue or a tongue with petechiae, and a hesitant or thready and rapid pulse.

Removal of blood stasis, dissolution of the obstruction and the clearing of the urinary tract is affected with Persica and Rhubarb Combination (tao he cheng qi tang).

If the patient's illness is prolonged, or should blood deficiency and a pale complexion develop, add 5 qian salvia (dan shen) and 3 qian astragalus (huang qi).

If the obstruction is only temporary, but distention and the "closure sensation" are accompanied by unbearable pain, add 0.02 qian musk (she xiang).

If the patient develops stones in the urinary tract, add 10 qian desmodium (jin qian cao) and 5 qian each of lygodium (hai jin sha) and abutilon (dong kui zi).

Common Acupuncture and Moxibustion Points

Basic Points for the Treatment of Uroschesis

- zhongji (CV 3) or qugu (CV 2)*
- lieque (L 7)
- baihuanshu (B 30)

* Great care should be taken when employing these two points in order to avoid puncturing of the urinary bladder.

Additional Points for Heat-dampness

- *pangguangshu* (B 28) • *sanyinjiao* (Sp 6)

Additional Points for Kidney Deficiency

- *mingmen* (GV 4) • *shenshu* (B 23)
- *yangchi* (TE 4)

Additional Points for the Descent of *Qi*

- *sanyinjiao* (Sp 6) • *shuidao* (S 28)
- *shuiquan* (K 5)

Section 26
Enuresis

Enuresis, or involuntary urination, is caused by spleen *qi* deficiency, *qi* deficiency of the middle energizer or kidney *qi* deficiency, any of which result in an inability to adequately control the kidneys and urinary bladder. The condition may be either complete or partial, diurnal or nocturnal and due to pathological or functional causes. Enuresis is often found in children or in the aged or weak.

Diagnosis and Herbal Treatment

Differentiation is made according to two patient types, namely, children or the aged or infirm.

Enuresis in Children

A pallid complexion, lucid and profuse urine, a thin tongue coating and a submerged, thready and weak pulse characterize enuresis in children.

Treatment replenishes *qi* and tonifies and warms kidney *yang* to halt enuresis. The recommended treatment is

Astragalus, Ginseng and Cinnamon Combination (*bao yuan tang*), plus 4 *qian* dragon bone (*long gu*) and 3 *qian* each of alpinia fruit (*yi zhi ren*), dioscorea (*shan yao*), cuscuta (*tu si zi*), cherokee rose (*jin ying zi*) and mantis (*sang piao xiao*).

Astragalus, Ginseng and Cinnamon Combination
Bao Yuan Tang
(Preserve the Basal Decoction)[2]

Ginseng	Ginseng radix	Ren shen	2.0
Astragalus	Astragali radix	Huang qi	3.0
Licorice	Glycyrrhizae radix	Gan cao	1.0
Cinnamon bark	Cinnamomi cortex	Gui pi	0.5

Urinary Incontinence in the Aged or Infirm

Pallor, soreness and weakness in the lower back and knees, cold limbs and a thready pulse generally accompany urinary incontinence in the aged or infirm. This type of enuresis is due to damage to a urinary bladder wracked by kidney *yang* deficiency.

Treatment tonifies and warms kidney *yang* with Rehmannia Eight Formula (*ba wei di huang wan*), plus 3 *qian* each of cuscuta (*tu si zi*) and rubus (*fu pen zi*).

If there are symptoms of *qi* deficiency, add 3 *qian* codonopsis (*dang shen*) and 1 *qian* baked licorice (*zhi gan cao*).

If there is *yin* deficiency, accompanied by heat, dark yellow urine, a feverish sensation in the palms and soles, and a thready and rapid pulse, Rehmannia and Schizandra Formula (*qi wei du qi wan*) can be given.

In the case of kidney deficiency with heat-dampness and frequent micturition of small amounts of yellow urine or dribbling urination, administer Anemarrhena, Phellodendron and

Rehmannia Formula (*zhi bo ba wei wan*) instead of Rehmannia and Schizandra Formula.

If *qi* in the middle energizer descends due to *qi* deficiency of the spleen and stomach and if this condition is accompanied by a poor appetite, loose stools, shortness of breath and listlessness, use Ginseng and Astragalus Combination (*bu zhong yi qi tang*) instead of Rehmannia and Schizandra Formula.

Acupuncture and Moxibustion Treatment

Points of First Choice

- *baihui* (GV 20)
- *shuigou* (GV 26)
- the *ye niao* point (located on the middle of the palm-side transverse crease of the second joint of the little finger)

Reserved Points

- *guanyuan* (CV 4)
- *zhongji* (CV 3)
- *sanyinjiao* (Sp 6)
- *zusanli* (S 36)
- *shenshu* (B 23)
- *huiyin* (CV 1)

Treatment Method

1. Use the points of first choice every other day for a total of 10 treatments.
2. If kidney *qi* deficiency is serious, add two or three of the reserved points.

Section 27
Xiao Ke

According to a TCM understanding, *xiao ke* can be translated as "wasting-away and thirst," though the term signifies both the syndrome and the disease. The former is characterized by severe and incessant thirst and the latter by polydipsia, polyphagia, polyuria and emaciation. The discussion which follows includes diabetes mellitus, diabetes insipidus and other similar syndromes of Western medicine.

The earliest record of *xiao ke* is found in *Nei Jing* (Internal Classic). Given the descriptions of the principal symptoms outlined in this ancient text, the disease was subsequently classified into upper, middle and lower *xiao*. TCM physicians continue to use these terms.

Diabetes may be induced by excessive consumption of alcohol or fatty, sweet, pungent or fried foods. The excess fat transforms into interior heat, accumulates and impairs *yin* fluid, and thereby prevents food essence from nourishing the muscles, skin, lungs and stomach. The onset of this form of *xiao ke* is slow.

Emotional disorders or prolonged anxiety may cause *qi* to stagnate and transform into fire, thereby impairing body fluids and causing *xiao ke*.

Sexual excess can impair *jing* in men and result in urinary infections in women, which, in turn, damage the kidneys. Excessive intake of hot herbs to tonify *yang* can consume and impair kidney *yin*. When *yin* essence becomes exhausted, *yang* cannot be curbed and *xiao ke* will develop.

Pathological changes resulting from *xiao ke* are primarily to the lungs, stomach and kidneys, and are exacerbated by *yin* deficiency and heat-dryness. *Yin* deficiency is the initial cause of the disease, and heat-dryness is a symptom, though both are interrelated. The more serious the heat-dryness, the more severely impaired is *yin* fluid, and this impairment prompts the formation of more heat-dryness.

Aside from herbal or drug therapy, it is also very important for the diabetic patient to restrict his or her diet to vegetables, fruits, lean meats, complex carbohydrates and other foods low in fat, salt and refined sugar. Food intake should be moderate and at regular intervals. Stress reduction is encouraged, and adequate rest, sleep and exercise are necessary to maintain good control.

Diagnosis and Herbal Treatment

Upper *Xiao*

Thirst, polydipsia, a dry mouth and tongue, polyuria, a red edge to the tongue, a red tongue tip, a thin, yellow tongue coating and a rapid pulse characterize upper *xiao*.

The condition is treated by removing heat, moistening the lungs and promoting the production of body fluids to quench thirst. Rehmannia and Trichosanthes Formula (*xiao ke fang*), less the honey, is recommended.

Rehmannia and Trichosanthes Formula*

Xiao Ke Fang[24]

(Proved Decoction for *Xiao Ke*)

Rehmannia, raw	*Rehmanniae radix*	*Sheng di huang*	5.0
Trichosanthes root	*Trichosanthis radix*	*Gua lou gen*	5.0
Coptis	*Coptidis rhizoma*	*Huang lian*	2.0
Lotus root juice	*Loti rhizoma*	*Ou zhi*	10.0
Honey	*Mel*	*Feng mi*	5.0

* Following decoction, some milk is added before administration.

Middle *Xiao*

This condition is characterized by polyphagia, polyuria, constipation, a dry, red, fissured tongue with a thin coating, and a slippery and rapid or thready and rapid pulse. In addition, the patient is often hungry, and though he or she may ingest a great deal of food, it cannot be properly metabolized and so the patient will gradually waste away.

Middle *xiao* is treated by clearing the stomach, purging fire, nourishing *yin* and tonifying body fluids with Rehmannia and Gypsum Combination (*yu nu jian*) and 10 *qian* jellywort (*xian cao*), also known as (*lian fen cao*).

Lower *Xiao*

This type of *xiao ke* is characterized by frequent and profuse urination; a dry mouth; polydipsia; fidgeting; a hot sensation in the chest, palms and soles; lower back pain; weak knees; dizziness; acratia; a red, dry tongue; and a thready, rapid pulse.

The condition is treated by nourishing *yin*, tonifying the kidneys and promoting the production of body fluids in order to remove heat. Rehmannia Six Formula (*liu wei di huang wan*) is recommended.

If there is an aversion to cold and a thready, weak pulse, indicating a kidney *yang* deficiency, use Rehmannia Eight Formula (*ba wei di huang wan*).

Complications Associated with *Xiao Ke*

Hearing loss and vision impairment are caused by a *yin* deficiency of the liver and kidneys, and are treated with Lycium, Chrysanthemum and Rehmannia Formula (*qi ju di huang wan*).

Furuncles, carbuncles and cellulitis are treated by expelling toxins, clearing heat and detoxifying with Angelica and Frankincense Combination (*xian fang huo ming yin*).

Angelica and Frankincense Combination[1]
Xian Fang Huo Ming Yin
(Sublime Formula for Sustaining Life)[2]

Pangolin scale	*Manitis squama*	*Chuan shan jia*	3.0
Trichosanthes root	*Trichosanthis radix*	*Gua lou gen*	3.0
Licorice	*Glycyrrhizae radix*	*Gan cao*	2.0
Frankincense	*Olibanum*	*Ru xiang*	3.0
Angelica	*Angelicae dahuricae radix*	*Bai zhi*	3.0
Peony, red	*Paeoniae rubra radix*	*Chi shao*	3.0
Fritillaria	*Fritillariae bulbus*	*Bei mu*	3.0
Siler	*Ledebouriellae bulbus*	*Fang feng*	3.0
Myrrh	*Myrrha*	*Mo yao*	3.0
Gleditsia spine	*Gleditsiae spina*	*Zao ci*	3.0
Tang-kuei	*Angelicae radix*	*Dang gui*	3.0
Citrus peel	*Citri pericarpium*	*Chen pi*	4.0
Lonicera	*Lonicerae flos*	*Jin yin hua*	5.0

Common Acupuncture and Moxibustion Points

Upper *Xiao*
- *chize* (L 5)
- *lianquan* (CV 23)
- *yuji* (L 10)
- *hegu* (LI 4)

Middle *Xiao*
- *pishu* (B 20)
- *zusanli* (S 36)
- *shangwan* (CV 13)
- *neiting* (S 44)

Lower *Xiao*
- *sanjiaoshu* (B 22)
- *taiyuan* (L 9)
- *guanyuan* (CV 4)
- *sanyinjiao* (Sp 6)

Section 28
Lumbago (Lower Back Pain)

Lumbago is a subjective manifestation of rheumatic arthritis, rheumatoid arthritis, lumbar muscle strain, lumbo-vertebral hypertrophy, nephrapostasis, nephritis, pyelonephritis, nephroptosis and trauma.

Lumbago may also be induced by living in a cold, damp environment or prolonged standing in water or exposure to the rain. Other possible causes include strain on the back due to lifting heavy objects, strenuous exercise or poor posture; an obstruction of the meridians; or an impairment of the circulation of blood and *qi* due to cold-dampness. Obstruction of the meridians due to heat-dampness pathogens, impairment of the meridians, *qi* or blood due to traumatic injuries, or the impairment of *qi* or blood flow due to an internal injury or prolonged illness can also result in lower back pain. Furthermore, obstruction of the meridians and collaterals as a result of *qi* stagnancy or blood stasis can also bring on lumbago.

Other causative factors include fatigue, overwork, age-related weakness, feebleness due to prolonged illness or emotional stress. All can cause a deficiency of kidney essence, which then can no longer properly nourish the meridians, thus inducing lumbago.

Treatment is determined according to whether the patient's conformation is one of excess or deficiency. The former is caused by cold-dampness, heat-dampness or blood stasis, whereas the latter is induced by kidney deficiency.

Diagnosis and Herbal Treatment

Cold-dampness

A cold, painful, heavy sensation in the lumbar region which is aggravated during rainy or cloudy weather, difficulty in turning over when lying supine and a white, greasy tongue coating characterize lumbago due to cold-dampness.

This type of lumbago is treated by dispelling cold, removing dampness, warming the meridians and opening the collaterals with Licorice and Ginger Combination (*gan cao gan jiang tang*) and Atractylodes and Hoelen Combination (*ling gui zhu gan tang*).

Licorice and Ginger Combination[1]

Gan Cao Gan Jiang Tang
(Licorice and Ginger Decoction)[2]

Licorice	*Glycyrrhizae radix*	Gan cao	4.0
Ginger, dried	*Zingiberis siccatum rhizoma*	Gan jiang	2.0

Heat-dampness

Lumbar pain with a distending, bearing-down and burning sensation; small amounts of dark urine; a yellow, greasy tongue coating; and a floating, soft and rapid pulse characterize lumbago due to heat-dampness.

Treatment consists in clearing heat and draining dampness with Phellodendron and Achyranthes Formula (*san miao wan*), plus 3 *qian* each of stephania (*fang ji*), tokoro (*bi jie*) and *tang-kuei* (*dang gui*).

Phellodendron and Achyranthes Formula
San Miao Wan[26]
(Three-marvel Pill)[2]

Phellodendron	*Phellodendri cortex*	*Huang bo*	120.0
Atractylodes	*Atractylodis lanceae rhizoma*	*Cang zhu*	180.0
Achyranthes	*Achyranthis radix*	*Niu xi*	60.0

The ingredients are ground into a powder and mixed with water to make 2-*qian* pills. One pill is taken twice daily.

Functions: clears heat; dries dampness.

Explanation: Bitter, cold-natured phellodendron clears heat and dries dampness, and bitter, warm-natured atractylodes also resolves dampness. Achyranthes guides the other two herbs downwards, while strengthening the lower back and knees and treating lumbago and numbness in the legs due to the descent of heat-dampness.

Kidney Deficiency

An aching lower back; lassitude; weakness in the legs, especially in the knees; cramps in the lower abdomen; a pale complexion; cold limbs; a pale tongue; and a submerged, thready pulse are characteristic of kidney *yang* deficiency; while restlessness, insomnia, a dry mouth and throat, a flushed complexion, dysphoria, a feverish sensation in chest, palms and soles, a red tongue and a thready, rapid pulse are typical signs and symptoms of kidney *yin* deficiency.

Treatment attempts to tonify the kidneys and strengthen the lower back. Eucommia and Rehmannia Formula (*you gui wan*) may be used to warm the kidneys and so treat kidney *yang* deficiency. Both Achyranthes and Rehmannia Formula (*zuo gui wan*) and Tang-kuei and Rehmannia Combination (*bu yin tang*) are recommended for nourishing *yin* and so treating kidney *yin* deficiency.

Tang-kuei and Rehmannia Combination[1]

Bu Yin Tang

(Nourish *Yin* Decoction)

Ginseng	Ginseng radix	Ren shen	2.0
Peony	Paeoniae radix	Shao yao	2.0
Rehmannia, cooked	Rehmanniae radix	Shu di huang	2.0
Citrus peel	Citri pericarpium	Chen pi	2.0
Achyranthes	Achyranthis radix	Niu xi	2.0
Psoralea	Psoraleae semen	Bu gu zhi	2.0
Eucommia	Eucommiae cortex	Du zhong	2.0
Tang-kuei	Angelicae radix	Dang gui	3.0
Hoelen	Poria sclerotium	Fu ling	3.0
Fennel	Foeniculi fructus	Xiao hui xiang	1.0
Anemarrhena	Anemarrhenae rhizoma	Zhi mu	1.0
Phellodendron	Phellodendri cortex	Huang bo	1.0
Licorice	Glycyrrhizae radix	Gan cao	1.0
Rehmannia, raw	Rehmanniae radix	Sheng di huang	2.0

Blood Stasis

Fixed, stabbing pain in the lower back which is aggravated by pressure, a dark purple tongue with achymosis, and a hesitant or wiry pulse characterize blood stasis.

Lumbago due to blood stasis is treated by promoting blood circulation to remove stasis, regulating *qi* circulation and alleviating pain with *Tang-kuei* and Persica Combination (*fu yuan huo xue tang*).

Acupuncture and Moxibustion Treatment

Points of First Choice

- *shenshu* (B 23)
- *qihaishu* (B 24)
- *weizhong* (B 40)

Reserved Points

- *yaoyangguan* (GV 3)
- *mingmen* (GV 4)
- *huantiao* (G 30)
- *yinmen* (B 37)
- *kunlun* (B 60)

Treatment Method

1. Cold-dampness conformation
   - warm needle
   - reinforcing method
   - moxibustion

2. Heat-dampness conformation
   - purging or cupping method

Section 29
Emission

There are two types of emission: nocturnal emission, which occurs during a dream; and spermatorrhea, which occurs when awake. If a sexually inactive man experiences emission two to three times a month without any other symptoms, this is considered normal; however, if the emission occurs as often as twice a week or if it is accompanied by dizziness, acratia, lower back pain, weakness in the legs and listlessness, the cause may be pathological and associated with prostatosis, neurosis or other chronic diseases.

According to TCM, the pathology of involuntary emission lies in the dysfunctioning of the kidneys, which cannot adequately store sperm, the reproductive essence. Specifically, emission is induced by fire due to *yin* deficiency, weakness of kidney *qi* or the descent of heat-dampness.

Deficiency-conformation emission which is not associated with a heat condition is caused by kidney deficiency and is treated by tonifying the kidneys. Deficiency-conformation emission which is heat-related is due to the excess fire associated with *yin* deficiency. This latter type is generally nocturnal and is treated by nourishing *yin* and removing fire. In the case of heat-dampness impairing the lower energizer, emission is treated by clearing heat and dissipating dampness.

Diagnosis and Herbal Treatment

In addition to the herbal treatments discussed below, the patient should also relax, as well as participate in some form of physical and mental training, such as *tai ji* boxing or *qi gong*. Furthermore, the patient should wash his legs with cold water before going to bed and sleep in a lateral recumbent position.

Kidney *Qi* Deficiency

Frequent nocturnal emission, as well as spermatorrhea, hyperaphrodisia, dizziness, tinnitus, weakness in the lower back and legs, a pale complexion, a pale tongue with a thin, white coating, and a submerged, weak pulse are characteristic of weak kidney *qi.*

This condition is treated by tonifying the kidneys and so controlling nocturnal emission with Lotus Stamen Formula (*jin suo gu jing wan*) or Hoelen and Cuscuta Formula (*fu tu dan*).

Hoelen and Cuscuta Formula[1]
Fu Tu Dan
(Poria and Cuscuta Special Pill)[2]

Cuscuta	Cuscutae semen	Tu si zi	4.0
Schizandra	Schizandrae fructus	Wu wei zi	2.0
Hoelen	Poria sclerotium	Fu ling	3.0
Lotus fruit	Nelumbinis fructus	Shi lian zi	3.0
Dioscorea	Dioscorea batatis rhizoma	Shan yao	4.0

The above ingredients are decocted, dried and made into 2-qian pills, one of which is taken t.i.d.

Fire Due to Yin Deficiency

Insomnia, drowsiness, hyperaphrodisia, frequent emission, dizziness, palpitation, listlessness, acratia, small quantities of dark urine, a red tongue and a thready, rapid pulse are associated with fire due to yin deficiency.

This constellation of symptoms is treated by nourishing yin, removing fire, tranquilizing shen (spirit) and thus controlling emission with Anemarrhena, Phellodendron and Rehmannia Formula (zhi bai ba wei wan).

If the patient is restless and has a red tongue tip, add 1 qian coptis (huang lian) and 3 qian gardenia (zhi zi).

If the patient is irritable and has a wiry, rapid pulse and conjunctival congestion, add 2 qian gentian (long dan cao) and 3 qian hoelen (fu ling).

If there is also a dry tongue, very little saliva and constipation, add 5 qian imperata (bai mao gen) and 3 qian each of scrophularia (xuan shen) and linum (ma zi ren) to the prescription given in the preceding paragraph. Mantis Formula (sang piao xiao san) may also be used to treat this particular constellation of symptoms.

Descent of Heat-dampness

Frequent emission, a bitter taste in the mouth, thirst, small amounts of dark urine, a thin, yellow and greasy tongue coating and a floating, soft and rapid pulse signal a descent of heat-dampness.

This condition is treated by clearing heat and dissolving dampness with Gentian Combination (*long dan xie gan tang*).

Acupuncture and Moxibustion Treatment

Nocturnal Emission

1. Points of first choice

   a. with acupuncture or moxibustion
   - *baihui* (GV 20)
   - *xinshu* (B 15)
   - *shenshu* (B 23)

   b. with acupuncture or moxibustion
   - *shuigou* (GV 26)
   - *shenmen* (H 7)
   - *guanyuan* (CV 4)

2. Reserved points
   - *qihaishu* (B 24)
   - *qihai* (CV 6)
   - *zhongji* (CV 3)
   - *sanyinjiao* (Sp 6)
   - *taixi* (K 3)
   - *zhaohai* (K 6)

Spermatorrhea

1. Points of first choice

   a. with acupuncture or moxibustion
   - *shenshu* (B 23)
   - *mingmen* (GV 4)
   - *taixi* (K 3)

   b. with acupuncture or moxibustion
   - *guanyuan* (CV 4)
   - *zhongji* (CV 3)
   - *sanyinjiao* (Sp 6)

2 Reserved points

- *qihaishu* (B 24)
- *henggu* (K 11)
- *fuliu* (K 7)
- *qugu* (CV 2)
- *dahe* (K 12)

Treatment Method

1 Employ the points from the a or b group on alternate days for a total of 10 days.

2 If the desired affect is not achieved, add the reserved points.

Section 30
Impotence

A weak erection or the failure to achieve an erection is known as sexual impotence. Impotence is sometimes due to physiological factors, such as excessive sex or frequent masturbation, both of which lead to a deficiency of kidney essence and a subsiding of fire from the gate of life. Fear, anxiety or the descent of heat-dampness can also impair heart and kidney functioning and so cause impotence.

If the impotence is caused by a deficiency of kidney essence and the decline of fire from the gate of life, the symptoms are manifested by a pale complexion, dizziness, listlessness, weakness in the lower back and legs, a pale tongue and a submerged, thready pulse.

This type of impotence is treated by tonifying the kidneys and strengthening *yang* with Eucommia and Rehmannia Formula (*you gui wan*).

If the impotence is caused by worry, anxiety or fear, heart and kidney functioning is impaired, and the symptoms are palpitation, susceptibility to fear, restlessness, dizziness, lower back pain and a thready, rapid pulse.

Fear- or anxiety-induced impotence is treated by reinforcing the kidneys, nourishing the heart and tranquilizing *shen* with Ginseng and Zizyphus Formula (*tian wang bu xin dan*) and Rehmannia Six Formula (*liu wei di huang wan*).

Impotence caused by the descent of heat-dampness is treated according to the patient's condition with herbs that reinforce the kidneys and tonify *yang*. Those commonly used to achieve these ends are:

deer horn (*lu rong*)	antler (*lu jiao*)
cistanche (*rou cong rong*)	curculigo (*xian mao*)
epimedium (*yin yang huo*)	cynomorium (*suo yang*)
morinda (*ba ji tian*)	fenugreek (*hu lu ba*)
cuscuta (*tu si zi*)	

Deer horn reinforces the vital functions of the kidneys and strengthens the bones and muscles for the treatment of the intolerance of cold, loss of strength, impotence, spontaneous seminal emission, leukorrhea in women and other symptoms due to deficiency of vital functions found in chronic diseases.

Antler is used for many of the same purposes as is deer horn, however, the former is not quite so effective. Furthermore, antler is used to remove blood stasis for the treatment of traumatic wounds and mastitis in women.

Cistanche reinforces the vital functions of the kidneys for the treatment of impotence and premature ejaculation. It is also effective as a mild laxative for chronic constipation in the elderly.

Curculigo warms the kidneys and strengthens the vital functions of the sex organs for the treatment of aching back and knees, intolerance of cold, impotence, urorrhea and climacteric hypertension.

Epimedium treats sexual neurasthenia.

Cynomorium reinforces the vital functions of the kidneys for the treatment of impotence and seminal emission.

Morinda reinforces the vital functions of the kidneys for the treatment of impotence and premature ejaculation in men and infertility in women.

Fenugreek warms the kidneys to disperse cold and relieve pain for the treatment of cold pain in the testes or abdominal pain due to gastrointestinal spasms.

Cuscuta replenishes the liver and kidneys, improves eyesight, corrects nocturnal emission, urorrhea and vertigo, and prevents miscarriages and threatened abortions.

Acupuncture and Moxibustion Treatment

Points of First Choice

1. Group #1

- *bai hui* (GV 20)
- *guanyuan* (CV 4)
- *sanyinjiao* (Sp 6)

2. Group #2

- *naohu* (GV 17)
- *ciliao* (B 32)
- *mingmen* (GV 4)

Reserved Points

- *shenmen* (H 7)
- *xinshu* (B 15)
- *pishu* (B 20)
- *shenshu* (B 23)
- *zhongji* (CV 3)
- *taibai* (Sp 3)
- *taixi* (K 3)

Treatment Method

1. The points from Group #1 and #2 are employed on alternate days for a total treatment course of 10 days.

2. To increase effectiveness, add two of the reserved points during each treatment session.

Section 31
Melancholia

Melancholia is severe, prolonged depression due to *qi* stagnancy. In Western medicine, neurosis and hysteria fall under the broad classification of melancholia.

Pathologically speaking, melancholia is induced by emotional disorders, dysfunctions of the liver or malfunctions of *qi*, all of which can induce liver *qi* stagnancy. General signs and symptoms are depression, chest fullness, frequent sighing, disturbances of the visceral functions and disharmony of the liver, which give rise to distention and pain in the hypochondrium.

If phlegm and *qi* accumulate in the throat, the patient will have a feeling of an obstruction in the throat which can neither be expectorated nor swallowed, known as plum pit *qi*, or globus hystericus in Western medicine.

If *qi* is stagnant, chest fullness occurs with great frequency. If liver *qi* becomes stagnant, causing liver *qi* to invade the stomach, stomach functioning will become impaired and stomach *qi* will descend, thus causing eructation and loss of appetite. If liver *qi* invades the spleen, disharmony between the liver and spleen occurs and abdominal pain and diarrhea will result. If the melancholia is not relieved, heart *qi* will become injured, leading to mental derangement, especially characterized by uncontrolled weeping and suicidal tendencies.

Diagnosis and Herbal Treatment
Liver *Qi* Stagnancy

Melancholy, chest fullness, pain in the hypochondrium, abdominal distention, eructation, loss of appetite, a thin, white tongue coating and a wiry pulse are characteristic of stagnant liver *qi*.

The condition is treated by dispersing liver *qi* with Bupleurum and Cyperus Combination (*chai hu shu gan tang*).

If the patient is troubled by indigestion, add 3 *qian* each of *shen-chu* (*shen qu*) and chicken gizzard lining (*ji nei jin*).

If pain develops in the hypochondrium, add 3 *qian* each of *tang-kuei* (*dang gui*) and salvia (*dan shen*).

If there is eructation and fullness in the chest, add 3 *qian* each of inula (*xuan fu hua*), hematite (*dai zhe shi*), citrus peel (*chen pi*) and tribulus (*ji li*).

If stagnant *qi* transforms into fire, add 2 *qian* gentian (*long dan cao*) and 3 *qian* coptis (*huang lian*).

Qi and Phlegm Stagnancy

Globus hystericus, the sensation of asphyxia, fullness or pain in the hypochondrium, a white, greasy tongue coating and a wiry, slippery pulse characterize stagnant *qi* and phlegm.

This condition is treated by dispersing phlegm, regulating *qi* and so alleviating depression with Pinellia and Magnolia Combination (*ban xia hou pu tang*).

Impairment of *Shen* (Spirit) Due to Prolonged Melancholy

Trance-like behavior or stupor, mental derangement, uncontrollable or continual weeping, repeated yawning, a pale tongue and a thready pulse characterize melancholia due to an impairment of *shen*.

Treatment nourishes the heart and tranquilizes *shen* with Licorice and Jujube Combination (*gan mai da zao tang*).

If the patient suffers from insomnia and is restless, irritated or dizzy, add 10 *qian* each of dragon teeth (*long chi*) and mother of pearl (*zhen zhu mu*).

Heart and Spleen Deficiency

Undue anxiety and worry, palpitation, timidity, insomnia, drowsiness, a pale complexion, listlessness, poor appetite or anorexia, a pale tongue and a thready, weak pulse characterize heart and spleen deficiency.

Treatment tonifies the heart and spleen with Ginseng and Longan Combination (*gui pi tang*).

If there is interior heat, Ginseng, Longan and Bupleurum Combination (*jia wei gui pi tang*) may be used.

Ginseng, Longan and Bupleurum Combination[1]
Jia Wei Gui Pi Tang
(Modified Strengthen the Heart and Spleen Decoction)

Ginseng	*Ginseng radix*	*Ren shen*	3.0
Atractylodes, white	*Atractylodis rhizoma*	*Bai zhu*	3.0
Hoelen	*Poria sclerotium*	*Fu ling*	3.0
Zizyphus	*Zizyphi spinosi semen*	*Suan zao ren*	3.0
Longan aril	*Longan arillus*	*Long yan rou*	3.0
Astragalus	*Astragali radix*	*Huang qi*	2.0
Tang-kuei	*Angelicae radix*	*Dang gui*	2.0
Polygala	*Polygalae radix*	*Yuan zhi*	1.0
Licorice	*Glycyrrhizae radix*	*Gan cao*	1.0
Saussurea	*Saussureae radix*	*Mu xiang*	1.0
Jujube	*Zizyphi fructus*	*Da zao*	1.0
Ginger, fresh	*Zingiberis rhizoma*	*Sheng jiang*	1.0
Bupleurum	*Bupleuri radix*	*Chai hu*	3.0
Gardenia	*Gardeniae fructus*	*Zhi zi*	2.0

Acupuncture and Moxibustion Treatment
Common Points

- *baihui* (GV 20)
- *shenmen* (H 7)
- *daduen* (Liv 1)
- *ganshu* (B 18)
- *xinjian* (Liv 2)

Treatment Method
Select three points for each treatment session.

Section 32
Manic-depressive Psychosis

Depressive psychosis is characterized by alternating bouts of complete silence, dementia, incoherent speech and unprovoked laughter, while mania is typified by ravings, greatly increased activity, euphoria and delusions of grandeur. If these states alternate, the condition is known as manic-depressive psychosis or simply manic depression.

Depressive psychosis is induced by prolonged melancholy, which prompts liver *qi* stagnancy and spleen *qi* deficiency, which, in turn, results in an inability of the spleen to adequately transport and transform nutrients. This disorder produces an accumulation of turbid phlegm, which impairs heart functioning and causes mental depression, silence and dementia, which in turn develop into depressive psychosis.

Alternately, excess anxiety impairs the heart and spleen and causes a deficiency of both *qi* and blood. This deficiency is the reason why the mind and heart do not receive adequate nourishment, thus causing mental derangement, which leads to incoherent speech, delusions and, eventually, depressive psychosis.

Unresolved anger or excessive or prolonged grief impair the functioning of the liver and gallbladder, thus prompting the formation of excess fire. This fire diminishes the body's fluids and transforms them into phlegm-fire which interferes with the proper functioning of the heart, thus causing mental confusion, restlessness, erratic behavior and, eventually, mania.

Diagnosis and Herbal Treatment

Apart from the conditions listed below, depressive psychosis and mania may also be due to interior obstructions manifested in blood stasis, a sallow complexion, a dark purple tongue with petechiae along the edges and varicosity of the sublingual veins.

This form of manic-depressive psychosis is treated by promoting blood circulation to remove stasis with Persica and Achyranthes Combination (*xue fu zhu yu tang*).

Depressive Psychosis

The principal aims of treatment are the soothing of the liver, the regulation of *qi* and the dissolution of phlegm.

1. Phlegm and *qi* accumulation

Depression, apastia, dementia, incoherent speech or muttering to oneself, moodiness, loss of appetite or anorexia, a greasy tongue coating and a wiry, slippery pulse are indicative of an accumulation of phlegm and *qi.*

This condition is treated by regulating *qi* and dissolving phlegm and, by so doing, alleviating depression. Hoelen and Bamboo Combination (*wen dan tang*), plus 3 *qian* each of acorus (*chang pu*) and polygala (*yuan zhi*), is recommended.

2. Heart and spleen deficiency

Trance-like behavior, insomnia, drowsiness, lack of strength to speak, palpitation, timidity, uncontrollable weeping, listlessness, weakness, loss of appetite, a pale tongue with a thin, white coating, and a thready, weak pulse indicate a deficiency of both the heart and spleen.

Such a deficiency is treated by nourishing the heart, strengthening the spleen and tranquilizing *shen* with Astragalus and Ziziphus Combination (*yang xin tang*).

Mania

Mania is treated by tranquilizing the heart, removing phlegm, clearing the liver and purging fire. If an interior obstruction occurs due to blood stasis, treatment promotes blood circulation in order to resolve the stasis. If there is a deficiency of *qi,* blood, *yin* or *yang, qi* should be reinforced, blood and *yin* nourished, and *yang* strengthened, respectively.

1. Disturbances due to the ascent of phlegm-fire

Irritability, susceptibility to anger, a red complexion, conjunctival congestion, fixed staring, frequent crying, restlessness, excessive aggressiveness which results in injury to others, greater-than-normal strength, a red tongue with a greasy, yellow coating and a wiry, slippery pulse are indicators of an ascent of phlegm-fire.

Treatment clears the liver, purges fire, subdues heart fire and dissolves phlegm with Iron Filings Combination (*sheng tie luo yin*).

Iron Filings Combination

Sheng Tie Luo Yin[22]
(Iron Filings Decoction)[2]

Asparagus	*Asparagi radix*	*Tian men dong*	3.0
Ophiopogon	*Ophiopogonis rhizoma*	*Mai meng dong*	3.0
Fritillaria	*Fritillariae bulbus*	*Bei mu*	3.0
Arisaema with bile	*Arisaema cum bile*	*Dan nan xing*	1.0
Orange peel	*Citri exocarpium rubrum*	*Ju hong*	1.0
Polygala	*Polygalae radix*	*Yuan zhi*	1.0
Acorus	*Acori rhizoma*	*Chang pu*	1.0
Forsythia	*Forsythiae fructus*	*Lian qiao*	1.0
Hoelen	*Poria sclerotium*	*Fu ling*	1.0
Fu-shen	*Poria cor*	*Fu shen*	1.0
Scrophularia	*Scrophulariae radix*	*Xuan shen*	2.0
Uncaria stem with hooks	*Uncariae ramulus cum uncus*	*Diao teng gou*	2.0
Salvia	*Salviae miltiorrhizae radix*	*Dan shen*	2.0
Iron filings*	*Pulveratum ferrum*	*Tie luo*	10.0

* The iron filings are decocted separately, then added to the other ingredients and decocted a second time.

Functions: tranquilizes the heart; eliminates phlegm; calms *shen*; clears the liver; purges fire.

Explanation: Asparagus and ophiopogon nourish *yin* and promote the ascent of phlegm-fire. Fritillaria, arisaema with bile, orange peel, polygala and acorus dissolve phlegm. Forsythia and uncaria stem with hooks clear the liver and purge fire. Hoelen and *fu-shen* tranquilize the mind, scrophularia purges fire, and salvia cools the blood. Iron filings subdue the heart and remove fire.

If there is liver fire, *Tang-kuei*, Gentian and Aloe Formula (*dang gui long hui wan*) may be added. A 3-*qian* dose of this patent medicine should be taken three times a day.

If there is phlegm-fire, Lapis and Scute Formula (*meng shi gun tan wan*) should be administered with Iron Filings Combination. Each dosage of the former weighs 3 *qian* and should be taken three times daily.

2. Impairment of *yin* due to fire

When mania persists for an extended period of time, the illness becomes less violent and may be accompanied by exhaustion, alternating spells of garrulousness and timidity, occasional mania, emaciation, a flushed complexion, dry mouth and lips, a red tongue with scant coating, and a thready, rapid pulse.

Yin impairment is treated by nourishing *yin*, quenching fire and tranquilizing *shen* with Scrophularia and Ophiopogon Combination (*zeng ye tang*) and Hoelen and Acorus Combination (*an shen ding zhi wan*).

Acupuncture and Moxibustion Treatment
Common Points for Treating Depressive Psychosis

- *xinshu* (B 15)
- *ganshu* (B 18)
- *pishu* (B 20)
- *shenmen* (H 7)
- *fenglong* (S 40)
- *neiguan* (P 6)

Common Points for Treating Mania

- *dazui* (GV 14)
- *fengfu* (GV 16)
- *shuigou* (CV 26)
- *neiguan* (P 6)
- *fenglong* (S 40)

Treatment Method

1. Use the reinforcing method for treating depressive psychosis.
2. Use the purging method for treating mania.

Section 33
Epilepsy

Epilepsy and epilepsia are nervous diseases characterized by convulsive spasms and a sudden loss of consciousness. The seizures may be accompanied by a frothing at the mouth, the upward fixation of the eyes, convulsions of the limbs or epileptic screams. Consciousness returns after a short while, and the patient feels as if he were waking from a normal sleep, though perhaps a little tired. There may be repeated attacks on the same day or at intervals which vary from several days to several months or years. Each onset lasts from several minutes to several hours. In Western medicine, epilepsy is classified into primary and secondary epilepsy. The etiology of primary epilepsy is not yet understood, but it appears to be related to hereditary factors. Secondary epilepsy is caused by cerebral cysts or trauma.

According to a TCM understanding, epilepsy can be induced by a disorder of the viscera due to mental, dietary or congenital factors, or by an obstruction of turbid phlegm. The disorder of the viscera occurs in the liver, spleen or kidneys and influences the heart, thus prompting the seizure. Fear can impair the liver and kidneys, causing *yin* deficiency of both organs. As *yin* fails to keep *yang* in check, heat and interior wind develop, consuming body fluids and transforming them into phlegm. Epilepsy can also be induced by improper diet, which injures the spleen and stomach, which in turn impairs the transportation and transformation of nutrients, thus causing an accumulation of turbid phlegm.

When repressed emotions or fatigue prompt stagnant phlegm to create interior wind, both phlegm and wind ascend and consequently invade and obstruct the heart. Sudden loss of consciousness with convulsions results.

Treatment of epilepsy depends on its origin, stage and symptoms. During the attack, treatments to induce resuscitation, alleviate convulsions and calm the patient are given. These are followed by treatments to regulate *qi*, subdue the heart and reduce phlegm. When the patient is not having a seizure, the systemic cause of the epilepsy should be treated by tonifying the liver and kidneys, strengthening the spleen, reducing phlegm, nourishing the heart and tranquilizing *shen*.

Diagnosis and Herbal Treatment

Attack Stage

During the attack, it is difficult and potentially dangerous to administer herbs. Medicine should be taken just prior to the seizure when the symptoms start to appear or after the seizure has subsided.

1. Turbid phlegm due to liver wind

Before the attack, the following may be observed: dizziness, a feeling of oppression in the chest and lassitude. However, often an attack occurs without warning. As the attack begins, the patient suddenly loses consciousness, may develop lockjaw, convulsions, frothing at the mouth, epileptic screams or urinary or fecal incontinence, as well as a tendency for the eyes to stare fixedly upwards. The patient may also behave as if in a trance and have no convulsions. The tongue has a greasy, white coating, and the pulse is wiry and slippery.

Treatment is focused on relieving the convulsions and calming the patient with Gastrodia and Amber Formula (*ding xian wan*).

Gastrodia and Amber Formula
Ding Xian Wan[22]
(Arrest Seizures Pill)[2]

Gastrodia	Gastrodiae rhizoma	Tian ma	30.0
Pinellia	Pinellia rhizoma	Ban xia	30.0
Hoelen	Poria sclerotium	Fu ling	30.0
Fu-shen	Poria cor	Fu shen	30.0
Arisaema with bile	Arisaema cum bile	Dan nan xing	15.0
Acorus	Acori rhizoma	Chang pu	15.0
Scorpion	Scorpio	Quan xie	15.0
Licorice	Glycyrrhizae radix	Gan cao	15.0
Silkworm	Bombyx batryticatus	Bai jiang can	15.0
Amber	Succinum	Hu po	15.0
Juncus	Junci caulis medulla	Deng xin cao	15.0
Citrus peel	Citri pericarpium	Chen pi	60.0
Polygala	Polygalae radix	Yuan zhi	60.0
Salvia	Salviae miltiorrhizae radix	Dan shen	60.0
Ophiopogon	Ophiopogonis rhizoma	Mai meng dong	60.0
Fritillaria	Fritillariae bulbus	Bei mu	30.0

The above herbs are combined with 120 *qian* of licorice (*gan cao*) and decocted, adding 100 ml bamboo juice (*zhu li*) and 50 ml juice of fresh ginger (*sheng jiang*). Six-*qian* pills are made from the above ingredients. One pill is taken with warm water, twice daily, preferably early in the morning and before retiring.

Functions: removes phlegm; calms interior wind.

Explanation: Bamboo juice clears heat, removes phlegm, relieves convulsions and induces resuscitation, while the warm-natured juice of fresh ginger aids in dissolving phlegm and inducing resuscitation. Arisaema with bile is specifically used to clear fire, dissolve phlegm, relieve convulsions and calm the patient, while pinellia, hoelen, citrus peel, ophiopogon and fritillaria remove phlegm, regulate the adverse flow of *qi* and prevent the impairment of *yin*. Acorus and salvia eliminate blood stasis and induce resuscitation, and scorpion and silkworm subdue interior wind and relieve spasms. Gastrodia dissolves phlegm and calms interior wind, while *fu-shen*, amber, juncus and polygala relieve convulsions and tranquilize *shen*. Licorice harmonizes the actions of the other herbs.

2. Heat-phlegm due to liver fire

During the attack, the patient may spasm, froth at the mouth or scream, as well as lose consciousness. Ordinarily, when the patient is not having a seizure, he or she is irritable, restless and constipated. Insomnia, a dry mouth, a bitter taste in the mouth, a red tongue with a yellow coating, and a wiry, rapid pulse may also be observed.

Treatment is focused on strengthening the liver, purging fire, dissolving phlegm and inducing resuscitation with Gentian Combination (*long dan xie gan tang*), plus 3 *qian* polygala (*yuan zhi*) and 2 *qian* acorus (*chang pu*).

If the patient is constipated, add 2 *qian* rhubarb (*da huang*) to the combination given in the preceding paragraph.

If the patient's mouth and lips are dry, add 4 *qian* raw rehmannia (*sheng di huang*) and 3 *qian* scrophularia (*xuan shen*).

Remission

1. Liver and kidney *yin* deficiency

Lower back pain, dizziness, hypomnesia, a dry mouth, insomnia, constipation, a red tongue and a thready, rapid pulse characterize a deficiency of liver and kidney *yin*.

Treatment is aimed at nourishing *yin* and tranquilizing *shen* with Achyranthes and Rehmannia Formula (*zuo gui wan*).

If the patient is restless and has a hot sensation in the chest, add 3 *qian* each of lotus embryo (*lian zi xin*) and gardenia (*zhi zi*).

If the patient is constipated, add 3 *qian* scrophularia (*xuan shen*) and 5 *qian* linum (*ma zi ren*).

2. Spleen and stomach deficiency

Dizziness, feebleness, poor appetite or anorexia, loose stools, a pale complexion and tongue, and a soft, thready pulse indicate a deficiency of the spleen and stomach.

Treatment consists in strengthening the spleen, dissolving phlegm, reinforcing *qi* and nourishing the heart with Saussurea and Cardamom Combination (*xiang sha liu jun zi tang*).

Common Acupuncture and Moxibustion Points

Paroxysm

- *shuigou* (GV 26)
- *hegu* (LI 4)
- *yongquan* (K 1)
- *dazhui* (GV 14)
- *baihui* (GV 20)

Remission

- *dazhui* (GV 14)
- *fengchi* (G 20)
- *hegu* (LI 4)
- *taicong* (Liv 3)

Section 34
Flaccidity (*Wei*) Conformation

Flaccidity conformation is associated with muscle feebleness and acratia of the limbs, which result in an inability to perform voluntary acts. Flaccidity in the legs is the most common manifestation. In a serious case, the patient is unable to walk or hold objects. Paralysis or myoatrophy may result.

Flaccidity was first mentioned in *Nei Jing* (Internal Classic) as "*wei bi*" (acratia of the limbs). "*Wei*" means feebleness of the limbs in general, and "*bi*" specifically refers to acratia in the legs. In short, the term as a whole connotes those who are unable to walk.

The clinical manifestations resemble those of polyneuritis, acute myelitis, progressive myoatrophy, myasthenia gravis, periodic paralysis, myodystrophy, hysterical paralysis or sequelae caused by pathologic changes to the central nervous system, all of which are manifested by flaccid paralysis, according to Western medicine.

Causes of flaccidity conformations fall into two broad categories: external pathogens and internal injuries. Flaccidity due to toxins, pathogenic heat or prolonged living in damp places is considered an exterior conformation, while flaccidity induced by a deficiency of the spleen and stomach or of the liver and kidneys is considered an internal injury.

Specifically, a deficiency of vital *qi* prompts an invasion of pathogenic heat. Alternately, pathogenic heat may not completely subside following an illness, and the patient will continue to have a low-grade fever. In either case, the lungs will become damaged by heat, and saliva and other body fluids will be unable to adequately lubricate the muscles, resulting in flaccidity.

An invasion by external heat-dampness or injury to the spleen and stomach as a result of excessive eating or drinking may lead to spleen and stomach deficiency and an impairment of the digestive and absorptive functions of these organs. Deficiencies of body fluids, *qi*, kidney essence or liver blood will then develop and, in turn, cause the muscles, bones and meridians to become dry and malnourished, thus leading to flaccidity conformation.

As regards the treatment of flaccidity, *Su Wen* (Plain Questions) points out: "Flaccidity is treated mainly through the *yang ming* meridian." According to this principle, flaccidity is corrected by reinforcing essence. Consequently, strengthening the stomach and nourishing *yin* are the primary concerns, especially if the flaccidity is caused by excess lung heat. If the illness is associated with heat-dampness conformation, however, it is treated by removing heat and draining dampness.

Diagnosis and Herbal Treatment

Injury to Body Fluids Due to Lung Heat

A fever at the onset, sudden weakness in the limbs, fidgeting, thirst, cough, a dry pharynx, small amounts of dark urine, constipation, a red tongue with a yellow coating and a thready, rapid pulse characterize injury of body fluids due to lung heat.

Treatment consists in removing heat, moistening dryness, nourishing the lungs and reinforcing the stomach with Eriobotrya and Ophiopogon Combination (*qing zao jiu fei tang*).

If there is a high fever and thirst, add 4 *qian* anemarrhena (*zhi mu*) and 5 *qian* each of lonicera (*jin yin hua*), forsythia (*lian qiao*) and fresh rehmannia (*xian shen di*).

If there is a cough with a very dry throat and only a little phlegm, add 4 *qian* trichosanthes peel (*gua lou pi*) and 3 *qian* morus bark (*sang bai pi*).

Heat-dampness

Flaccidity in the limbs, especially in the legs; fever; slight swelling; numbness; chest and stomach fullness; decreased micturition of yellow urine; a yellow, greasy tongue coating; and a soft, rapid pulse characterize an invasion by heat-dampness.

Treatment aims at removing heat and eliminating dampness with Phellodendron and Achyranthes Formula (*san miao wan*), plus 10 *qian* coix (*yi yi ren*) and 3 *qian* each of stephania (*fang ji*), tokoro (*bi jie*) and alisma (*ze xie*). This modification of Phellodendron and Achyranthes Formula is decocted in water for an oral dose.

If there is excess heat-dampness, add the following to the modification of Phellodendron and Achyranthes Formula given in the preceding paragraph: 3 *qian* each of elsholtzia (*xiang ru*), eupatorium (*pei lan*) and magnolia bark (*hou pu*).

If the patient develops excess heat, add 3 *qian* each of raw rehmannia (*sheng di huang*), ophiopogon (*mai men dong*) and tortoise shell (*gui ban*).

If there is blood stasis, add 5 *qian* salvia (*dan shen*) and 3 *qian* each of red peony (*chi shao*), persica (*tao ren*) and carthamus (*hong hua*).

Spleen and Stomach Deficiency

A gradual weakening of the legs, a poor appetite, shortness of breath, lack of energy to speak, a pale complexion, loose stools, a thin, white tongue coating and a thready, weak pulse characterize spleen and stomach deficiency.

Treatment consists in tonifying the liver, reinforcing the kidneys, nourishing *yin* and removing heat with Tiger Bone and Tortoise Shell Formula (*hu qian wan*) or Eucommia and Achyranthes Formula (*wei zheng fang*).

Tiger Bone and Tortoise Shell Formula
Hu Qian Wan[9]
(Hidden Tiger Pill)[2]

Phellodendron	Phellodendri cortex	Huang bo	150.0
Tortoise shell	Testudinis plastrum	Gui ban	120.0
Anemarrhena	Anemarrhenae rhizoma	Zhi mu	60.0
Rehmannia, cooked	Rehmanniae radix	Shu di huang	60.0
Citrus peel	Citri pericarpium	Chen pi	60.0
Peony	Paeoniae radix	Shao yao	60.0
Cynomorium	Cynomorii herba	Suo yang	45.0
Tiger bone	Os tigris	Hu gu	30.0
Ginger, dried	Zingiberis siccatum rhizoma	Gan jiang	15.0

The above ingredients are ground into a powder and made into 3.3-*qian* boluses with wine or honey. One bolus is taken b.i.d. (in the early morning and before retiring for the night) with salty soup or warm water. If the preparation is made into concentrated granules, the dose then becomes 2 *qian* t.i.d.

Functions: moistens *yin*; removes fire; consolidates the muscles and bones.

Explanation: Phellodendron and anemarrhena remove fire and clear heat, while tortoise shell, cooked rehmannia and peony moisten *yin* and nourish the blood in order to tonify liver and kidney *yin*. Cynomorium warms *yang*, enhances essence, nourishes the muscles and moistens dryness. Tiger bone strengthens the muscles and bones, and citrus peel and dried ginger warm the middle energizer, strengthen the spleen, regulate *qi* and harmonize the stomach.

Eucommia and Achyranthes Formula[1]
Wei Zheng Fang
(Flaccidity Decoction)

Tang-kuei	Angelicae radix	Dang gui	5.0
Peony	Paeoniae radix	Shao yao	2.0
Eucommia	Eucommiae cortex	Du zhong	1.0
Achyranthes	Achyranthis radix	Niu xi	3.0
Astragalus	Astragali radix	Huang qi	2.0
Atractylodes	Atractylodis lanceae rhizoma	Cang zhu	3.0
Rehmannia	Rehmanniae radix	Di huang	4.0
Phellodendron	Phellodendri cortex	Huang bo	1.0
Anemarrhena	Anemarrhenae rhizoma	Zhi mu	3.0

Blood Stasis

The manifestations are feebleness and acratia in the limbs, even disabled arms and legs; muscle numbness or swelling; a history of trauma; a submerged and hesitant pulse; and a dark-purple tongue with ecchymosis.

Blood stasis-associated flaccidity is treated by promoting blood circulation to remove stasis with Persica and Achyranthes (xue fu zhu yu tang).

Common Acupuncture and Moxibustion Points

Flaccidity in the Arms

- dazhui (GV 14)
- dashu (B 11)
- shenzhu (GV 12)
- quchi (LI 11)
- jianyu (LI 15)
- jianzhen (SI 9)
- waiguan (TE 5)
- wangu (SI 4)

Flaccidity in the Legs

- *yangguan* (GV 3)
- *yaoshu* (GV 2)
- *xuanzhong* (G 39)
- *yanglingquan* (G 34)
- *zusanli* (S 36)
- *xiajuxu* (S 39)
- *huantiao* (G 30)
- *fengshi* (G 31)
- *chengshan* (B 57)
- *sanyinjiao* (Sp 6)
- *yinlingquan* (Sp 9)
- *kunlun* (B 60)

Treatment Method

Three or four points should be selected for each daily or every-other-day treatment for a total treatment course of 10 days.

Section 35
Arthralgia Syndrome (*Bi* Conformation)

"*Bi*," which means stagnancy in Chinese, is the term used to describe the pain, numbness, swollen joints, heavy sensation in the legs and arms, and difficulty in bending and stretching of the limbs which result from an invasion of the body by external pathogenic factors and the subsequent impairment of *qi* and blood circulation.

Su Wen (Plain Questions), in its treatise on arthralgia syndrome, states: "Wind, cold and dampness come together to induce arthralgia. If wind holds a dominant position, migratory arthralgia develops. If cold dominates, aching arthralgia is induced. If dampness dominates, fixed and swelling arthralgia occurs." Furthermore, *Ji Shen Fang* (Life-preserving Prescriptions) notes: "Arthralgia is caused by wind, cold or dampness under the conditions of weakness and diminished resistance to disease."

There is also heat arthralgia, which is caused by a *yin* deficiency accompanied by interior heat. This type of arthralgia is manifested in acute attacks following an invasion of external pathogens. Heat arthralgia can also be caused by wind, cold or dampness retained in the meridians and collaterals which stagnates and transforms into heat.

Diagnosis and Herbal Treatment

Migratory Arthralgia

This type of arthralgia is not fixed and may involve any of the large joints of the shoulders, elbows, wrists, hips, knees or ankles. Exterior symptoms, such as fever and chills in the initial stage, as well as a thin, white tongue coating and a floating pulse, are common signs and symptoms.

Treatment dispels wind and removes dampness. Cinnamon and Angelica Formula (*shang zhong xia tong yong tong feng fang*) or Stephania and Carthamus Combination (*shu feng huo xue wan*) are recommended.

Cinnamon and Angelica Formula[1]

Shang Zhong Xia Tong Yong Tong Feng Wan
(Relieve Arthralgia Decoction)

Phellodendron	Phellodendri cortex	Huang bo	2.0
Atractylodes	Atractylodis lanceae rhizoma	Cang zhu	2.0
Arisaema	Arisaematis rhizoma	Tian nan xing	2.0
Shen-chu	Massa medicata fermentata	Shen qu	1.0
Cnidium	Cnidii rhizoma	Chuan xiong*	1.0
Persica	Persicae semen	Tao ren	1.0
Gentian	Gentianae scabrae radix	Long dan cao	1.0
Stephania	Aristolochiae fangchi radix	Fang ji	1.0
Angelica	Angelicae dahuricae radix	Bai zhi	1.0
Chiang-huo	Notopterygii rhizoma	Qiang huo	3.0
Clematis	Clematis radix	Wei ling xian	3.0
Cinnamon twig	Cinnamomi ramulus	Gui zhi	3.0
Carthamus	Carthami flos	Hong hua	2.0

Ligustici rhizoma, also known as *chuan xiong*, may be substituted for *Cnidii rhizoma*.

Stephania and Carthamus Combination[1]

Shu Feng Huo Xue Tang
(Disperse Wind and Invigorate the Blood Decoction)[2]

Tang-kuei	Angelicae radix	Dang gui	2.5
Cnidium	Cnidii rhizoma	Chuan xiong*	2.5
Clematis	Clematis radix	Wei ling xian	2.5
Angelica	Angelicae dahuricae radix	Bai zhi	2.5
Stephania	Aristolochiae fangchi radix	Fang ji	2.5
Phellodendron	Phellodendri cortex	Huang bo	2.5
Arisaema	Arisaematis rhizoma	Tian nan xing	2.5
Atractylodes	Atractylodis lanceae rhizoma	Cang zhu	2.5
Chiang-huo	Notopterygii rhizoma	Qiang huo	2.5
Cinnamon twig	Cinnamomi ramulus	Gui zhi	2.5
Carthamus	Carthami flos	Hong hua	1.0
Ginger, dried	Zingiberis siccatum rhizoma	Gan jiang	1.0

*Ligustici rhizoma, also known as chuan xiong, may be substituted for Cnidii rhizoma.

Aching Arthralgia

Severe, stabbing and fixed arthralgia which is aggravated by cold and relieved by heat, difficulty in the stretching and flexing of the joints, a cold sensation in the affected joints, a white tongue coating and a wiry, tense pulse characterize this type of arthralgia.

Treatment warms the meridians and dispels cold, wind and dampness with Wu-tou and Cinnamon Combination (wu tou gui zhi tang) or Cinnamon and Anemarrhena Combination (gui zhi shao yao zhi mu tang).

Wu-tou and Cinnamon Combination[1]
Wu Tou Gui Zhi Tang
(Aconite and Cinnamon Twig Decoction)[2]

Aconite root, Sichuan	*Aconiti radix*	*Wu tou*	0.5
Cinnamon twig	*Cinnamomi ramulus*	*Gui zhi*	1.0
Ginger, fresh	*Zingiberis rhizoma*	*Sheng jiang*	2.0
Jujube	*Zizyphi fructus*	*Da zao*	4.0
Peony	*Paeoniae radix*	*Shao yao*	3.0
Licorice	*Glycyrrhizae radix*	*Gan cao*	2.0

Cinnamon and Anemarrhena Combination[1]
Gui Zhi Shao Yao Zhi Mu Tang
(Cinnamon Twig, Peony and Anemarrhena Decoction)[2]

Cinnamon twig	*Cinnamomi ramulus*	*Gui zhi*	1.0
Peony	*Paeoniae radix*	*Shao yao*	3.0
Anemarrhena	*Anemarrhenae rhizoma*	*Zhi mu*	3.0
Ma-huang	*Ephedrae herba*	*Ma huang*	1.0
Siler	*Ledebouriellae radix*	*Fang feng*	3.0
Atractylodes, white	*Atractylodis rhizoma*	*Bai zhu*	4.0
Aconite, prepared	*Aconiti carmichaelii praeparata radix*	*Zhi fu zi*	1.0
Licorice	*Glycyrrhizae radix*	*Gan cao*	1.5
Ginger, fresh	*Zingiberis rhizoma*	*Sheng jiang*	2.0

Fixed and Swelling Arthralgia

Numbness and fixed pain in the joints; swelling and difficulty in stretching and flexing the joints; a white, greasy tongue coating; and a soft, floating and moderate pulse characterize this type of arthralgia.

Treatment focuses on strengthening the spleen and eliminating dampness, wind and cold. Either of the following three formulas may be used: Coix Combination (*yi yi ren tang*), Astragalus and Aconite Formula (*shi wei cuo san*) or Tang-kuei and Anemarrhena Combination (*dang gui nian tong tang*).

Coix Combination[1]

Yi Yi Ren Tang
(Coix Decoction)

Ma-huang	Ephedrae herba	Ma huang	4.0
Cinnamon twig	Cinnamomi ramulus	Gui zhi	3.0
Tang-kuei	Angelicae radix	Dang gui	4.0
Peony	Paeoniae radix	Shao yao	3.0
Atractylodes, white	Atractylodis rhizoma	Bai zhu	4.0
Licorice	Glycyrrhizae radix	Gan cao	2.0
Coix	Coicis semen	Yi yi ren	8.0

Astragalus and Aconite Formula[1]

Shi Wei Cuo San
(Ten Herbs, Including Astragalus and Aconite, Powder)

Tang-kuei	Angelicae radix	Dang gui	3.0
Peony	Paeoniae radix	Shao yao	3.0
Cnidium	Cnidii rhizoma	Chuan xiong*	3.0
Rehmannia	Rehmanniae radix	Di huang	3.0
Hoelen	Poria sclerotium	Fu ling	3.0
Atractylodes, white	Atractylodis rhizoma	Bai zhu	3.0
Astragalus	Astragali radix	Huang qi	3.0
Cinnamon twig	Cinnamomi ramulus	Gui zhi	3.0
Siler	Ledebouriellae radix	Fang feng	3.0
Aconite, prepared	Aconiti carmichaelii praeparata radix	Zhi fu zi	1.0

Ligustici rhizoma, also known as *chuan xiong*, may be substituted for *Cnidii rhizoma*.

Tang-kuei and Anemarrhena Combination[1]

Dang Gui Nian Tong Tang

(*Tang-kuei* Decoction for Relieving Pain)

Tang-kuei	Angelicae radix	Dang gui	2.5
Anemarrhena	Anemarrhenae rhizoma	Zhi mu	2.5
Chiang-huo	Notopterygii rhizoma	Qiang huo	2.5
Capillaris	Artemisiae capillaris herba	Yin chen hao	2.5
Scute	Scutellariae radix	Huang qin	2.5
Atractylodes, white	Atractylodis rhizoma	Bai zhu	2.5
Polyporus	Polyporus sclerotium	Zhu ling	2.5
Alisma	Alismatis rhizoma	Ze xie	2.5
Atractylodes	Atractylodis lanceae rhizoma	Cang zhu	2.0
Siler	Ledebouriellae radix	Fang feng	2.0
Pueraria	Puerariae radix	Ge gen	2.0
Ginseng	Ginseng radix	Ren shen	2.0
Sophora root	Sophorae radix	Ku shen	1.0
Cimicifuga	Cimicifugae rhizoma	Sheng ma	1.0
Licorice	Glycyrrhizae radix	Gan cao	1.0

When the arthralgia lingers over an extended period of time, the patient may develop *qi*, blood, liver or kidney deficiency. In such a case, not only must cold, wind and dampness be dispelled, but the liver, the kidneys, *qi* and blood must also be replenished. *Tu-huo* and Loranthus Combination (*du huo ji sheng tang*), *Chiang-huo* and Curcuma Combination (*juan bi tang*) or Major Siler Combination (*da fang feng tang*) can be used.

Tu-huo and Loranthus Combination[1]

Du Huo Ji Sheng Tang

(Angelica Pubescens and *Sangjisheng* Decoction)[2]

Pubescent angelica	Angelicae tuhuo radix	Du huo	3.0
Chin-chiu	Gentianae macro phyllae radix	Qin jiao	1.5
Siler	Ledebouriellae radix	Fang feng	3.0
Asarum	Asari herba cum radice	Xi xin	1.0
Loranthus	Loranthi ramulus	Sang ji sheng	4.5
Eucommia	Eucommiae cortex	Du zhong	3.0
Achyranthes	Achyranthis radix	Niu xi	3.0
Cinnamon bark	Cinnamomi cortex	Gui pi	1.0
Tang-kuei	Angelicae radix	Dang gui	3.0
Cnidium	Cnidii rhizoma	Chuan xiong*	1.5
Rehmannia	Rehmanniae radix	Di huang	3.0
Peony	Paeoniae radix	Shao yao	3.0
Ginseng	Ginseng radix	Ren shen	2.0
Hoelen	Poria sclerotium	Fu ling	3.0
Licorice	Glycyrrhizae radix	Gan cao	1.5

Ligustici rhizoma, also known as *chuan xiong*, may be substituted for *Cnidii rhizoma*.

Chiang-huo and Curcuma Combination[1]

Juan Bi Tang

(Remove Painful Obstruction Decoction)[2]

Chiang-huo	Notopterygii rhizoma	Qiang huo	1.5
Curcuma	Curcumae rhizoma	Jiang huang	2.0
Tang-kuei	Angelicae radix	Dang gui	3.0
Peony, red	Paeoniae rubra radix	Chi shao	3.0
Astragalus	Astragali radix	Huang qi	4.0
Siler	Ledebouriellae radix	Fang feng	1.5
Licorice	Glycyrrhizae radix	Gan cao	1.0
Ginger, fresh	Zingiberis rhizoma	Sheng jiang	1.0
Jujube	Zizyphi fructus	Da zao	9.0

Major Siler Combination[1]

Da Fang Feng Tang

(Major Ledebouriella Decoction)[2]

Tang-kuei	Angelica radix	Dang gui	3.0
Peony	Paeoniae radix	Shao yao	3.0
Rehmannia, cooked	Rehmanniae radix	Shu di huang	3.0
Astragalus	Astragali radix	Huang qi	3.0
Siler	Ledebouriellae radix	Fang feng	3.0
Eucommia	Eucommiae cortex	Du zhong	3.0
Atractylodes, white	Atractylodis rhizoma	Bai zhu	3.0
Cnidium	Cnidii rhizoma	Chuan xiong*	3.0
Ginseng	Ginseng radix	Ren shen	1.5
Chiang-huo	Notopterygii rhizoma	Qiang huo	1.5
Achyranthes	Achyranthis radix	Niu xi	1.5
Licorice	Glycyrrhizae radix	Gan cao	1.5
Jujube	Zizyphi fructus	Da zao	1.5
Ginger, fresh	Zingiberis rhizoma	Sheng jiang	1.5
Aconite, prepared	Aconiti carmichaelii praeparata radix	Zhi fu zi	1.0

Ligustici rhizoma, also known as *chuan xiong*, may be substituted for *Cnidii rhizoma*.

Heat Arthralgia

Heat arthralgia is relieved by cold and accompanied by a burning sensation, redness and swelling of the joints, impaired movement, fever, thirst, fidgeting, depression, a bright red tongue with a yellow coating, and a slippery, rapid pulse.

Treatment clears heat, dispels wind, resolves dampness and cools the *ying fen* with Gypsum Combination (*bai hu tang*), plus 1.5 *qian* each of cinnamon twig (*gui zhi*), lonicera (*ren dong teng*) and morus branch (*sang zhi*). As an alternative, Clematis and Carthamus Formula (*shu jin li an san*) can be used.

Clematis and Carthamus Formula[1]
Shu Jin Li An San
(Powder for Immediately Relaxing Muscles and Tendons)

Siler	Ledebouriellae radix	Fang feng	1.2
Chiang-huo	Notopterygii rhizoma	Qiang huo	1.2
Pubescent angelica	Angelicae tuhuo radix	Du huo	1.2
Hoelen	Poria sclerotium	Fu ling	1.2
Cnidium	Cnidii rhizoma	Chuan xiong*	1.2
Angelica	Angelicae dahuricae radix	Bai zhi	1.2
Rehmannia, raw	Rehmanniae radix	Sheng di huang	1.2
Atractylodes, white	Atractylodis rhizoma	Bai zhu	1.2
Carthamus	Carthami flos	Hong hua	1.2
Persica	Persicae semen	Tao ren	1.2
Arisaema	Arisaematis rhizoma	Tian nan xing	1.2
Citrus peel	Citri pericarpium	Chen pi	1.2
Pinellia	Pinellia rhizoma	Ban xia	1.2
Atractylodes	Atractylodis lanceae rhizoma	Cang zhu	1.2
Clematis	Clematis radix	Wei ling xian	1.2
Achyranthes	Achyranthis radix	Niu xi	1.2
Chaenomeles	Chaenomelis fructus	Mu gua	1.2
Stephania	Aristolochiae fangchi radix	Fang ji	1.2
Forsythia	Forsythiae fructus	Lian qiao	1.2
Scute	Scutellariae radix	Huang qin	1.2
Akebia	Akebiae caulis	Mu tong	1.2
Licorice	Glycyrrhizae radix	Gan cao	1.2
Aconite, prepared	Aconiti carmichaelii praeparata radix	Zhi fu zi	1.0
Bamboo shavings	Bambusae caulis in taeniis	Zhu ru	1.2
Gentian	Gentianae scabrae radix	Long dan cao	1.2

*Ligustici rhizoma, also known as chuan xiong, may be substituted for Cnidii rhizoma.

Herbs Commonly Used for Treating *Bi* Conformation

Herbs to Dispel Wind-dampness

siler (*fang feng*)	chiang-huo (*qiang huo*)
tu-huo (*du huo*)	cinnamon twig (*gui zhi*)
ma-huang (*ma huang*)	

Because wind can overpower dampness, these herbs for dispelling wind will also dispel dampness evils. Specifically, siler, cinnamon twig and *ma-huang* dispel wind-dampness throughout the body, while *chiang-huo* dispels wind-dampness from the upper body, particularly the arms, and *tu-huo* works on the lower body, especially the legs.

Other herbs for dispelling wind-dampness treat specific types of wind-dampness pain, such as pain in the lower legs or muscular pain. These less commonly prescribed herbs are: clematis (*wei ling xian*), chaenomeles (*mu gua*), acanthopanax (*wu jia pi*), stephania (*fang ji*), loranthus (*sang ji sheng*) and futokadsura (*hai feng teng*).

Herbs to Dispel Dampness

coix (*yi yi ren*)	atractylodes (*cang zhu*)
hoelen (*fu ling*)	polyporus (*zhu ling*)
capillaris (*yin chen hao*)	akebia (*mu tong*)

Coix effectively dispels wind-dampness from the joints, while atractylodes and hoelen strengthen the spleen and so aid in removing dampness. Mild-flavored polyporus, capillaris and akebia dispel dampness through diuresis.

Herbs to Warm the Meridians and Dispel Cold

prepared aconite (*zhi fu zi*)	cinnamon bark (*gui pi*)
Sichuan aconite root (*chuan wu*)	antler (*lu jiao*)

Prepared aconite and Sichuan aconite root dispel generalized cold, though the latter is much more potent and potentially toxic than the former, and so dosages should be adjusted accordingly. Cinnamon bark dispels localized cold. If cold is in the spine, where the *dumai* (GV) is located, tablets or powder of antler should be used.

Acupuncture and Moxibustion Treatment

Common Points

1. In the shoulders
   - *jianyu* (LI 15)
   - *jianliao* (TE 14)
   - *naoshu* (SI 10)

2. In the elbows and arms
   - *chize* (L 5)
   - *hegu* (LI 4)
   - *waiguan* (TE 5)
   - *quchi* (LI 11)
   - *tianjin* (TE 10)

3. In the wrists
   - *yangchi* (S 4)
   - *yangxi* (LI 5)
   - *waiguan* (TE 5)
   - *wangu* (SI 4)

4. In the back
   - *shenzhu* (GV 12)
   - *yiaoyangguan* (GV 3)

5. In the hips
   - *huantiao* (G 30)
   - *xuanzhong* (G 39)
   - *chengfu* (B 36)
   - *juliao* (G 29)
   - *zhibian* (B 54)
   - *yanglingquan* (G 34)

6. In the knees
   - *dubi* (S 35)
   - *yanglingquan* (G 34)
   - *liangqiu* (S 34)
   - *xiyangguan* (G 33)

7. In the ankles
   - *shenmai* (B 62)
   - *kunlun* (B 60)
   - *zhaohai* (K 6)
   - *qiuxu* (G 40)

Treatment Method

1. For migratory arthralgia

   a. reducing method or prick to induce bleeding

   b. add *geshu* (B 17) and *xuehai* (Sp 10)

2. For aching arthralgia

   a. acupuncture or moxibustion

   b. minimum of 15 minutes/point

   c. add *shenshu* (B 23) and *guanyuan* (CV 4)

3. For fixed and swelling arthralgia

   a. acupuncture or moxibustion

   b. cup or prick to induce bleeding

   c. add *zusanli* (S 36) and *shangqiu* (Sp 5)

4. For heat arthralgia

   a. reducing method or prick to induce bleeding

   b. add *dazhui* (GV 14) and *quchi* (LI 11)

Chapter 5

Differentiation of Conformations and Prescriptions for Common Diseases

Section 1
Bronchitis

Bronchitis can be classified into acute and chronic. The latter is further distinguished as either simple or asthmatic. The chief symptom of all forms of bronchitis is coughing, which transforms into asthma if it persists. In TCM, bronchitis belongs to one of three conformations: cough, phlegm and fluid retention, or cough and asthma.

This disease can be caused either by external pathogenic factors (seasonal external pathogens) or by interior pathogenic factors (such as a disorder of the internal organs). The latter is the more prevalent cause, especially in chronic cases, which often occur in elderly patients and consist of a deficiency complicated by an excess condition.

At the exterior stage, bronchitis can be diagnosed and treated according to wind-cold or wind-heat conformation, with the appropriate herbs added to relieve the cough and resolve the sputum. It is crucial to differentiate between the two conformations so that either warming and tonifying the healthy energy or clearing and eliminating the external pathogens may be accomplished. Furthermore, if a deficiency in the lungs or kidneys is observed, it must be determined whether it is a *yang* or *yin* deficiency, warming *yang* in the former case and nourishing *yin* in the latter.

Diagnosis and Herbal Treatment

Phlegm and Fluid Retention Due to Lung Cold

A cough with thin, white, frothy sputum which is easily expectorated, a preference for hot beverages, difficulty in lying supine because of the severe cough and asthma, a white, greasy tongue coating and a wiry, slippery pulse characterize phlegm and fluid retention. In addition, other symptoms of an exterior conformation may be present.

Treatment warms the lungs to eliminate fluid retention and relieve the cough and asthma. Minor Blue Dragon Combination (*xiao qing long tang*) can be given.

If the disease occurs in winter and persists until spring or summer and if stagnant cold has transformed into heat, some cool- or cold-natured herbs should be added. Major Blue Dragon Combination (*da qing long tang*) is just such a collection of herbs.

Major Blue Dragon Combination[1]

Da Qing Long Tang

(Major Bluegreen Dragon Decoction)[2]

Cinnamon twig	*Cinnamomi ramulus*	*Gui zhi*	3.0
Ma-huang	*Ephedrae herba*	*Ma huang*	6.0
Apricot seed	*Armeniacae semen*	*Xing ren*	5.0
Licorice	*Glycyrrhizae radix*	*Gan cao*	2.0
Gypsum	*Gypsum fibrosum*	*Shi gao*	10.0
Ginger, fresh	*Zingiberis rhizoma*	*Sheng jiang*	3.0
Jujube	*Zizyphi fructus*	*Da zao*	3.0

Turbid Phlegm Retention Due to Lung Heat

A cough with thick, yellow sputum which is expectorated with difficulty, chest fullness, shortness of breath, thirst and a preference for cold beverages, dark yellow urine, constipation, a yellow, greasy tongue coating or a yellow tongue coating that is sprinkled with white spots or a red tongue, and a wiry, slippery, rapid pulse characterize turbid phlegm retention due to lung heat. The patient may or may not have a fever.

Treatment clears phlegm and heat and relieves the cough and asthma. *Ma-huang* and Ginkgo Combination (*ding chuan tang*) can be used.

If there is fever and a bacterial infection, 10 *qian* each of dandelion (*pu gong yin*) and houttuynia (*yu xing cao*) should be added.

Ma-huang and Ginkgo Combination[1]
Ding Chuan Tang
(Arrest Wheezing Decoction)[2]

Ma-huang	Ephedrae herba	Ma huang	3.0
Apricot seed	Armeniacae semen	Xing ren	1.8
Perilla seed	Perillae semen	Zi su zi	1.8
Ginkgo	Ginkgo semen	Bai guo	4.8
Morus bark	Mori radicis cortex	Sang bai pi	1.8
Scute	Scutellariae radix	Huang qin	0.6
Pinellia	Pinellia rhizoma	Ban xia	3.0
Tussilago	Farfarae flos	Kuan dong hua	3.0
Licorice	Glycyrrhizae radix	Gan cao	0.6

Phlegm-dampness Accumulation Due to Spleen Deficiency

A cough; copious, turbid and white or gray sputum which is easily expectorated; abdominal fullness and distention following meals; an absence of the sense of taste; a preference for

331

warm beverages; a feeling of oppression in the chest; listlessness; heaviness in the torso and limbs; loose stools; a plump
tongue with teeth marks and a thin or greasy coating; and a
slippery pulse characterize phlegm-dampness accumulation
due to spleen deficiency.

Treatment strengthens the spleen, dispels dampness,
relieves the cough and resolves phlegm. Six Major Herb Combination (*liu jun zi tang*) can be used, or if phlegm-dampness is
severe, administer Magnolia and Ginger Formula (*ping wei
san*) and Perilla Fruit Combination (*su zi jiang qi tang*).

If the cough is severe, 3 *qian* each of aster (*zi wan*) and
stemona (*bai bu*) should be added to Six Major Herb Combination.

Perilla Fruit Combination[1]
Su Zi Jiang Qi Tang
(Perilla Fruit Decoction for Directing *Qi* Downward)[2]

Perilla seed*	*Perillae semen*	*Zi su zi*	3.0
Pinellia	*Pinellia rhizoma*	*Ban xia*	4.0
Magnolia bark	*Magnoliae officinalis cortex*	*Hou pu*	2.5
Peucedanum	*Peucedani radix*	*Qian hu*	2.5
Cinnamon bark	*Cinnamomi cortex*	*Rou gui*	1.0
Tang-kuei	*Angelicae radix*	*Dang gui*	2.5
Licorice, baked	*Glycyrrhizae radix*	*Zhi gan cao*	1.0
Citrus peel	*Citri pericarpium*	*Chen pi*	2.5
Perilla leaf	*Perillae folium*	*Zi su ye*	2.0
Ginger, fresh	*Zingiberis rhizoma*	*Sheng jiang*	1.5
Jujube	*Zizyphi fructus*	*Da zao*	4.5

*In some texts, perilla fruit is used, though the authors have found
perilla seed more effective.

Lung and Kidney *Yin* Deficiency

An aversion to heat, a flushed face, a dry mouth and throat, a cough with little sputum, insomnia, frequent, burning micturition of dark yellow urine, constipation, a red, fissured or denuded tongue, and a thready, rapid pulse characterize *yin* deficiency of the lungs and kidneys.

Treatment tonifies and moistens the lungs and kidneys and resolves phlegm. Eriobotrya and Ophiopogon Combination (*qing zao jiu fei tang*) can be used.

If there is copious sputum, Ophiopogon Combination (*mai men dong tang*) and Citrus and Pinellia Combination (*er chen tang*) can be used instead of Eriobotrya and Ophiopogon Combination.

If *yin* fails to check *yang* and kidney *qi* fails to regulate inhalation, thereby causing asthma, a flushed face and cold feet, Rehmannia and Schizandra Formula (*qi wei du qi wan*) can be used.

Spleen and Kidney *Yang* Deficiency

Chills; cold limbs; a cough with thin, copious sputum; shortness of breath; asthma aggravated following even minimal exertion; a feeling of oppression in the chest; abdominal fullness; a poor appetite; soreness and weakness in the lower back and legs; frequent, profuse and clear nocturia; diarrhea at dawn; a pale, plump tongue with deep teeth marks and a white coating; and a submerged, thready pulse characterize *yang* deficiency of the spleen and kidneys.

Treatment tonifies the spleen and warms the kidneys in order to improve inhalation and relieve asthma. Saussurea and Cardamom Combination (*xiang sha liu jun zi tang*) is the initial treatment. As soon as spleen functions have improved, it be replaced with Rehmannia Eight Formula (*ba wei di huang wan*).

For acupuncture and moxibustion treatment, please see the sections on cough and asthma in Chapter 4.

Section 2
Lobar Pneumonia

Lobar pneumonia is an acute infectious bacterial disease of the entire lung lobe which may occur any time during the year, but is more prevalent in the winter and spring. The disease occurs more often in men than in women and more often in the young and middle-aged than in the elderly. The onset is sudden and the main manifestations are chills, cough, high fever, dyspnea, chest pain, rusty-colored sputum, moist rales and congestion of the lungs. Pathological changes are considered atypical since mild lobar pneumonia occurs more frequently due to the wide application of antibiotics in modern societies. TCM herbs are very effective for this mild form, especially if the pneumonia is caused by some drug-resistant bacterial strain, in which case the use of antibiotics proves futile.

The major conformation of lobar pneumonia is excess heat-phlegm. Therefore, treatment aims to clear heat, detoxify and resolve phlegm, and promote the descent of lung *qi*. At the initial stage, the disease is associated with lung and *wei* (the superficial part of defensive energy) and should be treated by pungent, cool-natured herbs to dispel pathogenic factors from the exterior. When the accumulation of heat-phlegm is in the excess heat stage, the herbs to clear lung heat and resolve phlegm must be supplemented with other herbs which dispel the pathogenic factors. If heat-phlegm has dissipated, but residual pathogenic factors remain, the primary treatment should reinforce *qi*, nourish *yin* and moisten the lungs.

Diagnosis and Herbal Treatment

Attack by External Pathogens on the Lungs and *Wei*

This condition is characterized by an aversion to cold; fever; body aches; a cough with white or yellow sputum; a feeling of oppression and a low-level, nonspecific pain in the chest; thirst; redness along the edges of the tongue; a thin, white or yellow tongue coating; and a floating, rapid pulse.

Treatment dispels pathogenic factors from the exterior with pungent, cool-natured herbs which clear the lungs and resolve phlegm. Lonicera and Forsythia Formula (*yin qiao san*) and Morus and Lycium Formula (*xie bai san*) are recommended.

Heat-phlegm Accumulation in the Lungs

This condition is characterized by a high fever, with or without shivers; no aversion to cold; thirst; chest pain when coughing; thick, yellow or rusty-colored sputum; flared nostrils; labored breathing; dark yellow urine; a dry tongue with a yellow coating; and a surging, large pulse or a slippery, rapid pulse.

Treatment clears heat, detoxifies and ventilates the lungs, and resolves phlegm. *Ma-huang* and Apricot Seed Combination (*ma xing shi gan tang*) and Phragmites Combination (*wei jing tang*) can be given.

If the high fever does not subside, 10 *qian* each of houttuynia (*yu xing cao*) and polygonum (*kai jin suo*) and 5 *qian* dandelion (*pu gong ying*) can be added to help clear heat and detoxify the lungs.

To relieve severe chest pain, add 5 *qian* salvia (*dan shen*) and 3 *qian* red peony (*chi shao*) to the basic formula.

For constipation, add 1-2 *qian* rhubarb (*da huang*).

Qi and *Yin* Deficiency

In this case, heat-phlegm remains in the lungs. The characteristic symptoms are a cough, a slight fever, spontaneous sweating, a feverish sensation in the palms and soles, lassitude, a poor appetite, a red tongue with a thin coating, and a thready, rapid pulse.

Treatment replenishes *qi*, nourishes *yin*, moistens the lungs and resolves phlegm. Gypsum Combination (*bai hu tang*) and Ophiopogon Combination (*mai men dong tang*) can be used.

Section 3
Pulmonary Abscesses

According to TCM, pulmonary abscesses are usually caused by external pathogens attacking the lungs, which then become scorched, or the accumulation of heat-phlegm, which results in *qi* and blood stasis. If these conditions linger, the blood and tissues will become impaired and abscesses will form.

Pulmonary abscesses can also, at least to some degree, be related to the patient's constitution and diet. Either the impairment of *qi* and blood due to fatigue or overconsumption of spicy or greasy foods can prompt an accumulation of heat-dampness. If wind-heat evil then attacks the body, pulmonary abscesses are likely to occur.

Diagnosis and Herbal Treatment

Through an assessment of clinical manifestations, this disease is usually identified by the stage of its development and treated accordingly. In general, the primary treatment is clearing the lungs, resolving phlegm and purging the pathogen. The latter is especially important and, therefore, early tonification should be avoided in order to prevent the pathogenic factors from accumulating in the body and thereby making their removal extremely difficult.

Initial Stage

Chills, fever, cough, chest pain, small amounts of thick sputum, dyspnea, a dry mouth and nose, a thin, yellow tongue coating and a floating, slippery and rapid pulse characterize the initial stage.

Treatment expels wind and cold evils, clears the lungs and resolves phlegm. Lonicera and Forsythia Formula (*yin qiao san*) can be used.

If there is a severe headache, add 3 *qian* vitex (*man jin zi*).

For a severe cough with profuse sputum, add 1 *qian* fritillaria (*bei mu*).

If the patient is running a high fever, add 2 *qian* scute (*huang qin*).

Chest pain requires the addition of 3 *qian* each of red peony (*chi shao*) and turmeric (*yu jin*).

If the patient is prone to fidgeting and has a dry cough, add 3 *qian* each of glehnia root (*sha shen*) and ophiopogon (*mai men dong*).

Abscess-forming Stage

This stage is characterized by a high fever which is not relieved by sweating and which may or may not be accompanied by chills; a cough with dyspnea; asthma with chest fullness; the spitting up of thick, foul-smelling sputum which is sometimes mixed with blood; pain and a feeling of oppression in the chest; dry mouth, throat, lips and nose; a red tongue with a yellow, greasy coating; and a slippery, rapid pulse.

Treatment detoxifies accumulated pathogens, clears heat and dissipates blood stasis. Phragmites Combination (*wei jing tang*) and Platycodon Combination (*jie geng tang*) can be used.

If there is a high fever, add 10 *qian* houttuynia (*yu xing cao*), 5 *qian* dandelion (*pu gong ying*), 4 *qian* lonicera (*jin yin hua*) and 3 *qian* apricot seed (*xing ren*).

If excess heat is present, add 10 *qian* each of isatis leaf (*da qing ye*) and polyphylla (*qi ye yi zhi hua*) and 5 *qian* sargentodoxa (*hong teng*).

If the patient experiences hemoptysis, add 5 *qian* each of field thistle (*xiao ji cao*) and raw rehmannia (*sheng di huang*), 3 *qian* each of moutan (*mu dan pi*) and lotus root node (*ou jie*) and 10 *qian* imperata (*bai mao gen*).

If there is profuse sputum, add 3 *qian* morus bark (*sang bai pi*) and 5 *qian* lepidium (*ting li zi*).

Platycodon Combination[1]

Jie Geng Tang

(Platycodon Decoction)

Platycodon	*Platycodi radix*	Jie geng	2.0
Licorice	*Glycyrrhizae radix*	Gan cao	2.0

Diabrotic Stage

This stage is characterized by a lingering cough with profuse, foul-smelling sputum, with or without blood; pain and a feeling of oppression in the chest; dyspnea and difficulty in breathing when lying down; a general feeling of being unusually warm; a flushed face; extreme thirst; listlessness; gauntness; pallor; spontaneous sweating or night sweats; a red tongue with a yellow, greasy coating; and a rapid or thready and rapid pulse.

Treatment is aimed at detoxifying, draining pus and clearing heat-phlegm by using Platycodon and *Chih-shih* Formula (*pai* nong san) and Phragmites Combination (wei jing tang), plus 4 qian lonicera (jin yin hua), 10 qian houttuynia (yu xing cao) and 5 qian each of forsythia (lian qian), thlaspi (bai jiang cao), sargentodoxa (hong teng) and polygonum (kai jin suo).

Platycodon and *Chih-shih* Formula[1]
Pai Nong San
(Evacuate Pus Powder)

Platycodon	Platycodi radix	Jie geng	2.0
Chih-shih	Aurantii fructus immaturus	Zhi shi	3.0
Peony	Paeoniae radix	Shao yao	3.0

For *qi* deficiency, add 4-5 *qian* astragalus (*huang qi*).

For blood deficiency, add 3 *qian* each of *tang-kuei* (*dang gui*), gelatin (*a jiao*) and ophiopogon (*mai meng dong*).

Convalescent Stage

In this stage the pathogen withdraws and the body's resistance gradually recovers. The fever, cough and purulent sputum are gradually relieved, and the patient's physical strength and appetite slowly improve. The tongue is red with a thin coating, and the pulse is thready and weak.

Treatment moistens the lungs, resolves phlegm, replenishes *qi* and nourishes *yin*. Eriobotrya and Ophiopogon Combination (*qing zao jiu fei tang*) can be used.

Section 4
Coronary Atherosclerotic Cardiopathy

Coronary atherosclerotic cardiopathy (CAC), also known as coronary heart disease (CHD), is caused by atherosclerosis of the coronary artery. Stenosis or occlusion of the coronary artery impairs the cardiac muscle, preventing it from obtaining adequate blood and oxygen supplies. The clinical manifestations of CHD are angina pectoris, myocardiac infarction, arrhythmia, heart failure and cardiac dilation. Additionally, an electrocardiogram may show myocardial ischemia or other relevant changes.

Although the official name of the disease does not appear in ancient TCM literature, a disease with similar manifestations is found in many records. According to TCM, the conformations for CHD are obstruction of *qi* in the chest, chest pain, true angina pectoris and precordial pain with cold limbs. TCM theory contends that this disease is associated with old age and poor health. The latter may be attributed to one or both of the following factors: kidney *qi* deficiency or the excess consumption of rich or greasy foods, which impairs spleen and stomach functioning. Furthermore, this disease is related to both *qi* and blood stagnancy, caused by anxiety or long-term fatigue, as well as the invasion of the chest by cold evil, which results in obstruction and coagulation of *qi* and blood, pain and angina pectoris.

The spleen and kidneys are the deep-seated origin (*ben*) of the disease, while the stagnancy of *qi*, blood, phlegm or cold are the superficiality (*biao*).

Diagnosis and Herbal Treatment

CHD can be divided into two types: excess and deficiency. Clinically, both types can occur in the same patient, though the former is associated with *biao* and the latter with *ben*. When the excess is the more prominent conformation, it should be treated first. If the deficiency is dominant, the symptoms of *qi, yin* or kidney *yang* deficiency or of an exhaustion of kidney *yang* must be treated first.

Excess Conformations

In general, excess symptoms are similar to those of *qi* stagnancy, blood stasis, phlegm accumulation or dampness retention.

1. Obstruction of *yang* in the chest

Angina pectoris induced by cold is characterized by a shortness of breath, a sensation of oppression and suffocation in the chest, a greasy tongue coating and a wiry, slippery pulse. In a severe case, the angina pectoris radiates to the back.

Treatment activates *yang* and removes the obstruction. Trichosanthes, Bakeri and Pinellia Combination (*gua lou xie bai ban xia tang*) and Cinnamon and Ginseng Combination (*gui zhi ren shen tang*) can be used.

Cinnamon and Ginseng Combination[1]
Gui Zhi Ren Shen Tang
(Cinnamon Twig and Ginseng Decoction)[2]

Cinnamon twig	*Cinnamomi ramulus*	*Gui zhi*	2.0
Licorice	*Glycyrrhizae radix*	*Gan cao*	2.0
Ginseng	*Ginseng radix*	*Ren shen*	2.0
Ginger, dried	*Zingiberis siccatum rhizoma*	*Gan jiang*	2.0
Atractylodes, white	*Atractylodis rhizoma*	*Bai zhu*	3.0

2. Blood stasis in the heart and vessels

This condition is characterized by twinges in the heart and chest, distention and pain in the hypochondrium, shortness of breath, anxiety, petechiae on the tongue and a wiry, hesitant pulse.

Treatment activates blood circulation to remove stasis, soothes the liver and regulates the flow of *qi*. Bupleurum and Evodia Combination (*shu gan tang*) and Pteropus and Bulrush Formula (*shi xiao san*) can be used.

Bupleurum and Evodia Combination[1]

Shu Gan Tang
(Soothe the Liver Decoction)

Bupleurum	*Bupleuri radix*	*Chai hu*	5.0
Chih-ko	*Citri fructus*	*Zhi ke*	2.0
Tang-kuei	*Angelicae radix*	*Dang gui*	3.0
Persica	*Persicae semen*	*Tao ren*	3.0
Peony	*Paeoniae radix*	*Shao yao*	3.0
Immature citrus peel	*Citri immaturi pericarpium*	*Qing pi*	3.0
Cnidium	*Cnidii rhizoma*	*Chuan xiong**	3.0
Coptis	*Coptidis rhizoma*	*Huang lian*	1.0
Carthamus	*Carthami flos*	*Hong hua*	1.0
Evodia	*Evodiae fructus*	*Wu zhu yu*	0.5

**Ligustici rhizoma*, also known as *chuan xiong*, may be substituted.

Stagnancies of both *qi* and blood often appear simultaneously in clinical practice, with one usually more prominent than the other. Because *qi* controls blood circulation and *qi* stagnancy can induce blood stasis, *qi* stagnancy complicated by blood stasis should be treated with herbs to regulate the circulation of *qi*, with less of a focus on herbs to resolve the blood stasis. Herbs such as chinaberry (*chuan lian zi*), corydalis (*yan hu suo*), finger citron (*fo shou gan*), cyperus (*xiang fu zi*) and *chih-ko* (*zhi ke*) can be selected.

Alternately, blood stasis may obstruct *qi* circulation, and so a blood stasis conformation complicated by *qi* stagnancy should be treated with herbs to promote blood circulation, with less of a concentration on herbs to regulate *qi* circulation. Herbs such as cattail pollen (*pu huang*), pteropus (*wu ling zhi*), notoginseng (*san qi*), calamus gum (*xue jie*), myrrh (*mo yao*) and frankincense (*ru xiang*) are recommended.

3. Retention of turbid phlegm

This condition is characterized by pain or a feeling of oppression in the chest, obesity, a sensation of heaviness in the body, listlessness, a thick and greasy or dirty and greasy tongue coating and a slippery, excess pulse.

Treatment eliminates dampness through the use of aromatics and regulates spleen functioning to resolve phlegm. Styrax Formula (*su he xiang wan*) and Hoelen and Bamboo Combination (*wen dan tang*) can be used.

If there is heat-phlegm, add 1 *qian* coptis (*huang lian*).

If phlegm and *qi* stagnancies affect chest *yang*, add 3 *qian* each of long pepper (*pi bo*) and aristolochia (*qing mu xiang*), 2 *qian* santalum (*tan xiang*) and 1 *qian* aquilaria (*chen xiang*).

Deficiency Conformations

1. *Qi* and *yin* deficiency

This form of angina pectoris is characterized by a shortness of breath, palpitation, spontaneous sweating, a dry mouth with very little saliva, a red tongue with very little coating and a wiry, thready and weak pulse or a slow, uneven and intermittent pulse.

Treatment nourishes *qi* and *yin* with Ginseng and Ophiopogon Formula (*sheng mai san*) and Baked Licorice Combination (*zhi gan cao tang*).

If there is severe angina pectoris, add 1 *qian* aquilaria (*chen xiang*) and 3 *qian* turmeric (*yu jin*).

For reducing excess liver *yang* which is due to *yin* deficiency, add 3 *qian* each of uncaria stem with hooks (*gou teng*), morus leaf (*sang ye*) and gardenia (*zhi zi*).

Add 3 *qian* each of *fu-shen* (*fu shen*) and zizyphus (*suan zao ren*), 2 *qian* polygala (*yuan zi*) and 5 *qian* albizzia (*he huan pi*) for relief of irritability and anxiety.

2. Kidney *yang* deficiency

This variety of angina pectoris is characterized by shortness of breath, palpitation, chills, cold limbs, soreness in the lower back and knees, a pale tongue with a white coating, and a submerged, weak pulse or a slow, uneven and intermittent pulse.

Rehmannia Eight Formula (*ba wei di huang wan*) can be used for warming and replenishing kidney *yang.*

For relief of palpitation and insomnia, add 5 *qian* each of dragon bone (*long gu*) and oyster shell (*mu li*) and 3 *qian* of zizyphus (*suan zao ren*).

For treating impotence or premature ejaculation, add 3 *qian* each of curculigo (*xian mao*) and epimedium (*yin yang huo*).

For strengthening deficient spleen *yang*, add 3 *qian* each of codonopsis (*dang shen*) and white atractylodes (*bai zhu*), 1 *qian* dried ginger (*gan jiang*) and 2 *qian* licorice (*gan cao*).

3. *Yang* deficiency to the point of exhaustion

This form of angina pectoris is characterized by a shortness of breath, profuse sweating, cold limbs, pallor, a pale tongue with a white coating, an extremely submerged, faint pulse which can hardly be felt or a slow, uneven and intermittent pulse, and even syncope.

Treatment restores depleted *yang*, thereby rescuing the patient from total collapse. Dragon Bone, Oyster Shell, Ginseng and Aconite Combination (*shen fu long mu tang*), which is made by adding 3 *qian* each of ginseng (*ren shen*) and prepared aconite (*zhi fu zi*) to Dragon Bone and Oyster Shell

Combination (*long gu mu li tang*), should be given immediately.

Preventative Measures

1. Stress management which includes daily exercise.

2. Proper diet to prevent excess weight gain and a high cholesterol level.

3. Herbal therapy to lower the blood lipid level. The following herbs are recommended: *ho-shou-wu* (*he shou wu*), crataegus (*shan zha*), loranthus (*sang ji sheng*) and giant knotweed root (*hu zhang*).

4. Avoidance of smoking or of second-hand smoke.

5. Reduction in the intake of caffeinated or alcoholic beverages.

6. Control of hypertension through the use of TCM herbs or Western medicines.

7. Reduction of blood viscosity through the use of salvia (*dan shen*) tablets.

Acupuncture and Moxibustion Treatment

Points of First Choice

- *neiguan* (P 6)
- *zusanli* (S 36)
- *tanzhong* (CV 17, with moxibustion)
- *jujue* (CV 14, with moxibustion)

Reserved Points

- *xinshu* (B 15)
- *jueyinshu* (B 14)
- *ximen* (P 4)
- *jianshi* (P 5)
- *tongli* (H 5)
- *sanyinjiao* (Sp 6)

Coordinated Points

1. Paroxysmal auricular fibrillation or premature beat
   - *yinxi* (H 6)
   - *neiguan* (P 6)

2. Tachycardia
   - *xiabai* (L 4)
   - *shousanli* (LI 10)

3. Bradycardia
   - *tongli* (H 5)
   - *neiguan* (P 6)

Section 5
Hypertension

A distinction is made between primary hypertension, which is used to refer to a chronic vascular disease characterized by high artery blood pressure, especially with continuous high diastolic pressure, and secondary or symptomatic hypertension, which is only a symptom of some other disease. According to its clinical manifestations, hypertension can be classified into the TCM conformations of dizziness or headache.

The most common causes of the disease are fire due to liver *qi* stagnancy, which in turn is due to long-term mental stress, or kidney *yin* deficiency attributable to fatigue or old age. Kidney *yin* deficiency consumes body fluids and thus impairs the nourishment of the liver, causing an excess of liver *yang*. Furthermore, overconsumption of greasy or sweet foods or of alcoholic beverages can result in an accumulation of turbid phlegm. Any of the above can exacerbate the others, creating an imbalance of *yin* and *yang*, especially *yin* deficiency of the liver and kidneys, which can then give rise to excess liver *yang*. This imbalance can create a deficiency in the lower body and an excess in the upper body. Moreover, excess *yang* may transform into interior wind-fire, which, in turn, can transform body fluids into phlegm. In some severe cases, excess phlegm can induce apoplexy or syncope.

Diagnosis and Herbal Treatment

Liver Fire

Dizziness, headache, a flushed face, conjunctival congestion, a bitter taste in the mouth, fidgeting, constipation, red-tinged urine, a red tongue with a yellow coating, and a wiry pulse characterize liver fire.

Treatment soothes the liver and purges fire with Gentian Combination (*long dan xie gan tang*).

For constipation, add 2 *qian* rhubarb (*da huang*).

For a severe headache and dizziness, add 10 *qian* each of haliotis (*shi jue ming*) and nacre (*zhen zhu mu*).

For a dry mouth and tongue, add 3 *qian* scrophularia (*xuan shen*) and 5 *qian* dendrobium (*shi hu*).

Excess *Yang* Due to *Yin* Deficiency

This condition is characterized by headache, dizziness, soreness and weakness in the lower back and knees, tinnitus, memory loss or a poor memory, a feverish sensation in the palms, soles and heart area, palpitation, insomnia, a red tongue with a thin coating, and a wiry, thready and rapid pulse.

Treatment nourishes *yin* and suppresses excess *yang*. Lycium, Chrysanthemum and Rehmannia Formula (*qi ju di huang wan*), plus 10 *qian* oyster shell (*mu li*) and 3 *qian* tortoise shell (*gui ban*), can be given.

For severe dizziness, add 10 *qian* haliotis (*shi jue ming*) and 2 *qian* gastrodia (*tian ma*).

For *yin* deficiency resulting in constipation, add 3 *qian* each of linum (*ma zi ren*) and biota (*bo zi ren*).

Deficiency of Both *Yin* and *Yang*

Dizziness, headache, tinnitus, palpitation, shortness of breath even following the slightest physical activity, soreness and weakness in the lower back and legs, insomnia, drowsiness, muscular twitching and cramps, a pale or red tongue with a white coating, and a wiry, thready pulse are characteristic of deficiency of both *yin* and *yang*.

Treatment nourishes *yin* and strengthens *yang*. Curculigo and Epimedium Combination (*er xian tang*) can be used to meet these ends.

Curculigo and Epimedium Combination
Er Xian Tang[26]
(Two Immortal Decoction)[2]

Curculigo	*Curculiginis rhizoma*	*Xian mao*	3.0
Epimedium	*Epimedii herba*	*Yin yang huo*	3.0
Tang-kuei	*Angelicae radix*	*Dang gui*	3.0
Phellodendron	*Phellodendri cortex*	*Huang bo*	3.0
Anemarrhena	*Anemarrhenae rhizoma*	*Zhi mu*	3.0
Morinda	*Morindae radix*	*Ba ji tian*	3.0

For a dry mouth and throat and a feverish sensation in the palms and soles, add 5 *qian* dendrobium (*shi hu*) and 3 *qian* tortoise shell (*gui ban*).

For chills and cold limbs, add 3 *qian* each of antler (*lu jiao*) and eucommia (*du zhong*).

Accumulation of Phlegm-dampness

Dizziness, headache, a feeling of oppression in the chest, heavy-headedness, palpitation, a poor appetite, the spitting up of phlegm and fluids, a white, greasy tongue coating and a slippery pulse characterize phlegm-dampness accumulation.

Treatment aims at dispelling phlegm and resolving dampness with Pinellia and Gastrodia Combination (*ban xia bai zhu tian ma tang*).

For numbness in the limbs, add 3 *qian* each of uncaria stem with hooks (*gou teng*) and acorus (*chang pu*).

For palpitation and insomnia, add 3 *qian* each of zizyphus (*suan zao ren*) and anemarrhena (*zhi mu*).

Acupuncture and Moxibustion Treatment

Points of First Choice

- *baihui* (GV 20)
- *zusanli* (S 36, with moxibustion)
- *fengchi* (G 20)
- *xuanzhong* (G 39, with moxibustion)

Reserved Points

- *ganshu* (B 18)
- *taichong* (Liv 3)
- *shenshu* (B 23)
- *taixi* (K 3)

Treatment Method

1. Select two or three points of first choice, plus one or two reserved points for each treatment.
2. Administer a total of 10 treatments.

Section 6
Gastric or Duodenal Ulcer (Peptic Ulcer)

The most prominent symptom of a gastric or duodenal ulcer is pain in the mid-upper abdomen. For this reason, TCM generally refers to it as "the stomach disease." Alternately, it also belongs to the conformation of pain in the stomach area, pain in the liver and stomach due to irregular *qi* circulation, pain in the heart area or acid regurgitation.

The etiology of the disease is complicated. For example, stagnant liver *qi* due to persistent melancholy, anxiety or anger can attack the stomach and reverse the flow of stomach *qi*, or *qi* and blood circulation may become obstructed as a result of a spleen and stomach disorder caused by irregular eating habits or excess consumption of greasy foods or alcoholic beverages.

Yet another possibility is the excess consumption of raw or cold foods, which are difficult to digest. This results in deficiencies of spleen *yang*, stomach *qi* and kidney *yang*. These deficiencies impair digestion, as well as the transformation and transportation of fluids and nutrients. Turbid dampness results, which then obstructs the circulation of stomach *qi*.

Diagnosis and Herbal Treatment

Qi Stagnancy

Distended pain which is felt in the hypochondrium and relieved by eructation and the passing of flatus is the distinguishing symptom. Furthermore, fullness, distention and pain in the mid-upper abdomen, eructation, acid regurgitation, irritability, frequent sighing, poor appetite, a thin, white tongue coating and a submerged, wiry pulse characterize *qi* stagnancy.

Treatment regulates liver *qi*, harmonizes the stomach and relieves pain with Bupleurum and Cyperus Combination (*chai hu shu gan tang*).

If the patient feels cold in the mid-upper abdomen, add 1 *qian* each of evodia (*wu zhu yu*) and dried ginger (*gan jiang*).

For a burning sensation in the mid-upper abdomen, add 1 *qian* coptis (*huang lian*) and 3 *qian* gardenia (*zhi zi*).

Heat Stagnancy

Acute, severe pain with a burning sensation in the upper abdomen is the distinguishing characteristic of a heat stagnancy-induced peptic ulcer. This burning is not relieved by eating and may even be aggravated following meals. The patient has a preference for cold beverages, a dry mouth, a bitter taste in the mouth, constipation and gastric discomfort with acid regurgitation. The urine is dark yellow, the tongue is red with a greasy, yellow coating, and the pulse is wiry and rapid.

Treatment nourishes liver *yin* to harmonize the stomach and purge heat. Coptis and Rehmannia Formula (*qing wei san*) and Ophiopogon Combination (*mai men dong tang*) can be given.

If heat stagnancy in the liver and stomach causes bleeding, Coptis and Rhubarb Combination (*san huang xie xin tang*) should be used instead of the two above-mentioned formulas.

Deficiency-cold

A dull pain in the upper abdomen which is relieved by pressure, hot compresses and food, but aggravated by cold, is the predominant characteristic of a peptic ulcer induced by deficiency-cold. Other signs and symptoms include an aversion to cold, a sallow complexion, cold limbs, lassitude, regurgitation of watery fluids, loose stools, a pale tongue with a thin, white coating, and a soft, floating and thready pulse.

Treatment strengthens the spleen, harmonizes the stomach and warms the middle energizer in order to dispel the cold evil. Aconite and G.L. Combination (*fu zi li zhong tang*) or Astragalus Combination (*huang qi jian zhong tang*) can be used.

For fullness and distention in the mid-upper abdomen accompanied by a poor appetite, add 3 *qian* citrus (*chen pi*) and 1 *qian* amomum fruit (*sha ren*).

If the patient is troubled by frequent acid regurgitation, add 5 *qian* cuttlebone (*hai piao xiao*) and 10 *qian* calcined ark shell (*wa leng zi*).

For watery fluid regurgitation, add 1 *qian* clove (*ding xiang*) and 3 *qian* pinellia (*ban xia*).

Blood Stasis

Severe, fixed pain in the upper abdomen which feels as if the patient were being cut by a knife and which is aggravated by pressure is the distinguishing symptom of a peptic ulcer due to blood stasis. The pain may radiate to the chest and back and is often accompanied by cold limbs, sweating, repeated hematemesis, melena, a dark purple tongue with ecchymosis and a wiry or thready and hesitant pulse.

Treatment regulates *qi*, harmonizes the stomach and promotes blood circulation in order to remove blood stasis. Persica and Carthamus Combination (*ge xia zhu yu tang*) can be used.

Acupuncture and Moxibustion Treatment

Group #1
- *zhongwan* (CV 12)
- *liangmen* (S 21)
- *zusanli* (S 36)

Group #2
- *weishu* (B 21)
- *liangqiu* (S 34)
- *neiguan* (P 6)

Reserved Points
- *pishu* (B 20)
- *ganshu* (B 18)
- *taichong* (Liv 3)
- *gongsun* (Sp 4)
- *sanyinjiao* (Sp 6)

Treatment Method

1. Alternate the use of points from the first and second groups.
2. Treat every day or every other day for a total of 10 treatments.
3. If this treatment regimen is ineffective or not as effective as desired, add two reserved points during each treatment session.

Section 7
Chronic Gastritis

Chronic gastritis is one of the most common chronic stomach diseases. Its main pathogenic characteristic is a non-specific, chronic inflammation of the gastric mucosa, and its prominent clinical manifestations are dyspepsia and chronic pain in the upper abdomen. There is a high incidence in males between the ages of 20 and 40, however, the incidence of atrophic chronic gastritis is even higher in men older than 40.

According to TCM theory, chronic gastritis is generally caused by a dietary disorder aggravated by an emotional disturbance. Improper diet results in a disharmony between the spleen and stomach. *Zheng qi* (resistant energy) then becomes deficient, prompting an extreme emotional response, which, in turn, results in disharmony between the liver and spleen and, ultimately, liver *qi* stagnancy. This *qi* stagnancy can transform into fire and cause heat to accumulate in the liver and stomach, thereby exhausting stomach *yin* and impairing the stomach's ability to moisten and aid in the descent of *qi*.

Since the initial disease resides in *qi* and the persistent illness is located in the collaterals, if *qi* stagnancy injures the collaterals, blood stasis may occur. If the disease continues for a long time and results in a deficiency of the middle energizer, or if the spleen and stomach are deficient, or if excessive amounts of raw or cold foods have been consumed, spleen *yang* will become impaired. This, in turn, may impair the spleen's ability to transport nutrients, as well as a failure of stomach *qi* to descend, resulting in a deficiency-cold conformation.

Diagnosis and Herbal Treatment

Liver and Stomach *Qi* Stagnancy

This type of *qi* stagnancy is characterized by distention and pain in the mid-upper abdomen, fullness in the upper abdomen which is aggravated after meals or by emotional stress, pain which radiates to the hypochondrium, frequent eructation, pain relieved by passing flatus, nausea, vomiting, acid regurgitation, a thin, white tongue coating and a submerged, wiry pulse.

Treatment soothes the liver and harmonizes stomach *qi* with Bupleurum and *Chih-shih* Formula (*si ni san*) and Melia and Corydalis Formula (*jin ling zi san*).

Melia and Corydalis Formula
Jin Ling Zi San[26]
(Melia Toosendan Powder)[2]

Melia	*Meliae toosendan fructus*	*Chuan lian zi*	3.0
Corydalis	*Corydalis rhizoma*	*Yan hu suo*	4.0

To treat acid regurgitation, add 3 *qian* cuttlebone (*hai piao xiao*), 5 *qian* ark shell (*wa leng zi*) and Coptis and Evodia Formula (*zuo jin wan*).

To treat food retention in the stomach, poor appetite, fullness and distention in the upper abdomen and a thick, greasy tongue coating, add 3 *qian* each of *shen-chu* (*shen qu*) and crataegus (*shan zha*) and 5 *qian* malt (*mai ya*).

Severe, fixed pain which is aggravated by pressure indicates that the illness has affected the collaterals. In this case, Pteropus and Bulrush Formula (*shi xiao san*) should be added.

Stomach Heat Due to *Yin* Deficiency

Burning pain in the mid-upper abdomen which is aggravated in the afternoon or when the patient is hungry and relieved by meals is the primary symptom. Others include a dry, bitter-tasting mouth, fidgeting, irritability, poor appetite, a red tongue with a dry, yellow coating, and a wiry, thready and rapid pulse.

Treatment nourishes *yin* and clears the stomach. Coptis and Rehmannia Formula (*qing wei san*) and Rehmannia and Gypsum Combination (*yu nu jian*) are recommended.

If the heat is serious, add 10 *qian* of dandelion (*pu gong ying*).

If the patient is constipated, add 2 *qian* rhubarb (*da huang*).

Spleen and Stomach Deficiency

Vague pain in the mid-upper abdomen which is relieved by pressure, a preference for hot beverages, a poor appetite, distention and fullness in the stomach following meals, the spitting up of watery fluids, pallor, lassitude, cold limbs, a pale tongue with a white coating, and a submerged, thready and weak pulse characterize spleen and stomach deficiency.

Treatment reinforces spleen *qi* and warms and harmonizes the stomach. Saussurea and Cardamom Combination (*xiang sha liu jun zi tang*) or Astragalus Combination (*huang qi jian zhong tang*) can be used.

To treat poor appetite and severe distention in the upper abdomen following meals, add 3 *qian* chicken gizzard lining (*ji nei jin*), 5 *qian* each of malt (*mai ya*) and germinated rice (*gu ya*) and 1 *qian tsao-tou-kou* (*cao dou kou*).

If the patient's complexion, lips and tongue are pale, add 2 *qian* cnidium (*chuan xiong*) and 3 *qian* each of *tang-kuei* (*dang gui*) and peony (*shao yao*).

Acupuncture and Moxibustion Treatment

Points of First Choice
- *zhongwan* (CV 12)
- *neiguan* (P 6)
- *weishu* (B 21)
- *zusanli* (S 36)

Reserved Points
- *ganshu* (B 18)
- *taixi* (K 3)
- *gongsun* (Sp 4)
- *pishu* (B 20)
- *taichong* (Liv 3)

Treatment Method

1. Use moxibustion with the points of first choice in the case of a cold conformation.
2. Use the points of first choice every day or every other day for a total of 10 treatment sessions.
3. Add two reserved points if the points of first choice are not as effective as desired.

Section 8
Chronic Nonspecific Ulcerative Colitis

Chronic nonspecific ulcerative colitis is an inflammatory disease which primarily affects the mucosa and submucous layer of the rectum and descending colon, though in many instances the entire colon is involved. As a chronic disease, it goes through alternating periods of remission and exacerbation, the latter of which is characterized by rectal bleeding, diarrhea and abdominal pain which vary in severity and appear principally in persons between the ages of 30 and 40. Though there exists no specific treatment in Western medicine, TCM is very effective in combating mild cases.

According to TCM theory, the etiology of the disease is attributed to the spleen's inability to transport and transform fluids and nutrients because the spleen and stomach are attacked by external evils, thus accumulating dampness which is transformed into heat-dampness. The heat-dampness accumulates in the large intestine, blocking *qi* and blood circulation, and thereby forming pus. Abdominal pain, diarrhea and mucous or bloody stools may be observed.

Diagnosis and Herbal Treatment

Descent of Heat-dampness

This is usually seen in the initial episode and is manifested as fever, abdominal pain, diarrhea, tenesmus, bloody and mucous stools, a greasy, yellow tongue coating and a slippery, rapid pulse.

Treatment clears heat and eliminates dampness. Anemone Combination (*bai tou weng tang*) and Saussurea and Coptis Formula (*xiang lian wan*) can be given.

Saussurea and Coptis Formula[1]
Xiang Lian Wan
(Saussurea and Coptis Pill)

Saussurea	*Saussureae radix*	Mu xiang	3.0
Coptis	*Coptidis rhizoma*	Huang lian	12.0

Take one 1-*qian* pill, three times daily.

If there is a high fever, add 3 *qian* each of scute (*huang qin*) and lonicera (*jin yin hua*).

If dampness is excessive, add 3 *qian* each of magnolia bark (*hou pu*) and atractylodes (*cang zhu*).

Liver Excess and Spleen Deficiency

Diarrhea usually occurs after emotional stress or upset. Distention and pain in the chest and hypochondrium, fullness in the stomach, poor appetite, a thin, white tongue coating and a thready, wiry pulse are indicators of liver excess and spleen deficiency.

Treatment soothes the liver and strengthens the spleen. Siler and Atractylodes Formula (*tong xie yao fang*) can be used.

Spleen and Stomach Deficiency

Intermittent attacks, borborygmus, diarrhea with undigested stools, a poor appetite, a feeling of oppression in the chest, lassitude, a pale tongue with a white coating, and a floating, soft pulse characterize a deficiency of both the spleen and stomach.

Treatment tonifies the spleen and stomach with Ginseng and Atractylodes Formula (*shen ling bai zhu san*).

If there is residual heat, add Saussurea and Coptis Formula (*xiang lian wan*).

Kidney *Yang* Deficiency

This is commonly seen in lingering cases. An aversion to cold, pallor, lower back pain, cold knees, borborygmus and diarrhea at dawn and a submerged, thready and weak pulse are indicative of kidney *yang* deficiency.

Treatment warms kidney *yang* and arrests diarrhea with astringent herbs. Kaolin and Limonite Combination (*chi shi zhi yu yu liang tang*) and Psoralea and Myristica Formula (*si shen wan*) are recommended.

Kaolin and Limonite Combination[1]
Chi Shi Zhi Yu Yu Liang Tang
(Kaolin and Limonite Decoction)

Kaolin	*Halloysitum rubrum*	*Chi shi zhi*	5.0
Limonite	*Limonitum*	*Yu yu liang*	5.0

Acupuncture and Moxibustion Treatment

Points of First Choice

- *guanyuan* (CV 4)
- *tianshu* (St 25)
- *gongsun* (Sp 4)

Reserved Points

- *pishu* (B 20)
- *shenshu* (B 23)
- *mingmen* (GV 4)
- *zusanli* (S 36)

Treatment Method

1. Apply acupuncture or moxibustion during alternate treatment sessions.

2. Use the points of first choice with two or three reserved points daily or every other day for a total of 10 treatment sessions.

Section 9
Acute Edematous Pancreatitis

Acute edematous pancreatitis is a chemical inflammation due to the autodigestion of pancreatic tissue by pancreatic enzymes. The clinical manifestations are a sudden onset with severe pain in the epigastrium, fever, nausea, vomiting and elevated serum amylase and esterase levels.

Though no exact etiology has of yet been ascertained, the condition is usually associated with improper diet. Splenic functioning may become impaired by overeating, excess consumption of alcoholic beverages or excess intake of greasy or sweet foods, thus causing food retention in the middle energizer. This retained food is then transformed into heat-dampness, resulting in an excess conformation known as *yang ming*. Furthermore, stagnant liver *qi* can disturb the liver's ability to regulate *qi* flow, causing an accumulation of heat-dampness in the liver and gallbladder. Spleen and stomach functioning is thereby impaired, with acute edematous pancreatitis as the result.

Diagnosis and Herbal Treatment

Qi Stagnancy and Food Retention

Intermittent distention and pain in the epigastrium and hypochondrium, frequent eructation, nausea, constipation, a thin tongue coating and a wiry pulse characterize *qi* stagnancy aggravated by food retention.

Treatment soothes the liver, regulates *qi*, clears heat and voids the bowels by the purgation method. Major Bupleurum Combination (*da chai hu tang*), along with 3 *qian* saussurea (*mu xiang*) and 4 *qian* corydalis (*yan hu suo*), can be given.

Excess Heat in the Spleen and Stomach

Fullness, distention and pain in the mid-upper abdomen which is aggravated by pressure; constipation; a dry mouth; a greasy, thick and yellow or dry tongue coating; and a slippery, rapid pulse characterize excess heat in the spleen and stomach.

Treatment removes heat by the purgation method. Major Rhubarb Combination (*da cheng qi tang*), together with Bupleurum and *Chih-shih* Formula (*si ni san*), can be used.

Heat-dampness in the Liver and Gallbladder

Pain in the epigastrium and hypochondrium, fever, jaundice, a feeling of heaviness in the body, lassitude, a greasy, yellow tongue coating and a wiry, slippery and rapid pulse characterize heat-dampness in the liver and gallbladder.

Treatment clears the liver and gallbladder and removes heat-dampness. Gentian Combination (*long dan xie gan tang*) with Capillaris Combination (*yin chen hao tang*) can be given.

If the patient suffers from frequent episodes of acute pancreatitis, dyspepsia and fatty diarrhea will be observed. In this case, Bupleurum and Cyperus Combination (*shu gan san*) is recommended for the relief of symptoms and the prevention of relapses.

Common Acupuncture and Moxibustion Points

First Treatment

- *zhongwan* (CV 12)
- *liangmen* (S 21)

Second Treatment

- *zhongwan* (CV 12)
- *danshu* (B 19)
- *zusanli* (S 36)

Third Treatment

- *dadu* (Sp 2)
- *taibai* (Sp 3)

Section 10
Infectious Hepatitis

Infectious hepatitis is caused by the hepatitis virus and is divided into four types: A, B, D and non-A, non-B. Though it is not found in classic TCM literature, similar diseases have been recorded. *Nei Jing* (Internal Classic) points out that the chief symptoms of jaundice are "yellow-brown pigmentation of the sclera" and "dark yellow urine." In Hong Ge's works, written during the Jin dynasty, it is stated that "epidemic jaundice" is caused by "heat and toxic materials invading the interior." Finally, *Zhou Hou Bei Ji Fang* (A Handbook of Prescriptions for Emergencies) states that this disease is considered infectious.

According to TCM theory, infectious hepatitis is generally classified into the conformation of jaundice, pain in the hypochondrium and heat-dampness, and it is commonly held that heat-dampness pathogens are its primary cause. Although patient constitutions and degrees of toxicity of the virus vary greatly, there are two broad clinical types, namely, icteric and anicteric. Differentiation is often made as to whether dampness or heat is more severe or whether they are of comparable severity.

This disease primarily attacks the liver, as *Ling Su* (Miraculous Pivot--A Treatise on the Five Evils) points out: "If there is evil in the liver, there is pain on both sides of the hypochondrium." These pathologic changes, however, are also closely related to the spleen and stomach.

Diagnosis and Herbal Treatment

Heat-dampness Accumulation
1. Heat more severe than dampness

Dryness and pain in the throat, a dry mouth with a bitter taste, pain in the hypochondrium, abdominal distention, dry stools or constipation, dark yellow urine, facial acne, cutaneous pruritus, irritability, fidgeting, a feverish sensation, a feeling of oppression in the chest, a dry, red tongue with a white or greasy, yellow coating, and a wiry or rapid and large pulse characterize hepatitis in which heat is more severe than dampness.

2. Dampness more severe than heat

A feeling of oppression in the chest, nausea, vomiting, lassitude, a feeling of heaviness in the limbs, abdominal distention, hypochondriac pain, a poor appetite, loose stools, a pale tongue with a greasy, white or thick, greasy coating, especially on the root of the tongue, and a slow, soft and floating or wiry and thready pulse characterize hepatitis in which dampness is more severe than heat.

Heat-dampness conformation is often seen in acute icteric, acute anicteric and chronic active hepatitis, all of which are classifications from Western medicine.

In acute icteric hepatitis, heat-dampness attacks the spleen and disturbs its transportation and transformation functions. This causes an accumulation of dampness, which transforms into heat. The retention of heat-dampness in the spleen and stomach affects the liver and gallbladder and causes the bile to flow into the skin, resulting in jaundice.

Though most of the symptoms of heat-dampness conformation are present, in acute anicteric hepatitis, they are generally less severe than in acute icteric hepatitis. Furthermore, jaundice is not associated with the anicteric form.

Chronic active hepatitis, which includes some forms of chronic persistent hepatitis, can generally be categorized under the TCM conformation of deficiency in origin and excess in superficiality. The deficiency is caused by a lingering disease, while the excess is due to an accumulation of heat-dampness. Heat transforms into fire, impairing *yin*, thus creating excess interior heat and so a conformation of heat-dampness and interior heat with *yin* deficiency.

Treatment for all forms of heat-dampness-induced hepatitis aims at clearing heat and removing dampness. Capillaris Combination (*yin chen hao tang*) can be used when heat dominates dampness, while Capillaris and Hoelen Five Formula (*yin chen wu ling san*), along with Magnolia and Ginger Formula (*ping wei san*), can be used when dampness dominates heat. Gardenia and Phellodendron Combination (*zhi zi bo pi tang*), together with Hoelen Five Herb Formula (*wu ling san*), can be used when heat and dampness are equally troublesome.

To treat interior heat associated with *yin* deficiency, add 3 *qian* each of raw rehmannia (*sheng di huang*) and dendrobium (*shi hu*) to any of the therapies recommended in the preceding paragraph.

Gardenia and Phellodendron Combination[1]

Zhi Zi Bo Pi Tang
(Gardenia and Phellodendron Decoction)[2]

Gardenia	*Gardeniae fructus*	*Zhi zi*	3.0
Phellodendron	*Phellodendri cortex*	*Huang bo*	2.0
Licorice	*Glycyrrhizae radix*	*Gan cao*	1.0

Liver *Qi* Stagnancy

This is commonly seen in chronic nonactive hepatitis (hepatosplenomegaly with normal test levels for liver functioning) or in some cases of anicteric hepatitis. Liver *qi* stagnancy may be caused by a failure of the liver to regulate *qi* circulation and to harmonize with the stomach.

Pain in the hypochondrium, abdominal distention, pain in the mid-upper abdomen, a slight fever, dizziness, a feeling of oppression in the chest, irritability, nausea, eructation, a poor appetite, weak limbs, lassitude, a pale tongue with a thin, white coating or a thin, greasy coating on the root of the tongue, and a wiry, rapid pulse are all characteristics of liver *qi* stagnancy.

Treatment soothes the liver, regulates *qi* and harmonizes the stomach. *Tang-kuei* and Bupleurum Formula (*xiao yao san*) or Bupleurum and Cyperus Combination (*chai hu shu gan tang*) can be used.

Internal Heat Due to *Yin* Deficiency

This is common in chronic active hepatitis (including chronic persistent hepatitis), nonactive chronic hepatitis and the early stages of liver cirrhosis. Because of a lingering illness, dampness retention is transformed into heat, which then impairs *yin*. Consequently, *yin* deficiency (mainly in the liver and kidneys) aggravates interior heat, thereby exhausting body fluids and developing the conformation of interior heat due to *yin* deficiency.

This conformation is manifested in low-grade fever; dizziness; headache; insomnia; a feverish sensation in the palms and soles; a feeling of oppression in the chest; fidgeting; a dry, sore throat; a dry mouth; a bitter taste in the mouth; hypochondriac pain; lower back pain; and a red tongue with red prickles on the tip and edges, teeth marks, ecchymosis and a thin, yellow, greasy coating or a denuded coating.

Treatment nourishes *yin* and clears heat. Glehnia and Rehmannia Combination (*yi guan jian*) can be given.

To treat lassitude, add 3 *qian* astragalus (*huang qi*).

To treat pain in the right upper abdomen, add 3 *qian* each of cyperus (*xiang fu zi*) and corydalis (*yan hu suo*).

To treat nausea and vomiting, add 3 *qian* pinellia (*ban xia*).

If the abdomen is distended, add 3 *qian* each of magnolia bark (*hou pu*), saussurea (*mu xiang*) and *chih-ko* (*zhi ke*).

If the patient's appetite is poor, add 3 *qian* each of crataegus (*shan zha*), chicken gizzard lining (*ji nei jin*), germinated rice (*gu ya*) and malt (*mai ya*).

If the patient is constipated, add 2 *qian* rhubarb (*da huang*).

If the patient's gums or nose are prone to bleeding, add 10 *qian* fresh imperata (*bai mao gen*) and 3 *qian* moutan (*mu dan pi*).

To treat ascites, add 3 *qian* each of polyporus (*zhu ling*), hoelen (*fu ling*) and alisma (*ze xie*).

For cases of hepatosplenomegaly, add 3 *qian* each of turtle shell (*bie jia*), persica (*tao ren*) and zedoaria (*e zhu*).

Acupuncture and Moxibustion

Acute Hepatitis

- *danshu* (B 19)
- *zusanli* (S 36)
- *taichong* (Liv 3)

Chronic Hepatitis

- *gansu* (B 18)
- *zusanli* (S 36)
- *sanyinjiao* (Sp 6)

Additional Points for Jaundice

- *hegu* (LI 4)
- *houxi* (SI 3)

Additional Point for Abdominal Distention

- *guanyuan* (CV 4)

Additional Point for Distention in the Upper Abdomen

- *zhongwan* (CV 12)

Additional Point for Distention in the Lower Abdomen

- *tianshu* (S 25)

Additional Points for Hypochondriac Pain

- *dannang* (EX-LE6)
- *yanglingquan* (G 34)

Treatment Method

Treat once daily for two weeks.

Section 11
Aplastic Anemia (Aplasia Bone Marrow)

According to a Western medical perspective, aplastic anemia is caused by deficient red-cell production due to a bone-marrow disorder. The main clinical manifestation is pancytopenia. TCM views aplastic anemia as one aspect of the conformations of consumptive disease or blood problems. The disease is associated with disorders of the heart, liver, spleen and kidneys, though kidney deficiency is the most common malady.

As the storehouse of vital essence and the control center for bone-marrow production, the kidneys are crucial to the proper functioning of the body. If kidney essence becomes deficient and fails to aid in bone-marrow formation, the deficient marrow will not be able to regenerate blood cells in sufficient numbers. Since *qi*, blood and the five viscera are interdependent, if the kidneys become deficient, they will be unable to warm and nourish the other viscera, and thus the heart, liver and spleen will also become deficient.

Should a kidney *yang* deficiency occur, the spleen will not be warmed. Furthermore, if other factors are involved, such as improper diet or fatigue, spleen deficiency will result. Consequently, the transportation and transformation of food into vital essence will be impaired, thereby creating a deficiency of vital essence. This, in turn, will impair the regeneration of *qi* and blood, causing defensive energy to become deficient, in which case external pathogens are more likely to invade the body, thus exacerbating the *qi* and blood deficiencies. If unchecked, the deficiencies will transform into consumption.

Diagnosis and Herbal Treatment

As a consumptive disease related to blood deficiency, treatment focuses on tonification, though specific treatments for anemia, bleeding and fever should be designed according to the varying degrees, courses and dominant conditions of each. For example, bleeding with fever should be treated by first halting the bleeding and clearing heat, and after the patient is in relatively stable condition, by replenishing *qi* and blood or tonifying the spleen and kidneys.

Internal Heat Due to *Yin* Deficiency

This type of aplastic anemia is characterized by fever, fidgeting, a feverish sensation in the palms and soles, a dry throat and mouth, and a tendency to develop excess blood heat-induced hemorrhages.

Treatment nourishes *yin* and clears heat. *Chin-chiu* and Turtle Shell Formula (*qin jiao bie jia san*), together with Lycium, Chrysanthemum and Rehmannia Formula (*qi ju di huang wan*), can be used.

To treat fever and persistent massive hemorrhaging, 10 *qian* buffalo horn (*shui niu jiao*) and 3 *qian* gelatin (*a jiao*) can be added.

Qi and Blood Deficiency

The onset is usually insidious and the disease course is short. A pale or sallow complexion, dizziness, palpitation, shortness of breath, lassitude, a pink tongue and a soft, floating and thready pulse are common signs and symptoms.

Treatment replenishes *qi* and blood. Ginseng Nutritive Combination (*ren shen yang rong tang*) is recommended.

Spleen and Kidney *Yang* Deficiency

A prolonged disease course, pallor, a pale, thick tongue with a thin, white coating, an aversion to cold, cold limbs, insufficient strength to speak, spontaneous sweating, tinnitus, lower back pain, impotence and emission in men, irregular menstruation in women, and a submerged and slow or submerged and thready pulse indicate *yang* deficiency of the spleen and kidneys.

Treatment tonifies the spleen and kidneys with Four Major Herb Combination (*si jun zi tang*) and Eucommia and Rehmannia Formula (*you gui wan*).

Common Acupuncture and Moxibustion Points

First Treatment

- *dazhui* (GV 14)
- *ganshu* (B 18)
- *neiguan* (P 6)
- *zusanli* (S 36)

Second Treatment

- *dazhui* (GV 14)
- *geshu* (B 17)
- *mingmen* (GV 4)
- *zusanli* (S 36)

Third Treatment

- *xuanzhong* (G 39)
- *yinlingquan* (Sp 9)

Section 12
Iron Deficiency Anemia

Anemia is marked by reductions in hemoglobin and the number of circulating red blood cells. According to TCM theory, this disease is caused by the failure of nutrients to transform into blood, which, in turn, is due to spleen deficiency or repeated episodes of bleeding.

Diagnosis and Herbal Treatment

Spleen *Qi* Deficiency

A sallow, pale complexion, lassitude, a poor appetite, loose stools, a pale tongue with a thin, greasy coating, and a thready pulse characterize spleen *qi* deficiency.

Treatment reinforces spleen *qi* with Saussurea and Cardamom Combination (*xiang sha liu jun zi tang*).

To treat chills and cold limbs, add 1 *qian* prepared aconite (*zhi fu zi*) and 2 *qian* baked ginger (*pao jiang*).

Qi and Blood Deficiency

Pallor, lassitude, dizziness, palpitation, insufficient strength to speak, a pale, thick tongue with a thin coating, and a soft, floating and thready pulse characterize a deficiency of both *qi* and blood.

Treatment replenishes *qi* and blood with either *Tang-kuei* and Ginseng Eight Combination (*ba zhen tang*) or *Tang-kuei* and Astragalus Combination (*dang gui bu xue tang*).

Tang-kuei and Astragalus Combination[1]
Dang Gui Bu Xue Tang
(*Tang-kuei* Decoction to Tonify the Blood)[2]

Astragalus	Astragali radix	Huang qi	10.0
Tang-kuei	Angelica radix	Dang gui	2.0

To treat menorrhagia, add 3 *qian* each of gelatin (*a jiao*) and carbonized artemisia (*ai ye tan*). Alternately, Ginseng and Longan Combination (*gui pi tang*) can be given.

Common Acupuncture and Moxibustion Points

First Treatment

- *dazhui* (GV 14)
- *neiguan* (P 6)
- *ganshu* (B 18)
- *zusanli* (S 36)

Second Treatment

- *dazhui* (GV 14)
- *mingmen* (GV 14)
- *geshu* (B 17)
- *zusanli* (S 36)

Third Treatment

- *xuanzhong* (G 39)
- *yinlingquan* (Sp 9)

Section 13
Leukopenia

Leukopenia is an abnormal decrease in leukocyte (white blood corpuscle) levels to below 5000/mm^3. A great number of drugs may cause leukopenia, as can a bone-marrow disorder. In some instances, the reduction in the number of leukocytes is checked and the differential count remains normal. However, at times, neutrophils (also known as polymorphonuclear leukocytes, white blood cells possessing nuclei consisting of several parts or lobes) are disproportionately low and the terms "neutropenia" and "granulocytopenia" then become more descriptive of the condition. The disease can be divided into two types: the idiopathic variety, which is more prevalent, and the secondary type, which is becoming more common.

According to TCM theory, this disease is closely related to the spleen, which is the source of nutrients for growth and development, and the kidneys, which store vital essence and form bone marrow. If the patient's constitution is inherently weak or if weakness exists due to an illness, the consumption of any number of drugs or an attack by external pathogens, vital *qi* will become impaired, resulting in a deficiency of the spleen and kidneys, as well as deficiencies of *wei, qi, ying* and blood, all of which contribute to the onslaught of leukopenia.

Diagnosis and Herbal Treatment

Qi and *Yin* Deficiency

Pallor, lassitude, dizziness, fidgeting, a feverish sensation in the palms, soles and heart region, a pink tongue and a thready, weak pulse indicate a deficiency of *qi* and *yin*.

Treatment reinforces *qi* and nourishes *yin* with Four Major Herb Combination (*si jun zi tang*) and Rehmannia and Schizandra Formula (*qi wei du qi wan*).

To treat anemia, add 3 *qian ho shou wu* (*he shou wu*) and 5 *qian* millettia stem (*ji xue teng*).

To treat fidgeting and a feverish sensation in the palms, soles and heart region, add 3 *qian* anemarrhena (*zhi mu*).

Spleen and Kidney *Yang* Deficiency

This deficiency is marked by lassitude, insufficient strength to speak, chills, cold limbs, a poor appetite, loose stools, soreness and weakness in the lower back and knees, dizziness, tinnitus, a thin, white tongue coating and a thready, slow pulse.

Treatment tonifies the spleen and kidneys with Astragalus Combination (*huang qi jian zhong tang*) and Eucommia and Rehmannia Formula (*you gui wan*). Also, 0.6 *qian* of young deer horn (*lu rong*), taken twice daily, is effective at elevating leukocyte levels.

Common Acupuncture and Moxibustion Points

- *zusanli* (S 36)
- *guanyuan* (CV 4)
- *sanyinjiao* (Sp 6)
- *qihai* (CV 6)
- *baihui* (CV 20)

Section 14
Thrombocytopenic Purpura

Thrombocytopenic purpura is one of the most common hemorrhagic diseases. Incidence is high in childhood and in premenopausal women, though it may be seen in any age group. It is classified as either acute or chronic, with the latter being more common.

According to its clinical manifestations, it is similar to the TCM conformation of blood disorder. TCM theory holds that this disease is caused either by heat pathogens accumulated in the blood or *qi*, or by a blood deficiency in one of the internal organs.

Diagnosis and Herbal Treatment

Acute Type

Affected by unseasonable weather, external pathogens may enter the body and transform into heat or fire, either of which can accumulate in the stomach and invade *yin* and blood. As a result, the blood flows out of the vessels and permeates the muscles and skin, causing bleeding and ecchymosis. In some cases, the heat not only impairs the blood and its vessels, but also impairs *qi* and *yin*. In this way, an acute case of thrombocytopenic purpura can transform into a chronic one.

A sudden onset, severe hemorrhaging and a fever which is generally due to external pathogens are the chief manifestations of acute thrombocytopenic purpura.

1. Invasion by heat of *ying fen* and *xue fen*

A sudden onset, chills, fever, bright red or purple purpura and bleeding of the nose and gums characterize this type of heat invasion. In severe cases, the patient may experience anxiety, headache and even a loss of consciousness. A cardinal red tongue with scant coating and a slippery and rapid or large, wiry and rapid pulse may also be observed.

Treatment clears the *ying fen* and cools blood heat with Rhinoceros and Scrophularia Combination (*qing ying tang*).

2. Stomach fire

A sudden onset, dark purpura, a flushed face, thirst, preference for cold beverages, dark yellow urine, constipation, severe gum bleeding, a red tongue with a thin, yellow or dry, yellow coating, and a large and wiry or submerged and full pulse characterize stomach fire.

Treatment clears stomach heat and cools blood to halt bleeding. Gypsum Combination (*bai hu tang*), plus 10 *qian* buffalo horn (*shui niu jiao*) and 3 *qian* scrophularia (*xuan shen*), may be given. As an alternative, Gypsum, Coptis and Scute Combination (*san huang shi gao tang*) may also be given.

Chronic Type

An insidious onset, mild hemorrhaging, normal body temperature and more manifestations of a deficiency condition than of an excess one constitute a general description of chronic thrombocytopenic purpura. The disorder, which is closely related to the spleen and kidneys, is caused by an impairment of *qi* and blood, an imbalance of *yin* and *yang* or a deficiency of the viscera.

1. Excess fire due to *yin* deficiency

Large purple or red purpura, a flushed face, hectic fever, dizziness, tinnitus, bleeding nose and gums, a dry, red tongue with a thin coating, and a wiry, thready and rapid pulse characterize fire due to *yin* deficiency.

Treatment nourishes *yin* to reduce fire. Anemarrhena, Phellodendron and Rehmannia Formula (*zhi bo ba wei wan*), together with 3 *qian* each of tortoise shell (*gui ban*), ligustrum (*nu zhen zi*) and eclipta (*han lian cao*), can be given.

2. Descent of *qi* to maintain blood in the vessels

Intermittent, light purple purpura, a sallow complexion, lassitude, dizziness, general weakness, shortness of breath following activity, a poor appetite, hematochezia and uterine bleeding in women characterize this condition.

Treatment replenishes *qi* to stop bleeding. Ginseng and Longan Combination (*gui pi tang*) can be used.

To treat chills and cold limbs due to a *yang* and *qi* deficiency, add 3 *qian* each of antler (*lu jiao*), cistanche (*rou cong rong*) and epimedium (*yin yang huo*) to warm *yang* and thereby restrain *yin*.

Herb Selection According to Symptoms

For bleeding nose or gums resulting from an excess of *yang* or from a *yin* deficiency, add cimicifuga (*sheng ma*), scute (*huang qin*), gardenia (parched *zhi zi*) or imperata (*bai mao gen*) to supplement any of the above-recommended therapies.

If heat-induced hemoptysis impairs lung capillaries and makes the blood flow out of its vessels, add turmeric (*yu jin*), lotus root node (*ou jie*), gelatin (*a jiao*) or madder (*qian cao gen*).

To treat hematochezia and hematemesis, add notoginseng (*san qi*), bletilla (*bai ji*), sanguisorba (*di yu*) or sophora (*huai hua*).

To treat hematuria, add field thistle (*xiao ji*), cattail pollen (*pu huang*), lophatherum (*dan zhu ye*) or akebia (*mu tong*).

For uterine bleeding, add carbonized lotus receptacle (*lian fang tan*), palm bark (*zong shu pi*) or carbonized biota top (*ce bo ye tan*).

If blood stasis forms after the bleeding has stopped and if it is accompanied by purpura, hematoma, splenomegaly and a bluish purple tongue, add persica (*tao ren*), carthamus (*hong hua*), notoginseng (*san qi*) or other herbs which promote blood circulation to remove stasis.

Acupuncture and Moxibustion Treatment

Points of First Choice

- *quchi* (LI 11)
- *zusanli* (S 36)

Reserved Points

- *hegu* (LI 4)
- *xuehai* (Sp 10)
- *pishu* (B 20)
- *geshu* (B 17)

Treatment Method

Three points are selected each time for a total of 10 treatment sessions.

Section 15
Glomerulonephritis

Also called nephritis, glomerulonephritis may be classified into two types: acute and chronic.

Diagnosis and Herbal Treatment

Acute Nephritis

This is a disease of immunological mediated reactions to hemolytic streptococcus infection. The clinical manifestations are general edema, hypertension, hematuria and proteinuria. The highest incidence is in children. Acute nephritis belongs to the TCM conformation of *yang* edema.

According to TCM theory, the etiology of this disease is related, not only to invasion of the body by external evils, such as wind-cold, wind-heat or cold-dampness, but also to functional disturbances of the internal organs--particularly the lungs, spleen and kidneys. The disease can be caused by failure of the lungs to regulate water flow, failure of the spleen to transport and transform nutrients and fluids, or failure of the kidneys to govern the retention and discharge of fluids.

1. Wind edema

A sudden onset of edema which spreads from the eyelids to the face and then throughout the body, oliguria, dark yellow urine, soreness and heaviness in the limbs, a cough accompanied by a shortness of breath, fever, headache, sore throat, an aversion to drafts, a thin, white tongue coating and a floating, tense pulse or floating, rapid pulse characterize wind edema.

Treatment promotes diuresis by activating the dispersion function of the lungs. Atractylodes Combination (*yue pi jia zhu tang*), together with 4 *qian* phaseolus (*chi xiao dou*), 3 *qian* each of plantain (*che qian cao*) and alisma (*ze xie*), and 10 *qian* imperata (*bai mao gen*), should be used.

To treat a high fever and an aversion to drafts, add 1.5 *qian* each of *chiang-huo* (*qiang huo*) and siler (*fang feng*).

In the case of a severe sore throat or tonsillitis, add 3 *qian* lonicera (*jin yin hua*) and 4 *qian* dandelion (*pu gong yin*).

2. Wind-heat

In addition to edema and oliguria, the following may also be observed: fever with sweating, a dry mouth, thirst, pharyngitis, tonsillitis, a thin, yellow tongue coating and a floating and rapid or slippery and rapid pulse.

Treatment clears heat and induces diuresis through the administration of Lonicera and Forsythia Formula (*yin qiao san*), plus 3 *qian* polyporus (*zhu ling*) and 4 *qian* alisma (*ze xie*).

Gentian Combination (*long dan xie gan tang*) can be used for the treatment of liver or gallbladder fire.

Should the patient experience severe a headache and dizziness, supplement either of the above remedies with 10 *qian* nacre (*zhen zhu mu*) and 5 *qian* magnetite (*ci shi*).

3. Dampness edema

General edema, oliguria, a feeling of heaviness throughout the body, lassitude, a white, greasy tongue coating and a submerged, thready pulse characterize dampness edema.

Treatment activates *yang* to promote diuresis with Hoelen Five Herb Formula (*wu ling san*) and Hoelen and Areca Combination (*wu pi yin*).

If there is abdominal distention and a thick, greasy tongue coating, add 3 *qian* atractylodes (*cang zhu*) and 2 *qian* magnolia bark (*hou pu*).

If the patient has a poor appetite and edematous face in the morning, add 5 *qian* coix (*yi yi ren*), 1 *qian* amomum fruit (*sha ren*) and 3 *qian* codonopsis (*dang shen*).

4. Heat-dampness edema

During the febrile stage or just after the patient's temperature subsides, the following may be observed in the case of heat-dampness edema: bright red or dark red hematuria, oliguria, dry stools or constipation, irritability, fidgeting, thirst, mild edema, a red tongue tip, a thin, yellow tongue coating and a slightly rapid pulse.

Treatment clears heat, cools the blood and removes dampness by means of diuresis. Cephalanoplos Combination (*xiao ji yin zi*), plus 1 *qian* amber (*hu po*), can be given to achieve these ends.

During the convalescent stage, clinical symptoms of the disease disappear, though small amounts of protein and blood remain in routine urine tests. This means that some pathogens are still present and that kidney *qi* has failed to consolidate. In this case, Rehmannia Six Formula (*liu wei di huang wan*) and Anemarrhena, Phellodendron and Rehmannia Formula (*zhi bo ba wei wan*) can be given.

If the urine continues to contain protein, Achyranthes and Rehmannia Formula (*zuo gui wan*) can be used to strengthen vital energy and prevent the disease from becoming chronic.

If *qi* is deficient following the febrile stage and if the edema has subsided, administer Ginseng and Astragalus Combination (*bu zhong yi qi tang*).

Chronic Nephritis

Chronic nephritis is a common renal disease which develops from acute nephritis and is marked by edema of various degrees. Similar descriptions can be found in TCM literature under the category of *yin* edema. As Dan-qi Zhu described in his work *Zhen Yin Mai Zhi* (Treatment Based on Symptoms, Causes and Pulse): "A terribly pale complexion, edema and anuria occur now and then."

From a TCM viewpoint, this disease is caused by a functional disturbance of the spleen and stomach or by a deficiency of *yang* and *qi*, any of which can dissipate nutrients from food and disturb the functional activity of *qi*, with the end result of edema.

Generally speaking, when kidney *yang* deficiency is the dominant conformation, the clinical manifestation is termed "wild spreading of water and dampness," whereas when spleen *yang* deficiency is dominant, the clinical manifestation is known as "retention of water and dampness." In some severe cases of spleen and kidney *yang* deficiency, *yin* and the liver can also become impaired. This severe condition in which both *yin* and *yang* are deficient is called "excess in the upper and deficiency in the lower."

1. Wild spreading of water and dampness

A pale, lusterless complexion, listlessness, chills, an aversion to cold, poor appetite, nausea, vomiting, a feeling of oppression in the chest, abdominal distention, a cough with dyspnea, difficulty in lying down, oliguria, severe edema in the whole body and even hydrothorax and ascites, a pale or pale, thick tongue with a thin, white or white, slippery and greasy coating, and a submerged and thready pulse are all manifestations of wild spreading of water and dampness. The type involving a spleen and kidney *yang* deficiency mainly affects the kidneys.

Treatment warms the kidneys, reinforces the spleen and induces diuresis. Magnolia and Atractylodes Combination (*shi pi yin*), together with Hoelen Five Herb Formula (*wu ling san*), is the preferred remedy.

In case of severe chills, add 1 *qian* cinnamon bark (*gui pi*) or 2 *qian* cinnamon twig (*gui zhi*).

Should retained water and fluids ascend and attack the heart and lungs or should the accumulated phlegm induce a cough and asthma, *Ma-huang* and Asarum Combination (*ma huang fu zi xi xin tang*) and Hoelen Five Herb Formula (*wu ling san*) can be used.

If *yang* deficiency is mild and spleen *qi* deficiency dominates, spleen *qi* must be reinforced and diuresis induced with Stephania and Astragalus Combination (*fang ji huang qi tang*) and Hoelen Five Herb Formula (*wu ling san*).

2. Water and dampness retention

A slightly pale or sallow complexion, listlessness, mild chills, weak or cold limbs, a feeling of oppression in the chest, a poor appetite accompanied by nausea, distention and fullness in the upper abdomen which are relieved by heat or pressure, borborygmus, loose stools or stools with undigested food, mild, persistent edema, a pale tongue with a thin and white or greasy coating and a soft, floating and thready or submerged pulse characterize retention of water and dampness.

Treatment reinforces spleen *qi* in order to remove dampness and induce diuresis. Six Major Herb Combination (*liu jun zi tang*) and Stephania and Astragalus Combination (*fang ji huang qi tang*) can be used.

If *yang* deficiency is serious, add 1 *qian* prepared aconite (*zhi fu zi*) and 0.5 *qian* cinnamon bark (*rou gui*).

To treat chills and cold limbs due to kidney *yang* deficiency, add 3 *qian* each of curculigo (*xian mao*), epimedium (*yin yang huo*) and antler (*lu jiao*) and 2 *qian* morinda (*ba ji tian*).

If the patient's appetite is poor due to *qi* stagnancy, add 2 *qian* saussurea (*mu xiang*) and 1 *qian* cardamom (*suo sha ren*).

3. Spleen and kidney deficiency

Lassitude, weak limbs, dizziness, tinnitus, insomnia, sore and weak lower back and knees, impotence or emission, poor appetite, mild or no edema, a pale or sallow complexion, a thin tongue coating and a soft, floating and slippery or a weak pulse indicate a deficiency of the spleen and kidneys. In this type of chronic nephritis, the pathogens of water and dampness have subsided, but vital energy has not yet recovered, so there are features of *yang* deficiency of the spleen and kidneys, as well as those of *qi* and blood deficiency. This state is in some respects analogous to the remission stages of chronic and latent nephritis in Western medicine.

Tonification of the spleen and kidneys, as well as replenishment of *qi* and blood, are the most important aspects of treatment. Specific remedies follow.

a. deficiency of the spleen, kidneys, *qi* and blood

This can be treated with Four Major Herb Combination (*si jun zi tang*) and Eucommia and Rehmannia Formula (*you gui wan*).

If kidney *yang* deficiency is dominant, add 3 *qian* each of curculigo (*xian mao*) and morinda (*ba ji tian*).

If kidney *yin* deficiency is more prevalent, add 3 *qian* tortoise shell (*gui ban*) and 1 *qian* schizandra (*wu wei zi*).

In case of poor appetite accompanied by *qi* stagnancy, add 2 *qian* each of citrus peel (*chen pi*) and saussurea (*mu xiang*) and 1 *qian* cardamom (*suo sha ren*).

To treat emission due to kidney deficiency, add Lotus Stamen Formula (*jin suo gu jing wan*).

If fire of the vital gate, which controls sexual potency (*xiang huo*), is in excess, add Anemarrhena, Phellodendron and Rehmannia Formula (*zhi bo ba wei wan*).

b. spleen *qi* deficiency

If spleen *qi* deficiency dominates, Saussurea and Cardamom Combination (*xiang sha liu jun zi tang*) can be used.

If there is a blood deficiency, add 3 *qian* tang-kuei (*dang gui*) and 4 *qian* each of rehmannia (*di huang*) and peony (*shao yao*).

c. remission stage

When the patient's condition has improved, but there are still signs of a mild *qi* and blood deficiency, *Tang-kuei* and Ginseng Eight Combination (*ba zhen tang*) can be given.

In the case of a mild kidney *yin* deficiency, Rehmannia Six Formula (*liu wei di huang wan*) can be used.

To treat kidney *yang* deficiency, Rehmannia Eight Formula (*ba wei di huang wan*) can be selected.

To treat mild edema, Achyranthes and Plantago Formula (*niu che shen qi wan*) can be used.

4. Excess *yang* due to *yin* deficiency

A flushed face, a dry mouth, thirst, an occasional sore throat, headache, dizziness, palpitation, insomnia, lower back pain, spermatorrhea, urine with a reddish tinge and a hot sensation, constipation, a red tongue, a wiry and thready or slippery and rapid pulse, and high blood pressure indicate excess *yang* due to *yin* deficiency.

This type of chronic nephritis is analogous to hypertensive nephritis in Western medicine, but it is not very common in clinical practice. Because *yang* has not recovered and thereby impairs *yin*, liver and kidney *yin* become deficient, resulting in an excess of liver *yang*.

Treatment attempts to nourish kidney *yin* and soothe the liver to relieve excess *yang*. Rehmannia Six Formula (*liu wei di huang wan*), Pinellia and Gastrodia Combination (*ban xia bai zhu tian ma tang*) and 10 *qian* haliotis (*shi jue ming*) can be used.

To treat headache and dizziness, add 0.2 *qian* each of chrysanthemum (*ju hua*), nacre (*zhen zhu mu*), uncaria stem with hooks (*gou teng*) and antelope horn (powder of *ling yang*).

For palpitation and insomnia, add 3 *qian* each of dragon teeth (*long chi*) and zizyphus (*suan zao ren*).

To treat blurry vision, add 5 *qian* cassia seed (*jue ming zi*) and 4 *qian* ligustrum (*nu zhen zi*).

5. Body's resistance weakened by pathogenic factors

The clinical symptoms of this condition can be quite complex. A sallow, pale or dark gray complexion, listlessness, fidgeting, chills, edema or dehydration accompanied by gauntness, a sensation of oppression in the chest, shortness of breath, abdominal distention, a poor appetite, vomiting, nausea, oliguria or frequent, profuse urination, constipation or diarrhea, a thick, pale tongue with a white and greasy, yellow and greasy or black coating, and a submerged and thready or wiry and thready pulse describe the array of symptoms which characterize a body weakened by pathogenic factors. This constellation of signs and symptoms is analogous to those given in Western medicine for the azotemic or uremic stage of nephritis.

Dysfunctioning of the spleen and kidneys is the result of kidney *yin* and spleen *yang* deficiencies, with the latter dominating. When vital energy and fire from the gate of life are on the decline, turbid *yin* accumulates and then ascends, creating the symptoms outlined in the preceding paragraph.

Treatment attempts to strengthen resistance to eliminate turbid *yin*. Hoelen and Bamboo Combination (*wen dan tang*), along with Achyranthes and Plantago Formula (*niu che shen qi wan*), can be used.

Common Acupuncture and Moxibustion Points

First Treatment
- *shenshu* (B 23)
- *zhibian* (B 54)
- *fuliu* (K 7)

Second Treatment
- *shenshu* (B 23)
- *taixi* (K 3)
- *houxi* (SI 3)

Section 16
Pyelonephritis

Fever, lower back pain and paruria are the main clinical manifestations of pyelonephritis. In TCM it is categorized under the conformations of strangury or lumbago. As Jin-yue Zhang pointed out in his work on the diagnosis and treatment of lumbago, some of the causes are heat-dampness and "fire evil accumulation in the lower back and kidneys," the latter of which is always manifested by "a hot sensation and difficulty in urination and defecation." The acute stage of the disease is generally due to heat-dampness in the lower energizer, which disturbs the *qi*-transforming function of the urinary bladder. In the chronic stage, spleen and kidney deficiency with retained heat in the lower energizer is usually apparent.

According to a TCM understanding, the etiology of the disease can be traced to heat-dampness pathogens which accumulate in the lower energizer and impair its functioning. The most important organs of the lower energizer are the kidneys and urinary bladder, the former being *zang* (the solid organs) and the latter being *fu* (the hollow organs). As they are connected by meridians, their physiological functions are closely related. If deficient kidneys are unable to control fluid circulation, heat-dampness readily accumulates in the urinary bladder, thus giving rise to a number of urinary-disorder symptoms such as frequency of micturition, urgency of urination and lower back pain.

The disease can be divided into acute and chronic stages, according to its duration, the depletion of vital energy, the persistence of pathogenic factors, the nature of the excess or deficiency and the extent to which the internal organs have been affected. In the initial stage, the prominent pathogenic excess struggles with vital energy, and so there are a great number of excess-heat manifestations. Excess heat consumes body fluids, thus damaging vital energy and prompting the formation of kidney *yin* deficiency or spleen and kidney deficiency. When vital energy has been severely depleted and the pathogens have not been eliminated, the chronic stage has already set in.

Diagnosis and Herbal Treatment

Acute Stage

1. Heat-dampness in the urinary bladder

Chills, fever, frequency of micturition, urgency of urination, strangury, difficult and incontinent urination, distention and pain in the lower abdomen, lower back pain, a yellow and greasy or white and greasy tongue coating, and a soft, floating and rapid or slippery and rapid pulse characterize heat-dampness in the urinary bladder.

Treatment consists in clearing heat and toxic materials and inducing diuresis in order to alleviate strangury. Dianthus Formula (*ba zheng san*) is recommended.

2. Heat retention in the liver and gallbladder

Alternating spells of fever and chills, fidgeting, nausea, a bitter taste in the mouth, pain in the hypochondrium, lack of appetite, lower back pain, distention and pain in the lower abdomen, frequency of micturition with a hot sensation, a dark yellow tongue coating, and a wiry and rapid pulse indicate heat retention in the liver and gallbladder.

Treatment aims at clearing the liver and gallbladder, as well as clearing and regulating the passage of water through the body, with Gentian Combination (*long dan xie gan tang*) and Minor Bupleurum Combination (*xiao chai hu tang*).

3. Excess gastrointestinal heat

A persistently high fever which does not subside after sweating, foul breath, thirst, abdominal pain, constipation, headache, lower back pain, painful urination, turbid, red-tinged urine, a red tongue with a yellow, greasy coating, and a wiry, rapid pulse characterize excess gastrointestinal heat.

Treatment attempts to clear heat-dampness through purgation. Rehmannia and Akebia Formula (*dao chi san*) and Rhubarb Combination (*da huang huang lian xie xin tang*) are recommended.

Rhubarb Combination[1]
Da Huang Huang Lian Xie Xin Tang
(Rhubarb and Coptis Decoction)

Rhubarb	*Rhei rhizoma*	*Da huang*	2.0
Coptis	*Coptidis rhizoma*	*Huang lian*	1.0

Chronic Stage

Chronic pyelonephritis usually results when the sequelae of an acute urinary-tract infection persist, though, in some cases, the signs of the acute stage may not be observed until the disease is already in the chronic stage. Clinically, the symptoms of urinary irritation occur repeatedly, though irregularly, and are accompanied by deficiency symptoms of various kinds.

Treatment during the chronic stage must deal with both the primary and secondary causes simultaneously, that is to say, it should both tonify the kidneys and spleen and clear heat-dampness. Emphasis should be placed on the secondary symptoms (*biao*) only if the patient is experiencing an acute episode.

1. Kidney *yin* deficiency with accumulated heat-dampness

In addition to the symptoms of urinary irritation, the patient also experiences or evidences dizziness, tinnitus, a mild fever, night sweats, dry lips and throat, lower back pain, dark yellow urine, a red tongue with very little coating, and a wiry and thready or rapid pulse.

Treatment nourishes *yin* and clears heat. Anemarrhena, Phellodendron and Rehmannia Formula (*zhi bo ba wei wan*) can be used.

2. Spleen and kidney deficiency with dampness retention

In addition to the symptoms of urinary irritation, there are also "sinking symptoms" due to *qi* deficiency. Such things as edema in the face and limbs, a poor appetite, lower back pain, listlessness, a bearing-down sensation in the lower abdomen, a pale tongue with a thin, white coating, and a submerged, thready and weak pulse may be observed.

Treatment focuses on tonifying the spleen and kidneys. Ginseng and Astragalus Combination (*bu zhong yi qi tang*) and Rehmannia Six Formula (*liu wei di huang wan*) can be used.

3. Excess heat caused by heat-dampness accumulation

The functional activity of *qi* is disturbed through the accumulation of excess heat. Generally, this condition is corrected through the use of increased doses of herbs (at least four times daily) to clear heat and toxins. Should the large intake of bitter, cold-natured herbs impair the spleen and stomach, giving rise to frequent vomiting, the dose should be decreased appropriately or herbs for regulating and harmonizing stomach *qi* should be added.

Acupuncture and Moxibustion Treatment

First Treatment

- *fuliu* (K 7)
- *guilai* (S 29)
- kidney earpoint

Second Treatment

- *guanyuan* (CV 4)
- *feiyang* (B 58)
- urinary bladder earpoint

Third the Treatment

- *shenshu* (B 23)
- *sanyinjiao* (Sp 6)
- adrenal gland earpoint

Reserved Points

- *zhongji* (CV 3)
- *guanyuan* (CV 4)
- *sanyinjiao* (Sp 6)
- *pangguangshu* (B 28)

Treatment Method

1. Alternate points as indicated above, though some points may have to be used more often, depending on the patient's conformation.

2. Treat once daily for an acute case and twice weekly for a chronic case.

3. Use strong, stimulating and purging manipulation to treat excess heat and mild, tonifying manipulation in the case of a deficiency.

Section 17
Hyperthyroidism

Hyperthyroidism is a common endocrinopathy caused by an excess concentration of thyroxin hormones in the blood. The basic pathophysiological changes it induces are an acceleration of the oxidation process, an increased rate of tissue metabolism and certain disturbances of the neuromuscular system. The main manifestations are thyroid enlargement, an increase in appetite, weight loss, tachycardia with an irregular heartbeat, irritability, an aversion to heat, profuse sweating, exophthalmus and a slight trembling of the fingers.

This disease is often seen in women, with affected females outnumbering males 4:1. People of any age can become afflicted, though the young and middle-aged are much more likely than the elderly to do so.

According to TCM theory, hyperthyroidism belongs to the conformation of goiter and, at least to some extent, relates to the patient's emotions and constitution. When, due to long-term depression or sudden psychic trauma, the liver no longer properly regulates the flow of vital energy and blood, liver *qi* stagnates and fails to transport fluids. The fluids accumulate and transform into phlegm, which then obstructs the neck with *qi* and gradually induces goiter. Lingering liver *qi* transforms into fire, which is manifested in fidgeting and irritability.

If fire consumes body fluids and stomach *yin*, the resulting *yin* deficiency produces heat. Even though this heat overstimulates appetite, the patient still loses weight. If the spleen is impaired, it will be unable to transport or transform nutrients, thereby giving rise to diarrhea, gauntness and lassitude.

If heart *yin* is deficient, palpitation or severe palpitation with fear, fidgeting, insomnia and profuse sweating can be observed. If liver *yin* deficiency affects kidney *yin*, interior wind will be formed by excess *yang*. Furthermore, if a *yin* deficiency and *qi* stagnancy occur simultaneously, liver fire can result in *yin* impairment, making recovery all the more difficult.

In its initial stage, this disease is generally considered an excess condition, the main pathogen being *qi* stagnancy with liver fire, phlegm retention and blood stasis. The persistent stage is often associated with *yin* deficiency, which is manifested in pathological changes in the liver, kidneys, heart and spleen.

Diagnosis and Herbal Treatment

Since the pathological changes induced by the disease are primarily *qi* stagnancy and phlegm retention, regulating *qi*, resolving phlegm and softening the hard masses are the principal therapies. If the goiter is hard and persists for a long time, it is categorized as blood stasis. Treatment focuses on promoting blood circulation to remove stasis. If the main pathogenic change is an increase in liver fire, clearing the liver and purging fire take precedence. Should excess fire consume *yin*, methods of nourishing *yin* can be selected.

Qi Stagnancy and Phlegm Retention

Goiter which is soft and painless in the anterior cervical region, a feeling of oppression in the chest, pain in the hypochondriac region, frequent sighing, a thin, greasy tongue coating and a wiry, slippery pulse indicate *qi* stagnancy and phlegm retention.

Treatment regulates *qi,* resolves phlegm, and softens and removes the mass. Forsythia and *Kun-pu* Combination (*san zhong kui jian tang*), 10 *qian* oyster shell (*mu li*) and 5 *qian* cyclina (*hai ge fen*) can be used.

Forsythia and *Kun-pu* Combination[1]

San Zhong Kui Jian Tang

(Dissipate Hard Mass Decoction)

Tang-kuei	Angelicae radix	Dang gui	1.5
Peony	Paeoniae radix	Shao yao	1.5
Bupleurum	Bupleuri radix	Chai hu	1.5
Scute	Scutellariae radix	Huang qin	1.5
Coptis	Coptidis rhizoma	Huang lian	1.5
Forsythia	Forsythiae fructus	Lian qiao	1.5
Phellodendron	Phellodendri cortex	Huang bo	1.5
Anemarrhena	Anemarrhenae rhizoma	Zhi mu	1.5
Trichosanthes root	Trichosanthis radix	Gua lou gen	1.5
Platycodon	Platycodi radix	Jie geng	1.5
Gentian	Gentianae scabrae radix	Long dan cao	1.5
Pueraria	Puerariae radix	Ge geng	1.5
Sparganium**	Sparganii rhizoma	San ling	1.5
Zedoaria	Zedoariae rhizoma	E zhu	1.5
Kun-pu***	Ecklonia kurome	Kun bu	1.5
Seaweed	Sargassum	Hai zao	1.5
Cimicifuga	Cimicifugae rhizoma	Sheng ma	1.5
Ginger, fresh	Zingiberis rhizoma	Sheng jiang	1.5
Licorice	Glycyrrhizae radix	Gan cao	1.5

* This formula is also known as Forsythia and Laminaria Combination.

** Some books give the common name as scirpus.

*** The nomenclature for this herb is rather complex and so some confusion surrounds it. *Kun-pu* (or in *pinyin*, *kun bu*) has been used to describe all of the following species: *Laminariae japonica* Aresch. (with the *pinyin* name of *hai dai*), *Ecklonia kurome* Okam. (*pinyin* name of *kun bu*) and *Undaria pinnatifida* (Harv.) Sur. (known by the *pinyin* name of *qundai cai*). Since *kun bu* is both the collective *pinyin* name and the name used to describe one of the three species, *kun bu* has been incorrectly associated with the individual name for *Laminariae japonica*, rather than only its more general name.

If the goiter is hard and nodular, add 2 *qian* cnidium (*chuan xiong*) and 3 *qian* each *tang-kuei* (*dang gui*), persica (*tao ren*) and carthamus (*hong hua*).

To treat loose stools and lassitude, add herbs to strengthen the spleen and resolve dampness, specifically, 3 *qian* of one of the following: white atractylodes (*bai zhu*), dolichos (*bai pian dou*) or coix (*yi yi ren*).

Liver Fire

This condition is characterized by goiter, exophthalmus, ir-ritability, a flushed face, an aversion to heat, profuse sweating, a bitter taste in the mouth, conjunctival congestion, a thin, yellow tongue coating and a wiry, rapid pulse.

Treatment is aimed at clearing the liver and purging fire. Gentian Combination (*long dan xie gan tang*) can be used.

To purge heat from the middle energizer, add 1 *qian* coptis (*huang lian*) and 5 *qian* gypsum (*shi gao*).

To treat constipation, add 2 *qian* rhubarb (*da huang*).

Heart and Liver *Yin* Deficiency

Palpitation, restlessness accompanied by fear or anxiety, fidgeting, insomnia, pain in the hypochondrium, a dry mouth, a red tongue and a thready, rapid pulse characterize *yin* deficiency of the heart and liver.

Treatment nourishes the heart in order to calm the mind, as well as nourishes the liver and *yin*. Ginseng and Zizyphus Formula (*tian wang bu xin dan*) and Glehnia and Rehmannia Combination (*yi guan jian*) can be given.

If there is lower back pain and tinnitus, add 5 *qian* ligustrum (*nu zhen zi*) and 3 *qian* each of *ho-shou-wu* (*he shou wu*) and tortoise shell (*gui ban*).

To treat a flushed face and a slight trembling of the fingers, add 10 *qian* nacre (*zhen zhu mu*), 3 *qian* uncaria stem with hooks (*gou teng*) and 5 *qian* oyster shell (*mu li*).

Common Acupuncture and Moxibustion Points

- *naohui* (TE 13)
- *hegu* (LI 4)
- *zusanli* (S 36)
- *tianrong* (SI 17)
- *tianding* (LI 17)
- *tiantu* (CV 22)

Section 18
Diabetes Mellitus

Diabetes mellitus is a systematic disease generally caused by a disturbance of carbohydrate metabolism which has resulted from either absolute or partial hypoinsulinism. The main clinical manifestations are polydipsia, polyphagia, polyuria, gauntness, hyperglycosuria and hyperglycosemia. It may be accompanied by disturbances in protein and fat metabolism, the latter of which can give rise to ketosis, dehydration, coma or even death. This disease is commonly seen in persons aged 40 to 60, and only five percent of the cases occur in persons 10 years or younger, while only three percent of the cases occur in persons 80 years and older. Between the ages of 40 and 70, diabetes is more common in women than in men, though slightly more males under 40 are afflicted than females of the same age group.

According to TCM theory, three factors can cause the disease: improper diet, emotional distress or kidney *yin* deficiency. All three factors give rise to interior heat and the impairment of *yin*, both of which consume nutrients and fluids, thereby inducing disease onset. If the disease remains untreated or is poorly controlled, *yin* deficiency can affect *yang*, giving rise to kidney *yang* deficiency.

Diagnosis and Herbal Treatment

Although diabetes can be divided into that of the upper, middle and lower energizers, and though it can be differentiated according to lung heat, stomach heat or kidney deficiency, respectively, the three sets of manifestations generally appear at the same time with the only difference being varying degrees of severity. Heat-dryness due to *yin* deficiency is the basic pathological mechanism.

Treatment clears heat and nourishes the kidneys. If *yin* deficiency affects *yang*, *yin* and *yang* should be reinforced at the same time to restore their proper balance.

Heat-dryness in the Lungs and Stomach

Fidgeting, thirst, polyphagia, gauntness, a dry mouth and tongue, a red tongue tip and edges, and a slippery, rapid pulse characterize heat-dryness in the lungs and stomach.

Treatment attempts to nourish *yin* and clear heat. Ginseng and Gypsum Combination (*bai hu jia ren shen tang*) and Phellodendron Combination (*zi yin jiang huo tang*) can be used.

Ginseng and Gypsum Combination[1]
Bai Hu Jia Ren Shen Tang
(White Tiger plus Ginseng Decoction)[2]

Ginseng	Ginseng radix	Ren shen	3.0
Gypsum	Gypsum fibrosum	Shi gao	15.0
Anemarrhena	Anemarrhenae rhizoma	Zhi mu	5.0
Rice	Oryzae semen	Jing mi	10.0
Licorice	Glycyrrhizae radix	Gan cao	2.0

To treat excessive thirst, add 10 *qian* trichosanthes root (*gua lou gen*).

For constipation, add 1 *qian* rhubarb (*da huang*).

An ulcerated mouth or tongue should be treated by adding 3 *qian* lonicera (*jin yin hua*) and 1 *qian* coptis (*huang lian*).

Kidney *Yin* Deficiency

Frequent and profuse urination in which a fatty film may float on the surface of the toilet bowl, lower back pain, lassitude, a dry mouth, a red tongue and a submerged, thready and rapid pulse indicate kidney *yin* deficiency.

Treatment nourishes kidney *yin* with Rehmannia Six Formula (*liu wei di huang wan*).

In the case of lassitude due to *qi* and *yin* impairment, add 1.5 *qian* ginseng (*ren shen*) and 3 *qian* each of astragalus (*huang qi*) and white atractylodes (*bai zhu*). Alternately, Trichosanthes and Ophiopogon Formula (*yue quan wan*) can be used.

If there is dizziness, blurred vision or tinnitus, add 3 *qian* each of lycium (*gou qi zi*) and mulberry (*sang shen zi*) and 5 *qian* ligustrum (*nu zhen zi*).

Trichosanthes and Ophiopogon Formula
Yue Quan Wan[9]
(Jade Spring Water Pill)

Trichosanthes root	*Trichosanthis radix*	Gua lou gen	3.0
Pueraria	*Puerariae radix*	Ge gen	3.0
Ophiopogon	*Ophiopogonis rhizoma*	Mai men dong	2.0
Ginseng	*Ginseng radix*	Ren shen	2.0
Hoelen	*Poria sclerotium*	Fu ling	2.0
Plum	*Mume fructus*	Wu mei	2.0
Licorice	*Glycyrrhizae radix*	Gan cao	2.0
Astragalus, raw	*Astragali radix*	Shen huang qi	1.0
Astragalus, baked	*Astragali radix*	Zhi huang qi	1.0

The above ingredients are ground into a powder and made into 3-*qian* boluses, one of which is taken t.i.d. Alternately, 2 *qian* of concentrated extract should be taken t.i.d.

Functions: nourishes *yin*; promotes salivation; tonifies *qi*.

Explanation: Trichosanthes root, pueraria, ophiopogon and plum nourish *yin* and promote salivation, thereby alleviating thirst. Ginseng, hoelen, licorice and astragalus strengthen *qi* and improve the spleen's transformation and transportation functions, thereby controlling diabetes.

Deficiency of Both *Yin* and *Yang*

Frequent and profuse urination in which a fatty film may float on the surface of the bowl, a sallow or pale complexion, edema, diarrhea, impotence, an aversion to cold, a pale tongue with a white coating, and a submerged, thready and weak pulse characterize a deficiency of both *yin* and *yang*.

Treatment nourishes the kidneys and warms *yang*. Rehmannia Eight Formula (*ba wei di huang wan*) can be used.

Acupuncture and Moxibustion Treatment

See Chapter 4, Section 27.

Section 19
Carcinoma of the Stomach

Carcinoma of the stomach accounts for a full 50 percent of carcinomas involving the digestive system, and it is three times more likely to occur in men than in women.

It is generally categorized as one of the following TCM conformations: dysphagia, regurgitation, pain in the mid-upper abdomen or mass in the abdomen. According to a TCM understanding, anxiety can impair the spleen, giving rise to spleen *qi* stagnancy, which disturbs the fluid flow, causing accumulated fluids to transform into phlegm. Alternately, anger impairs the liver, resulting in liver *qi* stagnancy, which in turn disturbs blood circulation. Phlegm accumulation and blood stasis result in the obstruction of stomach *qi*, bringing about dysphagia while eating or vomiting following a meal.

Vital *qi* deficiency is the interior causal agent for the formation of stomach tumors. Moreover, the occurrence of stomach carcinoma usually follows a deficiency of *qi* and blood or a deficiency of the spleen and stomach. If, in addition to the above conditions, the person is emotionally distraught or has an improper diet, phlegm and stagnant *qi* will combine with excess heat and blood stasis, thereby consuming and exhausting blood and other fluids. As a result, carcinoma of the stomach occurs.

Diagnosis and Herbal Treatment

Treatment is based on an analysis of the cancer's development and severity. In the initial stage, it is classed as an exterior-excess conformation, specifically an accumulation of *qi*, blood, food, phlegm or dampness. In the later stages, it is best classified as a deficiency of *qi* and blood.

Disharmony Between the Liver and Spleen

Distention, fullness and pain in the mid-upper abdomen which radiates to the hypochondrium, eructation with fetid odor, hiccuping, vomiting, regurgitation, a pink tongue with a thin, white coating or thin, yellow coating, and a wiry pulse indicate disharmony of the liver and spleen.

Treatment regulates liver *qi* in order to harmonize the stomach and relieves pain to maintain the downward flow of *qi*. Bupleurum and Cyperus Combination (*chai hu shu gan tang*) and Inula and Hematite Combination (*xuan fu hua dai zhe shi tang*) can be given.

When persistent *qi* stagnancy transforms into fire and *yin* is thereby consumed, or when accumulated heat in the stomach impairs *yin*, there is a hot, burning sensation in the stomach, as well as thirst, gastric discomfort with acid regurgitation, a poor appetite, a preference for cold foods, fidgeting, a feverish sensation in the palms, soles and heart region, dry stools, a bright red tongue without coating, and a slippery and rapid or thready and rapid pulse.

Treatment nourishes *yin* and clears heat, for which Phellodendron Combination (*zi yin jiang huo tang*) can be administered.

Phlegm and Food Accumulation

Distention and fullness in the chest and upper abdomen, loss of appetite, difficulty in swallowing, expectoration of sticky sputum, vomiting of retained food, abdominal distention, loose stools, a white, greasy tongue coating and a wiry, slippery pulse indicate an accumulation of phlegm and food.

Treatment regulates *qi*, resolves phlegm, promotes digestion and eliminates the retained mass. The following should be used: Lithospermum and Oyster Shell Combination (*zi gen mu li tang*), plus 3 *qian* each of pinellia (*ban xia*), fritillaria (*bei mu*) and arisaema (*tian nan xing*) and 5 *qian* each of crataegus (*shan zha*), shen-chu (*shen qu*) and jelly seed (*mu man tou*).

Lithospermum and Oyster Shell Combination[1]

Zi Gen Mu Li Tang
(Lithospermum and Oyster Shell Decoction)

Tang-kuei	Angelicae radix	Dang gui	5.0
Peony	Paeoniae radix	Shao yao	3.0
Rhubarb	Rhei rhizoma	Da huang	1.5
Cnidium	Cnidii rhizoma	Chuan xiong*	3.0
Cimicifuga	Cimicifugae rhizoma	Sheng ma	2.0
Oyster shell	Ostreae testa	Mu li	4.0
Astragalus	Astragali radix	Huang qi	2.0
Licorice	Glycyrrhizae radix	Gan cao	1.0
Lonicera stem	Lonicerae caulis et folium	Ren dong teng	1.5
Lithospermum	Lithospermi radix	Zi cao gen	3.0

*Ligustici rhizoma, also known as chuan xiong, may be substituted.

Phlegm Accumulation and Blood Stasis

Fixed spasms in the mid-upper abdomen which are aggravated by pressure, a palpable mass, abdominal fullness, loss of appetite, vomiting of brown, watery substances, tarry stools, a dark purple tongue with ecchymosis or a thin, white tongue coating, and a thready and hesitant pulse characterize phlegm accumulation aggravated by blood stasis.

Treatment promotes blood circulation to remove stasis, resolves phlegm and softens the hard masses. Forsythia and Kun-pu Combination (san zhong kui jian tang), plus 3 qian pinellia (ban xia) and 5 qian crataegus (shan zha), can be given.

Deficiency-cold in the Spleen and Stomach

A vague sense of pain in the mid-upper abdomen which is relieved by heat and pressure, the vomiting of retained food the morning following ingestion or during the night from a meal eaten earlier in the day, dyspepsia, watery regurgitation, a sallow complexion, diarrhea, a pale tongue with a thin, white coating, and a submerged and slow or thready and weak pulse characterize deficiency-cold in the spleen and stomach.

Treatment warms the middle energizer in order to dissipate cold and strengthen the spleen and stomach. Ginseng and Ginger Combination (*ren shen tang*) and Six Major Herb Combination (*liu jun zi tang*) can be used.

If there is a *yang* deficiency of the spleen and kidneys which is marked by chills and cold limbs, add 1 *qian* cinnamon bark (*gui pi*) and 3 *qian* each of psoralea (*bu gu zhi*) and epimedium (*yin yang huo*).

A *qi* and blood deficiency may result from a spleen and stomach deficiency, which impairs the transformation of nutrients into *qi* and blood. This condition is marked by pallor, lassitude, palpitation, shortness of breath, spontaneous sweating, dizziness, a pale tongue and a submerged, thready and weak pulse.

Treatment replenishes *qi* and blood with Ginseng and *Tang-kuei* Ten Combination (*shi quan da bu tang*).

In the diagnosis and treatment of the four types of stomach cancer mentioned above, traditional Chinese herbs with anti-cancer properties can be selected and added to the above prescriptions. These herbs include:

lyrate nightshade (*bai ying*)   Chinese sage (*shi jian chuan*)
sago cycas leaf (*tie shu ye*)   oldenlandia (*bai hua she she cao*)
black nightshade (*long kui*)   Chinese actinidia root (*teng li gen*)
duchesnea (*she mei*)   smilax China root (*ba qi*)
scute (the whole plant)
(*ban zhi lian*)

Acupuncture and Moxibustion Treatment

See Chapter 4, Section 6.

Section 20
Whooping Cough

Whooping, or paroxysmal, cough is spasmodic and followed by an echo which sounds something like a cock's crow. It may persist for up to 100 days, and so is sometimes known as the hundred-day cough. Because a sick child may stretch his or her neck while coughing as does a cormorant, it is also called the cormorant cough.

A common infectious disease in children under five years old, whooping cough occurs in winter and spring. Its infectivity is the most severe in the first two to three weeks. Because of latent phlegm which is difficult to expectorate, the disease course is protracted and recovery difficult. Whooping cough can be very harmful to the health of young children, especially those who are already feeble. If there are no complications, however, the prognosis is good. When cured, the sick child can acquire a persistent immunity, and few suffer repeated attacks. The disease develops if the child's viscera are delicate or if he or she receives inadequate care, either of which can result in an accumulation of latent phlegm or of seasonal external pathogens in the mouth and nose which can affect the lungs.

Diagnosis and Herbal Treatment

Initial Stage

This stage lasts one to two weeks and, at first, the cough is like that of the common cold. Gradually, it worsens and is accompanied by sneezing, nasal discharge and a mild fever. The cough often is aggravated at night and accompanied by thin sputum, nasal and eye discharge, pale lips, a pale tongue with a white coating, and a floating, weak pulse. Alternately, a flushed face, red lips, thick sputum, a dry mouth, a red tongue with a yellow coating, and a floating, rapid pulse may be observed.

Treatment ventilates the lungs, relieves exterior symptoms, stops the cough and dispels phlegm with Platycodon and Schizonepeta Formula (*zhi sou san*), plus 3 *qian* plantago (*che qian zi*) and 1 *qian* licorice (*gan cao*).

If the whooping cough is accompanied by excess cold, add 1 *qian* each of *ma-huang* (*ma huang*) and asarum (*xi xin*) to the above modification of Platycodon and Schizonepeta Formula.

Should excess heat be present, add 3 *qian* each of morus bark (*sang bai pi*) and forsythia (*lian qiao*) and 1 *qian* fritillaria (*bei mu*) to the Platycodon and Schizonepeta Formula modification.

Platycodon and Schizonepeta Formula[1]
Zhi Sou San
(Stop Coughing Powder)[2]

Aster	*Asteris radix et rhizoma*	*Zi wan*	3.0
Stemona	*Stemonae radix*	*Bai bu*	3.0
Cynanchum	*Cynanchi stauntoni rhizoma et radix*	*Bai qian*	3.0
Citrus peel	*Citri pericarpium*	*Chen pi*	2.0
Schizonepeta	*Schizonepetae herba*	*Jing jie*	1.5
Platycodon	*Platycodi radix*	*Jie geng*	1.5
Licorice	*Glycyrrhizae radix*	*Gan cao*	1.0

Intermediate (Spasmodic-cough) Stage

This stage lasts four to six weeks and is characterized by severe cough paroxysms, congested face and eyes, clenched fists, a bent-over body, a protruded tongue, discharge from the nose and eyes during coughing fits, thick sputum, expectoration of sputum mixed with fluids or food, and hemoptysis or epistaxis. After a short pause, the cough resumes. It becomes worse at night and is aggravated by the accompanying signs of a dry mouth, thirst, a dry tongue coating and a slippery, rapid pulse.

Treatment clears the lungs, purges heat, promotes the descent of *qi* and resolves sputum. Morus and Platycodon Formula (*dun sou san*) is recommended.

If there is frequent vomiting, add 3 *qian* each of eriobotrya (*pi pa ye*) and hematite (*dai zhe shi*).

To treat distention and fullness in the chest and hypochondrium, add 1 *qian* gentian (*long dan cao*) and 3 *qian* each of trichosanthes peel (*gua lou pi*) and scute (*huang qin*).

To treat hemoptysis, add 5 *qian* each of imperata (*bai mao gen*) and agrimony (*xian he cao*).

If expectoration is especially difficult, add 3 *qian* trichosanthes fruit (*gua lou*) and 2 *qian* arisaema with bile (*dan nan xing*).

If the patient's throat is dry, add 3 *qian* asparagus (*tian meng dong*) and 3 *qian* ophiopogon (*mai men dong*).

Morus and Platycodon Formula[1]

Dun Sou San
(Relieve Spasmodic-cough Powder)

Bupleurum	*Bupleuri radix*	Chai hu	5.0
Platycodon	*Platycodi radix*	Jie geng	3.0
Scute	*Scutellariae radix*	Huang qin	3.0
Morus bark	*Mori radicis cortex*	Sang bai pi	3.0
Gardenia	*Gardeniae fructus*	Zhi zi	2.5
Licorice	*Glycyrrhizae radix*	Gan cao	1.0
Gypsum	*Gypsum fibrosum*	Shi gao	5.0

Late (Convalescent) Stage

This stage lasts two to three weeks. During this time, the coughing fits abate, and the echo and deep inhalation subside. There is only now a weak coughing sound, which is accompanied by smaller amounts of thin sputum, lassitude, sweating, pale lips, a pale tongue with very little coating, and a submerged, excess pulse.

Treatment ventilates the lungs, tonifies the spleen and alleviates the cough with astringent herbs. Four Major Herb Combination (*si jun zi tang*) and Fritillaria and Platycodon Formula (*ning sou wan*) can be given.

If there is a feverish sensation in the palms and soles, 3 *qian* each of glehnia root (*bei sha shen*) and lycium bark (*di gu pi*) should be added.

If there is a *yang* deficiency, 3 *qian* each of astragalus (*huang qi*) and cinnamon twig (*gui zhi*) should be added.

Fritillaria and Platycodon Formula[1]

Ning Sou Wan

(Relieve Cough Pill)

Platycodon	*Platycodi radix*	Jie geng	2.0
Fritillaria	*Fritillariae bulbus*	Bei mu	2.0
Morus bark	*Mori radicis cortex*	Sang bai pi	1.5
Dendrobium	*Dendrobii caulis*	Shi hu	2.0
Perilla seed	*Perillae semen*	Zi su zi	2.0
Citrus peel (exterior)	*Citri exocarpium rubrum*	Ju hong	1.0
Pinellia	*Pinellia rhizoma*	Ban xia	2.0
Hoelen	*Poria sclerotium*	Fu ling	2.0
Malt	*Hordei germinatus fructus*	Mai ya	1.0
Mentha	*Menthae herba*	Bo he	1.5
Licorice	*Glycyrrhizae radix*	Gan cao	0.5
Apricot seed	*Armeniacae semen*	Xing ren	1.5

Acupuncture and Moxibustion Treatment

Points of First Choice

- *dazhui* (GV 14)
- *sifeng* (EX-VE10)*

Reserved Points

- *shaoshang* (L 11)
- *shangyang* (LI 1)

Prick to induce bleeding.

- *chize* (L 5)
- *hegu* (LI 4)

Treatment Method

Treat once daily for a total of nine treatments.

* Prick point to withdraw a few drops of clear yellow fluid.

Chapter 6

Surgical and Skin Diseases

Section 1
Furuncle

A furuncle is an acute pyogenic infection in the outer tissue of the skin. It involves a single hair follicle and its sebaceous glands and frequently spreads to the subcutaneous tissue. Its diameter is no more than 3 cm. Furuncles often develop in the head, face, neck, back or buttocks. They are characterized by redness, burning, a sensation of heat, pain, a projection with a shallow base and a linited swelling area. Healing involves draining the pus.

The disease is induced by an accumulation of toxins due to heat in the muscles and skin. Excess consumption of alcohol or heat in the viscera can result in a disorder of *qi* and blood, which then creates a stagnancy in the meridians and collaterals. In hot weather, when perspiration cannot dissipate, summer dampness is retained in the muscles and skin, thereby inducing an infection when the skin is scratched.

Diagnosis and Herbal Treatment

The initial clinical manifestation is a small, hard, red nodule accompanied by burning pain. The nodule gradually enlarges, and a white or yellow, purulent core is formed. After several days the furuncle softens and festers. In most cases, when the pus is drained, the redness and swelling dissipate and the furuncle begins to heal. Most cases have no general symptoms, but in a severe case, an aversion to cold, fever, headache, a dry throat, constipation, dark yellow urine, a yellow tongue coating and a rapid pulse may be observed.

Treatment clears heat and toxins, cools the blood and removes blood stasis. Angelica and Frankincense Combination (*xian fang huo ming yin*) can be used.

If there is fever and an aversion to cold, 2 *qian* schizonepeta (*jing jie*) should be added.

In the case of high fever, fidgeting or thirst, add 4 *qian* raw rehmannia (*sheng di huang*) and 10 *qian* gypsum (*shi gao*).

If there is severe summer dampness, add 3 *qian* each of agastache (*huo xiang*) and eupatorium (*pei lan*).

If the furuncles are on the buttocks, add 3 *qian* each of achyranthes (*niu xi*) and phellodendron (*huang bo*).

When pus has formed, the furuncle should be incised for drainage or the purulent core should be removed. Squeezing can result in the proliferation of toxins and is, therefore, discouraged.

Common Acupuncture and Moxibustion Points

Group #1

- *fengchi* (G 20)
- *quchi* (LI 11)
- *dazhui* (GV 14)

Group #2

- *dazhui* (GV 14)   • *dashu* (B 11)
- *weizhong* (B 40)

Use the points from Groups #1 and #2 on alternate days.

Section 2
Carbuncle

A carbuncle is a serious purulent infection in the skin or deep tissue. The affected area (10-13 cm) is larger than that of a furuncle. A carbuncle is characterized by redness and swelling, though often without a purulent core. The onset is abrupt and accompanied by heat and pain. If the carbuncle does not fester, it easily subsides, but if it does, it is liable to break. Carbuncles are known as acute cellulitis in Western medicine.

According to a TCM understanding, carbuncles are associated with a *yang* conformation. If *qi* and blood are impeded by pathogens, stagnancy occurs and toxins accumulate in the skin and subcutaneous tissue, causing carbuncles. This condition is generally induced by excess consumption of fats or meat, which leads to an accumulation of heat-dampness or fire toxins. Deficiency of vital *qi,* caused by prolonged diabetes or invasions of pathogens into the broken skin, give rise to *qi* stagnancy and blood stasis, and the festering tissue becomes a carbuncle.

Diagnosis and Herbal Treatment

Initial Stage

The carbuncle has a purulent core and is red, swollen, localized and similar to a furuncle, with a white or yellow core. As inflammation and pain develop, the mass spreads rapidly to the adjacent tissue. Likewise, a carbuncle without a purulent core will also be red, swollen, inflamed and painful, with a clear margin and a rapid development. To varying degrees, both types share some general manifestations, namely, chills, fever, headache, thirst, dry stools, dark yellow urine, a red tongue with a dry, yellow coating, and a slippery, rapid pulse. The conformation which includes both types of carbuncle is overabundance of heat toxins, leading to an obstruction of the meridians.

Treatment clears heat and toxins, while promoting blood circulation to remove stasis. Angelica and Frankincense Combination (*xian fang huo ming yin*) can be used.

If there is a high fever, fidgeting or thirst, add 10 *qian* gypsum (*shi gao*) and 5 *qian* isatis leaf (*da qing ye*).

When dealing with a carbuncle in the upper body, add 3 *qian* wild chrysanthemum (*ye ju hua*). To treat one in the midsection, add 20 *qian* gentian (*long dan cao*) and 3 *qian* scute (*huang qin*). To treat a carbuncle in the lower body, add 3 *qian* each of achyranthes (*niu xi*) and phellodendron (*huang bo*).

Add 2 *qian* rhubarb (*da huang*) to relieve constipation.

Suppurative Stage

The red, swollen center turns soft and suppurates in a honeycomb pattern. Manifestations include severe pain, persistent fever, a dry mouth, thirst, constipation, dark yellow urine, a thick, yellow tongue coating and a surging, rapid pulse. Gleditsia Combination (*tuo li xiao du yin*) can be used.

Gleditsia Combination[1]

Tuo Li Xiao Du Yin

(Drain Pus and Expulse Toxin Decoction)

Tang-kuei	Angelicae radix	Dang gui	5.0
Hoelen	Poria sclerotium	Fu ling	5.0
Ginseng	Ginseng radix	Ren shen	3.0
Peony	Paeoniae radix	Shao yao	3.0
Cnidium	Cnidii rhizoma	Chuan xiong*	3.0
Platycodon	Platycodi radix	Jie geng	3.0
Atractylodes, white	Atractylodis rhizoma	Bai zhu	3.0
Gleditsia thorn	Gleditsiae spina	Zao ci	2.0
Astragalus	Astragali radix	Huang qi	1.5
Lonicera	Lonicerae flos	Jin yin hua	1.0
Angelica	Angelicae dahuricae radix	Bai zhi	1.0
Licorice	Glycyrrhizae radix	Gan cao	1.0

Ligustici rhizoma, also known as *chuan xiong*, may be substituted.

Post-festering Stage

Following pus drainage, swelling gradually subsides, new tissue regenerates, the carbuncle heals and general symptoms disappear. If the patient's constitution is weak and the pus is thin, however, granulation grows slowly or remains hard at the base and fails to dissipate. In this case, Astragalus Combination (*huang qi jian zhong tang*) should be used for strengthening the spleen and stomach.

If the carbuncle does not completely drain, surgical means may become necessary.

Acupuncture and Moxibustion Treatment

Common Points

- *shenzhu* (GV 12)
- *lingtai* (GV 10)
- *hegu* (LI 4)
- *weizhong* (B 30)

Treatment Method

Needle with the reducing method or prick the points to induce bleeding.

Section 3
Erysipelas

As the onset of this illness is sudden, its spread rapid, and the skin color red, erysipelas is known as "red poison" (*dan du*). When it occurs in the face and head, it is called "fire-redness around the head" (*bao tou huo dan*); if it develops in the legs, it is known as "flowing fire" (*liu huo*); and if it migrates over the entire body, it is "wandering erysipelas" (*chi you dan*).

When the skin is broken, fire pathogens invade the skin and muscles. Alternately, blood stasis and excess heat can cause a blockage of the meridians and collaterals, as well as a disorder of *ying* and *wei*, a stagnation of *qi* and blood, or an accumulation of external toxic pathogens--all of which can induce the illness. If erysipelas occurs in the face, it is caused by wind-heat; when it develops in the hypochondrium, waist or hips, it is induced by liver heat; and if it occurs in the legs, heat-dampness is the culprit.

Diagnosis and Herbal Treatment

Onset is abrupt. At first there are chills, fever, headache, thirst, a poor appetite, constipation, red-tinged urine, a red tongue with a thin, white or greasy, yellow coating, and a rapid or slippery and rapid pulse. The erythema is slightly raised when compared to the adjacent skin and is delineated by clear, irregular margins. Hot pain and blisters in the red, swollen area may also be present. The erythema spreads rapidly and, after five or six days, turns from bright to dark red, then desquamates and gradually heals. In some cases, the inflammation invades the subcutaneous tissues, resulting in erysipelas of the cellulitis.

Treatment clears heat and toxins, cools the blood and removes blood stasis. Specific formulas are selected according to the location of the disease. Erythema of the face is treated with Scute and Cimicifuga Combination (*pu ji xiao du yin*). When erythema is located in the legs, Coptis and Rhubarb Combination (*huang lian jie du tang*) and Lonicera and Rehmannia Formula (*bai du san*) are recommended.

Scute and Cimicifuga Combination[1]
Pu Ji Xiao Du Yin
(Universal Benefit Decoction to Eliminate Toxin)[2]

Scute	Scutellariae radix	Huang qin	3.0
Coptis	Coptidis rhizoma	Huang lian	2.0
Arctium	Arctii fructus	Niu bang zi	3.0
Scrophularia	Scrophulariae radix	Xuan shen	3.0
Licorice	Glycyrrhizae radix	Gan cao	1.0
Platycodon	Platycodi radix	Jie geng	1.0
Cimicifuga	Cimicifugae rhizoma	Sheng ma	1.0
Bupleurum	Bupleuri radix	Chai hu	2.0
Puffball	Lasiosphaera	Ma bo	1.0
Citrus peel	Citri pericarpium	Chen pi	1.0
Mentha	Menthae herba	Bo he	1.5
Silkworm	Bombyx batryticatus	Bai jiang can	2.0
Isatis root	Isatidis rhizoma et radix	Ban lan gen	4.0
Forsythia	Forsythiae fructus	Lian qiao	4.0

Lonicera and Rehmannia Formula[1]
Bai Du San
(Antiphlogistic Powder)

Rehmannia, raw	*Rehmanniae radix*	*Sheng di huang*	4.5
Platycodon	*Platycodi radix*	*Jie geng*	2.5
Forsythia	*Forsythiae fructus*	*Lian qiao*	2.5
Moutan	*Moutan radicis cortex*	*Mu dan pi*	2.0
Trichosanthes root	*Trichosanthis radix*	*Gua lou gen*	2.5
Scrophularia	*Scrophulariae radix*	*Xuan shen*	2.5
Lonicera	*Lonicerae flos*	*Jin yin hua*	2.5
Bupleurum	*Bupleuri radix*	*Chai hu*	2.0
Licorice	*Glycyrrhizae radix*	*Gan cao*	1.0
Phellodendron	*Phellodendri cortex*	*Huang bo*	1.5
Mentha	*Menthae herba*	*Bo he*	1.5
Peony, red	*Paeoniae rubra radix*	*Chi shao*	1.5
Gypsum	*Gypsum fibrosum*	*Shi gao*	3.0
Arctium	*Arctii fructus*	*Niu bang zi*	2.5

Common Acupuncture and Moxibustion Points

- *hegu* (LI 4)
- *quchi* (LI 11)
- *zusanli* (S 36)
- *jiexi* (S 41)
- *yinlingquan* (Sp 9)
- *xuehai* (Sp 10)
- *weizhong* (B 40)

Section 4
Mumps

Also known as "swollen cheeks" or "toad's cheeks" in TCM, mumps is an acute infectious disease characterized by fever and pain in the cheeks and the area beneath the ears. Mumps can occur at any time during the year, but it is most common in spring and winter. For the most part, the illness develops in young school-age children, but only rarely in infants.

Mumps is caused by wind-heat pathogens, which invade the body through the mouth and nostrils, block the *shao yang* meridians and accumulate in the cheeks, thereby causing them to become swollen, hard and painful. *Shao yang* disease alternates with *jue yin* disease, in which a pathogenic invasion of the *jue yin* meridians can result in a red scrotum and painful, red, swollen testes in older boys.

Diagnosis and Herbal Treatment

The main symptom is swelling of the cheeks and the area beneath the ears. In mild cases, the swelling involves one or both sides of the parotid glands with accompanying soreness and difficulty in chewing. In severe cases, the swelling worsens in the first two to three days and extends to the side of the neck, with general symptoms such as fever, an aversion to cold, fidgeting, thirst, a poor appetite and listlessness.

Ascent of Wind-heat

An aversion to cold, fever, headache, a slight cough, swelling with soreness in one or both sides of the cheeks and subaural regions, difficulty in opening the mouth and chewing, occasional redness in the cheeks, a thin, white or yellow tongue coating and a slippery, rapid pulse characterize mumps due to an ascent of wind-heat.

Mild cases heal spontaneously in three to four days, but severe cases require the use of Lonicera and Forsythia Formula (*yin qiao san*), which dispels wind, clears heat, softens the affected area and reduces swelling. In addition, cotton rose leaf (*fu rong ye*) can be made into a paste and applied topically to the affected areas.

Excess Toxic Heat

This type of mumps is characterized by an aversion to cold, a high fever, headache, fidgeting, thirst, a poor appetite, vomiting, diffuse, hard swelling in the cheeks with hot pain and tenderness, redness and swelling in the throat, difficulty in swallowing and chewing, dry stools, small amounts of dark yellow urine, a red tongue with a yellow coating, and a slippery, rapid pulse.

Scute and Cimicifuga Combination (*pu ji xiao du yin*) can be used to clear heat and toxins, soften the tissue and reduce swelling.

If the swelling is diffuse and hard, add 3 *qian* each of prunella (*xia ku cao*) and kun pu (*kun bu*).

To treat constipation, add 2 *qian* rhubarb (*da huang*).

If the disease affects the testes, they will become swollen and painful. Three *qian* each of citrus seed (*ju he*), litchi seed (*li zhi he*) and corydalis (*yan hu suo*) should be added.

Acupuncture and Moxibustion Treatment

Points of First Choice

- *yifeng* (TE 17)
- *jiache* (S 6)
- *hegu* (LI 4)

Reserved Points

To treat fever, add *quchi* (LI 11) and *dazhui* (GV 14).

Treatment Method

Needle with the reducing method, retaining the needle for 20-30 minutes.

Treat once daily until the swelling subsides.

Chapter 7

Gynecological Disorders

Section 1
Abnormal Menstruation

Abnormal menstruation refers to abnormalities in duration of cycle or the amount, color or quality of blood. Clinical classifications are advanced menstruation, retarded menstruation, menorrhagia, oligomenorrhea, dysmenorrhea, amenorrhea and uterine bleeding.

It should be noted that it is not abnormal for a woman to experience symptoms such as mild pain in the lower abdomen, lower back pain, lassitude, a poor appetite, distention of the breasts or fidgeting, either during or just prior to the menstrual period. In a normal patient, these symptoms disappear naturally after menstruation has ceased. Furthermore, there is always a period of irregular menstruation or even amenorrhea after menophania, however, this is also self-correcting.

Advanced menstruation generally belongs to the blood heat or *qi* deficiency conformation, whereas retarded menstruation to the blood cold or blood deficiency conformation.

Menstruation is further differentiated into blood deficiency, when the color of the blood is light; blood heat conformation, when the color is deep red; and deficiency-cold, when the color is dark red or black. Profuse menstruation belongs to blood heat or *qi* deficiency, and scanty menstruation to blood deficiency or blood cold conformation. Lower abdominal pain which can be alleviated with pressure or warmth is generally caused by deficiency-cold, whereas pain which is aggravated by pressure and feels as if there were a hard, small mass in the abdomen is characteristic of blood stasis. Continual pain that is aggravated before or following menstruation is due to blood stasis and excess heat, while a distending pain in the lower abdomen during menstruation is due to *qi* stagnancy.

In general, the *ben* (origin or root) is of primary concern when treating abnormal menstruation. A patient suffering from a particular disease should have the disease administered to first, since the menstruation will be spontaneously corrected following recovery. Of course, if there is no accompanying disease, the patient should be treated to normalize her periods.

Diagnosis and Herbal Treatment

Regardless of whether the menstruation is advanced or retarded, treatment should be given after the period is finished in order to affect a radical cure according to the patient's constitution, the severity of the ailment and its differentiation as to cold or heat and deficiency or excess.

Advanced Menstruation

When the menstrual cycle is less than 25 days or when menstruation begins at least a week early for three consecutive months, the condition is known as advanced menstruation. When the woman's period is only occasionally early and she has no other symptoms, her menstrual cycle is not considered advanced.

Advanced menstruation is due to *yin* deficiency of the liver and kidneys, which results in blood heat, excess internal *qi* and fire, and/or dysfunctions of the *chongmai* (flush vessel, FV) and *renmai* (conception vessel, CV). Occasionally, fatigue can also impair these vessels and thereby induce advanced menstruation.

According to TCM, advanced menstruation is due to heat and blood deficiency. The manifestations are: profuse amounts of bright red blood, occasional abdominal pain and lower back soreness, a pale red and thorny tongue, and a weak and somewhat rapid pulse.

Treatment nourishes blood and clears heat with *Tang-kuei Four Combination* (*si wu tang*), 3 *qian* scute (*huang qin*) and 2 *qian* parched schizonepeta (*jing jie tan*). This modification is known as Decoction of Scute, Schizonepeta and Four Herbs (*qin jing si wu tang*).

If there is abdominal pain, add 3 *qian* each of melia (*chuan lian zi*) and cyperus (*xiang fu zi*).

For lower back pain, add 3 *qian* each of dipsacus (*xu duan*) and eucommia (*du zhong*).

To treat fullness of the breasts, add 2 *qian* bupleurum (*chai hu*).

If menstrual flow is profuse, causing anemia, the tongue coating will be light and the pulse weak. Should this occur, Ginseng and Longan Combination (*gui pi tang*) may be added.

Retarded (Late) Menstruation

A menstrual cycle which exceeds 35 days for three consecutive cycles and for which early pregnancy has been ruled out is known as retarded menstruation. The ailment is usually due to a constitutional deficiency, lack of proper care following an illness, a deficiency of *qi* and blood, a deficiency of the *chongmai* (FV) and *renmai* (CV), or the effects of consuming very cold drinks during the menstrual period, getting soaked in the rain or standing in water for a long time. In any of the above scenarios, the end result is cold-dampness accumulation in the uterus and, consequently, retarded menstruation.

The conformation of retarded menstruation belongs to uterine cold and blood deficiency. Key manifestations are monthly delayed menstruation with small quantities of dark- or light-colored blood, abdominal and lower back pain, a light-colored tongue coating and a thready pulse.

Treatment nourishes blood and warms the meridians with *Tang-kuei* Four Combination (*si wu tang*), plus 2 *qian* artemisia (*ai ye*) and 3 *qian* cyperus (*xiang fu zi*).

For abdominal pain, add 3 *qian* corydalis (*yan hu suo*).

For cases of severe cold pain, add 0.5 *qian* cinnamon bark (*rou gui*).

For patients with lower back pain, add 3 *qian* each of dipsacus (*xu duan*) and eucommia (*du zhong*).

If the menstrual flow is heavy and the blood is light-colored, thereby indicating anemia, Ginseng and Longan Combination (*gui pi tang*) can also be used.

Amenorrhea

Physiological amenorrhea is the normal absence of menstruation during pregnancy or lactation or following menopause. Amenorrhea occurring at any other time is considered pathogenic. Primary amenorrhea is the absence of menarche in a female 16 years or older. Secondary amenorrhea is a failure to menstruate for at least three consecutive months at some time following menarche. Because primary amenorrhea is often due to anatomic or congenital deformities or endocrine disturbances, only secondary amenorrhea will be discussed here.

According to a TCM understanding, amenorrhea is usually due to a deficiency of the spleen and kidneys which impedes blood flow in the uterus, or to cold coagulation, blood stasis and the blockage of the *chongmai* (FV) and *renmai* (CV), so that the menstrual blood cannot be properly or adequately discharged from the body.

1. Spleen and kidney deficiency

Manifestations include dizziness, a poor appetite, lassitude, palpitation, shortness of breath, abdominal distention, loose stools, lower back pain, weak legs, a pale tongue with a thin, white coating, and a submerged and thready or thready and weak pulse.

Treatment tonifies the liver and kidneys and nourishes and warms the *chongmai* and *renmai*. The following is recommended: Ginseng and *Tang-kuei* Ten Combination (*shi quan da bu tang*), plus 4 *qian* cuscuta (*tu si zi*), 3 *qian* cistanche (*rou cong rong*) and 5 *qian* leonurus (*yi mu cao*).

2. Cold coagulation and blood stasis

Cold pain in the lower abdomen, distending pain in the breasts, lower back soreness, loose stools, cold limbs, a purple tongue with petechiae, and a thready pulse characterize cold coagulation aggravated by blood stasis.

Treatment warms the meridians, dispels cold, stimulates blood circulation and eliminates blood stasis. *Tang-kuei* and Evodia Combination (*wen jing tang*) can be used.

Tang-kuei and Evodia Combination[1]
Wen Jing Tang
(Warm the Menses Decoction)[2]

Evodia	Evodiae fructus	Wu zhu yu	1.0
Cinnamon twig	Cinnamomi ramulus	Gui zhi	2.0
Tang-kuei	Angelicae radix	Dang gui	3.0
Cnidium	Cnidii rhizoma	Chuan xiong*	2.0
Peony	Paeoniae radix	Bai shao yao	2.0
Gelatin	Asini gelatinum	A jiao	2.0
Ophiopogon	Ophiopogonis rhizoma	Mai men dong	5.0
Moutan	Moutan radicis cortex	Mu dan pi	2.0
Ginseng	Ginseng radix	Ren shen	2.0
Pinellia	Pinellia rhizoma	Ban xia	5.0
Ginger, dry	Zingiberis rhizoma	Gan jiang	1.0
Licorice	Glycyrrhizae radix	Gan cao	2.0

*Ligustici rhizoma, also known as chuan xiong, may be substituted.

For patients with lower back pain, add 3 qian each of dipsacus (xu duan) and psoralea (bu gu zhi).

To treat profuse leukorrhea, add 3 qian each of cuscuta (tu si zi) and hoelen (fu ling).

For patients with a poor appetite, add 1.5 qian citrus peel (chen pi) and 3 qian crataegus (shan zha).

Should blood stasis become severe, add 3 qian each of persica (tao ren) and carthamus (hong hua) and 5 qian of leonurus (yi mu cao).

If amenorrhea lasts more than three months and there are no other symptoms or complications and the patient has a normal tongue and pulse, the problem may be emotional distress or a change in the weather or the patient's environment. For such a case, qi and blood must be nourished in order to improve the functioning of the liver and kidneys. Tang-kuei and

Ginseng Eight Combination (*ba zhen tang*) or *Tang-kuei* and Bupleurum Formula (*xiao yao san*) can be used.

Beng Lou (Uterine Bleeding)

Beng lou is the condition, as well as the corresponding conformation, of persistent, irregular menstrual bleeding, which may be scanty or copious and is characterized by short, intermittent periods in which the blood flow ceases. "*Beng*" refers to sudden, profuse uterine bleeding, while "*lou*" refers to mild, persistent vaginal bleeding known as spotting in the United States. Though the two are dissimilar, either can transform into the other during the course of the disease, and there are some similarities in the methods of treatment. When the blood flow is sometimes profuse and sometimes scanty, thereby making exact categorization into *beng* or *lou* impossible, the condition is called *beng lou* in TCM. *Beng lou* is most often seen in puberal or climacteric women and can be a manifestation of many functional and organic diseases.

The etiology of uterine bleeding can, for the most part, be traced to the derangement of the *chongmai* and *renmai* and their consequent inability to stop menstruation. Specifically, *beng lou* can be attributed to four causes: spleen *qi* deficiency, kidney deficiency, blood heat or blood stasis.

Diagnosis and Herbal Treatment

Spleen *Qi* Deficiency

A failure of spleen *qi* to keep blood circulating within the vessels is characterized by irregular vaginal bleeding which may be continuous in small amounts or sudden and profuse or may alternate between these two extremes; light-colored, dilute menstrual blood with no blood clots; lassitude; a pale complexion; shortness of breath; sweating; edema in the face and feet; a poor appetite; loose stools; a light-colored, thick tongue with teeth marks along the edges and a thin, white coating; and a soft and floating pulse or thready and weak pulse.

Treatment reinforces *qi* and controls blood with Ginseng and Longan Combination (*gui pi tang*).

If the blood is a "fresh" red, add 3 *qian* each of sanguisorba (*di yu*) and biota top (*ce bo ye*).

In the case of massive bleeding, add 3 *qian* each of cattail pollen (*pu huang*) and sanguisorba (*di yu*).

To improve a poor appetite, add 3 *qian* each of citrus peel (*chen pi*) and germinated rice (*gu ya*).

Kidney *Yin* Deficiency

This deficiency is manifested in irregular vaginal bleeding which is sometimes profuse and sometimes scanty (though profuse bleeding is more commonly seen); "fresh" red menstrual blood; dizziness; tinnitus; insomnia; thin, dry skin; lower back pain; painful heels; a sore throat; a dry mouth; constipation; a cardinal red tongue with a thin, dry coating; and a thready, rapid pulse.

Treatment reinforces the kidneys, nourishes *yin*, consolidates the meridians and controls bleeding. Anemarrhena, Phellodendron and Rehmannia Combination (*zhi bo ba wei wan*) can be used.

In case of massive bleeding, 3 *qian* each of sanguisorba (*di yu*) and madder (*qian cao gen*) should be added.

To treat a general *yin* deficiency, add 3 *qian* each of tortoise shell (*gui pan*) and gelatin (*a jiao*).

To treat dizziness, add 3 *qian* each of ligustrum (*nu zhen zi*) and eclipta (*han lian cao*).

In the case of a dry mouth and sore throat, add 3 *qian* each of scrophularia (*xuan shen*) and ophiopogon (*mai men dong*).

Kidney *Yang* Deficiency

This deficiency is characterized by irregular but persistent vaginal bleeding which is sometimes profuse and sometimes scanty (though profuse bleeding is more common); light-colored and dilute or dark purple menstrual blood; chills; an aversion to cold; cold limbs; lower back pain; cold pain in the lower abdomen; frequent, clear urination or dripping after urination; a light-colored tongue with a thin coating; and a submerged, thready and weak pulse.

Treatment reinforces the kidneys and warms *yang*. Eucommia and Rehmannia Formula (*you gui wan*) can be used.

Blood Heat

This condition is marked by profuse, irregular, bright red vaginal bleeding; a flushed face; a dry mouth and throat; thirst with a preference for cold beverages; fidgeting; insomnia; constipation; a dark red tongue with a thin, yellow coating or a red tongue with little coating; and a thready, wiry and rapid pulse.

Treatment clears heat, cools the blood, consolidates the meridians and thereby controls bleeding with Tortoise Shell and Scute Combination (*gu jing tang*).

Tortoise Shell and Scute Combination
Gu Jing Tang[18]
(Menorrhagia Decoction)[18]

Tortoise shell	*Testudinis plastrum*	*Gui ban*	4.0
Peony	*Paeoniae radix*	*Shao yao*	3.0
Scute	*Scutellariae radix*	*Huang qin*	3.0
Phellodendron	*Phellodendri cortex*	*Huang bo*	3.0
Ailanthus root	*Ailanthi cortex*	*Chun pi*	2.0
Cyperus	*Cyperi rhizoma*	*Xiang fu zi*	3.0

Functions: eliminates heat; nourishes *yin*; consolidates the meridians to stop bleeding.

Explanation: Tortoise shell and peony nourish *yin*, while scute, phellodendron and ailanthus root clear heat, stop bleeding and consolidate the meridians. Cyperus adjusts the flow of *qi* and relieves stagnancy.

Blood Stasis

Blood stasis, as it relates to menstrual disorders, is marked by mild, persistent vaginal discharge or sudden, profuse blood flow with black clots; lower abdominal pain which is aggravated by pressure and alleviated by the discharge of clots; a purple tongue with a thin, white coating and petechiae along its edges; and a submerged, hesitant pulse.

Treatment normalizes bleeding by eliminating blood stasis and alleviates pain by regulating the flow of *qi. Tang-kuei* Four Combination (*si wu tang*) and Pteropus and Bulrush Formula (*shi xiao san*) can be used.

If the discharge of blood clots is impeded, 3 *qian* each of crataegus (*shan zha*) and corydalis (*yan hu suo*) can be added. However, if the discharge is profuse and purple, add 3 *qian* sophora (*huai hua*) instead.

Acupuncture and Moxibustion Treatment

Advanced Menstruation

- *qihai* (CV 6)
- *taichong* (Liv 3)
- *sanyinjiao* (Sp 6)
- *taixi* (K 3)

Retarded Menstruation

- *qihai* (CV 6)
- *xuehai* (Sp 10)
- *sanyinjiao* (Sp 6)
- *guilai* (S 29)

Amenorrhea

1. Spleen and kidney deficiency
   - *pishu* (B 20)
   - *zusanli* (S 36)
   - *shenshu* (B 23)
   - *qihai* (CV 6)

2. Cold coagulation and blood stasis
   - *zhongji* (CV 3)
   - *xuehai* (Sp 10)
   - *xingjian* (Liv 2)
   - *hegu* (LI 4)
   - *sanyinjiao* (Sp 6)

Beng Lou (Uterine Bleeding)

1. Common points
   - *guanyuan* (CV 4)
   - *yinbai* (Sp 1)
   - *sanyinjiao* (Sp 6)

2. Additional points for the treatment of excess heat
   - *xuehai* (Sp 10)
   - *shuiquan* (K 5)

3. Additional points for the treatment of *yin* deficiency
   - *neiguan* (P 6)
   - *taixi* (K 3)

4. Additional points for the treatment of *qi* deficiency
   - *pishu* (B 20)
   - *zusanli* (S 36)

Section 2
Dysmenorrhea

The main symptom of dysmenorrhea, or painful menstruation, is pain in the lower abdomen and lower back which appears just before and just following menstruation or for a few hours during the menstrual period or throughout the entire period for at least three consecutive menstrual cycles. In severe cases, nausea, vomiting, loss of appetite or poor appetite, diarrhea, sweating, cold limbs, a pale complexion, and headache and backache which adversely affect daily activities may also be present. Dysmenorrhea can be classified into primary and secondary types, the former of which may begin shortly after menarche and is not associated with any organic disease, and the latter of which is always accompanied by an organic disease. Slight discomfort just prior to or during menstruation is not considered dysmenorrhea.

Etiologically, dysmenorrhea is mainly due to the impeded flow of *qi* and blood. For example, *qi* and blood deficiency or *qi* stagnancy aggravated by blood stasis may cause the retardation of the menstrual flow and result in dysmenorrhea.

The pain is usually located in the lower abdomen. In TCM, the middle part of the lower abdomen, or *xiao fu*, belongs to the *renmai* (CV) and is subordinate to the kidneys, while the outer part of the lower abdomen, or *shao fu*, belongs to the *chongmai* (FV) and is subordinate to the liver. In the former case, the pain generally results from blood stasis, while in the latter, it is the result of *qi* stagnancy. In a severe case, the pain may radiate to the lower back, pudendum and anus, or even upwards to the epigastrium, prompting nausea and vomiting.

Lower abdominal pain is excess in nature if it is aggravated by pressure and deficient if it is reduced by pressure. When there are intermittent cramps, the pain is categorized as excess, while persistent, lingering pain is considered deficient.

The pain is associated with a heat conformation when it is aggravated by heat and with a cold conformation when it is alleviated by heat.

When abdominal distention surpasses the pain, *qi* stagnancy is the causative agent, while blood stasis is the underlying cause when the pain is more acute than the distention. When distention and pain are of the same degree, both *qi* stagnancy and blood stasis are involved.

If the lower abdominal pain and distention are intermittent, *qi* stagnancy is to blame, but if paroxysmal pain is alleviated by the discharge of clots, blood stasis is involved. If the pain is accompanied by a bearing-down sensation, *qi* deficiency is the cause, whereas persistent, fixed pain may be traced to blood stasis.

Pain prior to and during menstruation is induced by *qi* stagnancy or blood stasis, both of which are associated with an excess syndrome, while pain following menstruation is caused by a deficiency of *qi* or blood. According to the principle "there is no pain when there is circulation," treatment attempts to remove the obstruction to the flow of *qi* and blood and thereby halt the pain. If the dysmenorrhea is cold-natured, the warming method should be applied, but if it is deficient in nature, tonification is necessary.

Diagnosis and Herbal Treatment

Qi and Blood Stagnancy

Distending or paroxysmal pain in the lower abdomen before or during menstruation; scanty, impeded menstrual flow which is dark purple or contains blood clots; pain which is alleviated following the discharge of clots; distending pain in the chest, breasts and hypochondrium prior to menstruation; a dark purple tongue with a thin, white coating and petechiae or spots along the edge; and a submerged, wiry or submerged, hesitant pulse characterize *qi* stagnancy aggravated by blood stasis.

Treatment regulates *qi*, tonifies blood, removes blood stasis and halts pain. Persica and Achyranthes Combination (*xue fu zhu yu tang*) can be used.

If the distention is worse than the pain, add 3 *qian* each of cyperus (*xiang fu zi*) and turmeric (*yu jin*).

To treat distending pain in the breasts, add 4 *qian* each of prunella (*xia ku cao*) and horse chestnut (*suo luo zi*).

If the discharge of clots is difficult, add 3 *qian* each of sparganium (*san ling*) and zedoaria (*e shu*).

For the treatment of severe pain, also administer Pteropus and Bulrush Formula (*shi xiao san*).

Cold Coagulation and Blood Stasis

Severe, cold or cramping pain in the lower abdomen before or during menstruation; an aversion to cold in the painful region; alleviation of pain after the application of hot compresses; impeded, scanty, dark purple menstruation with blood clots; an aversion to cold; loose stools; a dark purple tongue with petechiae and spots; a thin or thin, white and greasy tongue coating; and a submerged, wiry pulse characterize cold coagulation complicated by blood stasis.

Treatment warms the meridians, dispels cold, activates blood circulation and stops the pain, for which *Tang-kuei* and Evodia Combination (*wen jing tang*) can be used.

In case of abdominal pain and vomiting, add 2 *qian* galanga (*gao liang jiang*) and 1 *qian* evodia (*wu zhu yu*).

For patients with blood stasis which is not confined to menstrual disorders, add 3 *qian* each of sparganium (*san ling*) and lycopus (*ze lan*).

To treat diarrhea and cold limbs, add 2 *qian* each of psoralea (*bu gu zhi*) and zanthoxylum (*jiao mu*).

Should the patient experience lower abdominal pain, add 1.5 *qian* fennel (*xiao hui xiang*) and 3 *qian* artemisia (*ai ye*).

_Qi_ and Blood Deficiency

Lingering, persistent lower abdominal pain during or following menstruation which is accompanied by a bearing-down sensation and distention in the vulva and which can be alleviated by warmth and pressure; scanty, light-colored menstrual flow with no clots; a pale complexion; lassitude; a soft voice; a light-colored, thick tongue with a thin, white coating and teeth marks along the edges; and a thready, weak and submerged pulse characterize *qi* and blood deficiency.

Treatment reinforces *qi*, nourishes blood, regulates the meridians and alleviates pain with Ginseng and *Tang-kuei* Ten Combination (*shi quan da bu tang*).

In case of thin, light-colored menstrual blood, 3 *qian* gelatin (*a jiao*) and 2 *qian* artemisia (*ai ye*) should be added.

For severe pain, also give the patient Pteropus and Bulrush Formula (*shi xiao san*).

To treat diarrhea during menstruation, add 2 *qian* psoralea (*bu gu zhi*) and 3 *qian shen-chu* (*shen qu*).

For patients with lower back pain, add 3 *qian* eucommia (*du zhong*).

To treat a bearing-down sensation in the vulva, add 3 *qian* each of cimicifuga (*sheng ma*), bupleurum (*chai hu*) and *chih-ko* (*zhi ke*).

Acupuncture and Moxibustion Treatment

Common Points

- *zhongji* (CV 3)
- *sanyinjiao* (Sp 6)

Additional Point to Treat *Qi* and Blood Stagnancy

- *ligou* (Liv 5)

Additional Points to Treat Cold Coagulation

- guanyuan (CV 4)
- sanyinjiao (Sp 6)
- *zusanli* (S 36)

Apply the warming needle with moxibustion.

ional Points to Treat *Qi* and Blood Deficiency

- *qihai* (CV 6)
- *dahe* (K 12)
- *sanyinjiao* (Sp 6)

Section 3
Leukorrhea

A certain amount of vaginal discharge is normal during the reproductive years. It usually appears in small amounts and is nonpurulent, white or clear and without blood. There is no itching or irritation, no abnormal lesions can be found on examination, and no abnormal cells appear on a vaginal cytological smear. The amount of discharge may increase during menarche, pregnancy or ovulation, as well as in women on birth control hormones, but it is still considered normal.

Leukorrhea may be creamy, white or yellow mucoid or a thick, yellow, frothy, foul-smelling discharge or a watery discharge without appreciable mucous or a bloody discharge. According to TCM, leukorrhea can be classified into five types: yellow, red, green, white and black. In clinical practice, however, it becomes more practical to use the following categories.

Colorless, Transparent and Mucous Leukorrhea

This variety is similar to normal vaginal discharge. Dilute, discharged in large amounts and with no particular foul smell, it generally results from a deficiency of the spleen and/or kidneys.

Creamy, White, Curd-like Leukorrhea

Often discharged in large amounts and in white pieces which resemble curds, this leukorrhea is characterized by an itching or burning sensation in the vulva and is usually due to an invasion of the lower energizer by cold-dampness.

Purulent Leukorrhea

Manifested by large amounts of thick, purulent, foul-smelling, yellow or yellow-green vaginal discharge, as well as burning pain or itching in the vulva, this type of leukorrhea is most often due to heat-dampness or dampness toxins invading the lower energizer.

Bloody Leukorrhea

Generally induced by blood heat or heat-dampness, bloody leukorrhea is red, red and white or yellow and white.

Watery, Yellow Leukorrhea

Having as its primary cause the invasion of heat-dampness or dampness toxins, this type of leukorrhea is marked by a distinctive foul smell and a watery, yellow or yellow and white appearance.

Diagnosis and Herbal Treatment

The primary interior causes of leukorrhea are deficiencies of the spleen, kidneys or liver, while the key exterior factor is invasion of the body by dampness evil or dampness toxins.

Spleen Deficiency and Dampness Retention

Persistent, white or slightly yellow, dilute and odorless leukorrhea; a sallow complexion; cold limbs; lassitude; a poor appetite; loose stools; edema of the face or lower limbs; a light-colored tongue with a white, creamy coating; and a weak pulse characterize spleen deficiency exacerbated by dampness retention.

Treatment reinforces spleen *qi* and removes dampness to halt leukorrhea with Lotus Seed Combination (*qing xin lian zi yin*).

To treat lower back pain, add 3 *qian* each of eucommia (*du zhong*) and dipsacus (*xu duan*).

Should the patient have yellow leukorrhea, add 3 *qian* phellodendron (*huang bo*).

To treat watery leukorrhea, add 3 *qian* each of cuscuta (*tu si zi*) and euryale (*qian shi*).

Kidney Deficiency

Profuse, lingering, white, dilute leukorrhea with no foul smell; a pale complexion; severe lower back pain; clear, profuse or frequent urination; loose stools; cold pain in the lower abdomen; an aversion to cold; a light-colored tongue with a thin, white coating; and a submerged, slow pulse are characteristic of leukorrhea due to kidney deficiency.

Treatment warms *yang,* tonifies the kidneys and strengthens the belt vessel (*daimai*). Eucommia and Rehmannia Formula (*you gui wan*), plus 3 *qian* each of tribulus (*ji li*) and astragalus (*huang qi*), can be administered.

To treat *qi* deficiency, add 3 *qian* each of codonopsis (*dang shen*) and white atractylodes (*bai zhu*) and 1 *qian* licorice (*gan cao*).

For patients with diarrhea, add 2 *qian* psoralea (*bu gu zhi*) and 3 *qian* dioscorea (*shan yao*). If the diarrhea is watery, add 3 *qian* euryale (*qian shi*) and 5 *qian* each of dragon bone (*long gu*) and oyster shell (*mu li*).

Descent of Heat-dampness

Large amounts of thick, foul-smelling, yellow-green or purulent leukorrhea which is sometimes mixed with blood or accompanied by itching and a burning sensation in the vulva; fidgeting; irritability; yellow- or red-tinged urine; constipation; a bitter taste in the mouth; a dry throat; conjunctival congestion; headache; a bright red tongue; a red lingual tip and edge; a thin, yellow or greasy, yellow tongue coating; and a wiry, rapid pulse are the constellation of signs and symptoms which signal a descent of heat-dampness.

Treatment clears heat and removes dampness through diuresis with Gentian Combination (*long dan xie gan tang*).

In case of excess heart and liver fire, add 1 *qian* coptis (*huang lian*).

To treat bloody leukorrhea, add 3 *qian* each of moutan (*mu dan pi*) and red peony (*chi shao*).

To correct constipation, give the patient *Tang-kuei* Eight Herb Formula (*ba wei dai xia fang*) in addition to Gentian Combination.

Tang-kuei Eight Herb Formula[1]

Ba Wei Dai Xia Fang

(Decoction with Eight Herbs for Leukorrhea)

Tang-kuei	Angelicae radix	Dang gui	5.0
Cnidium	Cnidii rhizoma	Chuan xiong*	3.0
Hoelen	Poria sclerotium	Fu ling	3.0
Akebia	Akebiae caulis	Mu tong	1.5
Smilax	Smilacis glabrae rhizoma	Tu fu ling	4.0
Citrus peel	Citri pericarpium	Chen pi	2.0
Lonicera	Lonicerae flos	Jin yin hua	3.0
Rhubarb	Rhei rhizoma	Da huang	1.0

Ligustici rhizoma, also known as *chuan xiong*, may be substituted.

Acupuncture and Moxibustion Points

- *daimai* (G 26)
- *qihai* (CV 6)
- *yanglingquan* (G 34)
- *baihuanshu* (B 30)
- *xingjian* (Liv 2)

Section 4
Excessive Movement of the Fetus

Continuous or intermittent bloody discharge from the uterus is known as *tai lou* (vaginal bleeding during pregnancy). Fetal movement is accompanied by a bearing-down and distending sensation, as well as occasional lower abdominal pain-- all of which are warning signs of a possible miscarriage.

A spontaneous abortion occurring prior to 12 weeks is called an early abortion, while one occurring between 12 and 28 weeks is known as a late abortion, and the term "miscarriage" covers any spontaneous abortion prior to 28 weeks. *Hua tae* (habitual abortion) is the term used to describe a pregnancy which terminates in spontaneous abortion when at least three previous pregnancies have ended similarly.

The causes of miscarriage and habitual abortion are manifold, though, by and large, they are induced by the failure of the *chongmai* and *renmai* to assimilate the blood and nourish the fetus. According to TCM theory, the *chongmai* is the known as the "blood sea" and the *renmai* is in charge of the fetus. When the fetus is not properly nourished, bloody uterine discharge, lower back and lower abdominal pain and, ultimately, miscarriage will result.

The inability of the *chongmai* and *renmai* to adequately nourish the fetus is most often due to one or more of the following factors: *qi* and blood deficiency, sexual intemperance during pregnancy, injuries or accidents which impair *qi* and blood flow, acute febrile diseases or a disturbance of the fetus by heat toxins.

Diagnosis and Herbal Treatment

Qi and Blood Deficiency

During pregnancy, *qi* and blood deficiency is manifested by lassitude, a sallow complexion, a poor appetite, continual fetal movement, a bearing-down sensation in the lower abdomen and vulva, small amounts of bloody discharge, mild lower back and lower abdominal pain, a thready, weak pulse and a thick, light-colored tongue with a thin, white coating.

Treatment nourishes *qi* and blood and thereby tranquilizes the fetus. *Tang-kuei* and Cuscuta Combination (*an tai yin*) can be used.

Tang-kuei and Cuscuta Combination[1]
An Tai Yin
(Tranquilize the Fetus Decoction)

Tang-kuei	Angelicae radix	Dang gui	4.5
Cnidium	Cnidii rhizoma	Chuan xiong*	4.5
Peony	Paeoniae radix	Shao yao	6.0
Magnolia bark	Magnoliae officinalis cortex	Hou pu	2.0
Ginger, fresh	Zingiberis rhizoma	Sheng jiang	2.0
Chih-ko	Citri fructus	Zhi ke	1.8
Fritillaria	Fritillariae bulbus	Bei mu	3.0
Astragalus	Astragali radix	Huang qi	2.4
Artemisia	Artemisiae argyi folium	Ai ye	2.0
Schizonepeta	Schizonepetae herba	Jing jie	2.4
Cuscuta	Cuscutae semen	Tu si zi	3.0
Licorice	Glycyrrhizae radix	Gan cao	1.5
Chiang-huo	Notopterygii rhizoma	Qiang huo	1.5

Ligustici rhizoma, also known as *chuan xiong*, may be substituted.

Kidney Deficiency

During pregnancy, kidney deficiency is manifested in lower back pain, a bearing-down and distending sensation in the lower abdomen, bloody discharge, dizziness, tinnitus, a thready, weak pulse and a thin, white tongue coating.

Treatment reinforces the kidneys and calms the fetus. Loranthus and Cuscuta Combination (*shou tai wan*) can be used.

Loranthus and Cuscuta Combination
Shou Tai Wan[23]
(Fetus Longevity Pill)[2]

Loranthus	*Loranthi ramulus*	*Sang ji sheng*	4.0
Cuscuta	*Cuscutae semen*	*Tu si zi*	4.0
Dipsacus	*Dipsaci radix*	*Xu duan*	4.0
Gelatin	*Asini gelatinum*	*A jiao*	3.0

In case of abdominal pain, add 2 *qian* artemisia (*ai ye*), 3 *qian* perilla stalk (*su geng*) and 4 *qian* peony (*bai shao yao*).

If the patient also manifests *qi* deficiency, add 5 *qian* each of astragalus (*huang qi*) and codonopsis (*dang shen*).

To more effectively treat bloody discharge, add 3 *qian* sanguisorba (*di yu*) and 4 *qian* cattail pollen (*pu huang*).

Blood Heat

During pregnancy, blood heat is manifested in bloody vaginal discharge, the continual movement of the fetus with a bearing-down and distending sensation, lower abdominal pain, a dry mouth and throat, constipation, a red tongue with a thin, yellow coating, and a rapid, slippery pulse.

Treatment nourishes *yin*, tonifies blood, clears heat and stabilizes the fetus. *Tang-kuei* Formula (*dang gui san*) is recommended.

Tang-kuei Formula[1]
Dang Gui San
(Tang-kuei Powder)[2]

Teng-kuei	Angelicae radix	Dang gui	1.5
Peony	Paeoniae radix	Shao yao	3.0
Cnidium	Cnidii rhizoma	Chuan xiong*	3.0
Scute	Scutellariae radix	Huang qin	3.0
Atractylodes, white	Atractylodis rhizoma	Bai zhu	1.5

Ligustici rhizoma, also known as *chuan xiong*, may be substituted.

Section 5
Climacteric Syndrome

Menopause is a transitional time in a woman's life when her menstrual periods cease. Usually, it is a natural part of the aging process and has its onset between the ages of 40 and 50. Menopause may be either asymptomatic or with symptoms prompted by an estrogen deficiency or adverse responses of the autonomic nervous system.

The etiology of climacteric syndrome is mostly attributed to kidney deficiency because the kidneys govern reproduction and are the source of congenital essence and vital energy. When a woman is in her forties, her kidney *qi* becomes impaired, as do the functions of the *chongmai* and *renmai*. In addition, kidney *yin* and *yang* become imbalanced and influence the other organs, and so bring on the climacteric stage.

Diagnosis and Herbal Treatment

Kidney *Yin* Deficiency

Lower back pain, a flushed face, a feverish sensation in the palms and soles, painful heels, a slight fever, night sweats, palpitation, restlessness, dizziness, tinnitus, thirst, a thin, red tongue with a thin coating, and a thready, wiry pulse are characteristic of kidney *yin* deficiency during menopause.

Treatment nourishes *yin* and reinforces kidneys, for which Achyranthes and Rehmannia Formula (*zuo gui wan*) can be used.

If kidney *yin* deficiency affects the liver and results in liver *yin* deficiency, manifested in irritability, melancholy or even weeping, add 3 *qian* anemarrhena (*zhi mu*) and 5 *qian* each of haliotis (*shi jue ming*) and oyster shell (*mu li*).

To treat lower back pain, add 3 *qian* each of eucommia (*du zhong*) and dipsacus (*xu duan*).

To treat profuse sweating, add 5 *qian* light wheat (*fu xiao mai*) and 4 *qian* dragon bone (*long gu*).

Kidney *Yang* Deficiency

Lower back pain, an aversion to cold, cold limbs, lassitude, a poor appetite, a pale complexion, clear and frequent urination, a pale tongue with a thin, white coating, and a thready, submerged pulse are characteristic of kidney *yang* deficiency during menopause.

Treatment reinforces the kidneys and warms *yang*. Eucommia and Rehmannia Formula (*you gui wan*) can be used, though, in our experience, Curculigo and Epimedium Combination (*er xian tang*) has proved very useful, however, the dose of the individual herbs must be adjusted. In the case of kidney *yin* deficiency, double the doses of anemarrhena and phellodendron, and in the case of *yang* deficiency, double the doses of curculigo, epimedium and morinda.

Acupuncture and Moxibustion Treatment

Points of First Choice

- *guanyuan* (CV 4)
- *sanyinjiao* (Sp 6)
- *houxi* (SI 3)
- *taixi* (K 3)
- *shenmen* (H 7)
- *taiyang* (EX-HN5)
- *zusanli* (S 36)
- *qihai* (CV 6)

Treatment Method

1. Select three or four points for each treatment session.
2. Retain the needles for 15-20 minutes.
3. Treat once daily for a total of 10 treatments.

References

1. Hsu, H. and Hsu, C.S. *Commonly Used Chinese Herb Formulas With Illustrations*. First edition. Los Angeles: Oriental Healing Arts Institute, 1980.

2. Bensky, D. and Barolet, R. *Chinese Herbal Medicine: Formulas and Strategies*. Seattle: Eastland Press, 1990.

3. Hu, G.C. *New Viewpoint on Symptom-complexes and the Treatment of Miscellaneous Diseases* (in Chinese). Chengdu: Sichuan People's Publishing House, 1958.

4. Yu, G.C. *Popular Treatise on Febrile Diseases* (in Chinese). Taipei: Round Wind Publishing House, 1971.

5. World Health Organization. *Standard Acupuncture Nomenclature, Parts I and II*. Manila: WHO Regional Office for the Western Pacific, 1984, 1988.

6. Wang, M.Y. *Compendium of Epidemic Febrile Diseases* (in Chinese). Beijing: People's Health Publishing Co., 1964.

7. Wu, T. *Discrimination of Feverish Diseases* (in Chinese). Chengdu: Sichuan People's Publishing House, 1957.

8. Wang, G.R. *Corrections of Errors in the Medical Literature* (in Chinese). Taipei: Chi-wen Publishing House, 1975.

9. Wang, Y.K. et al. *Traditional Chinese Medical Dictionary: Formula Volume* (in Chinese). Beijing: People's Health Publishing House, 1983.

10. Zheng, Z.J. *Chin Kuei Yao Lueh* (Prescriptions from the Golden Chamber). Trans. from the Chinese by Hong-yen Hsu et al. Los Angeles: Oriental Healing Arts Institute, 1983.

11. Zhang, J.Y. *Complete Works of Jing-yue* (in Chinese). Shanghai: Shanghai People's Publishing House, 1958.

12. Wang, S.X. *The Professional Essay of Liu Zhou* (in Chinese). Shanghai: Dadong Publishing House, 1937.

13. Yan, Y.H. *Life-preserving Prescriptions* (in Chinese). Revised edition. Beijing: People's Health Publishing House, 1980.

14. Zhu, D.X. *Dan Xi's Experiential Therapy* (in Chinese). Shanghai: Shanghai Science and Technology Publishing House, 1959.

15. Li, N.J. *The Formula Can be Preserved Forever Like a Seal* (in Chinese). Beijing: Beijing University Press, 1985.

16. Han, M. *Han's Book on Medicine* (in Chinese). Shanghai: Shanghai Health Publishing House, 1958.

17. Ye, G. *Therapy Handed Down Secretly* (in Chinese). Shanghai: Shanghai Science and Technology Publishing House, 1963.

18. Chen, Z.M. *The Complete Book of Effective Prescriptions for Women* (in Chinese). Nanchang: Jiangxi People's Publishing House, 1983.

19. Li, G. *Explanations for the Puzzles of Endogenous and Exogenous Injuries* (in Chinese). Shanghai: Shanghai Ancient Books Publishing House, 1959.

20. Chen, S.W. et al. *Formulas of the People's Welfare Pharmacy* (in Chinese). Beijing: People's Health Publishing House, 1959.

21. Li, D.Y. *Secret Collection of the Orchid House* (in Chinese). Shanghai: Shanghai Ancient Books Publishing House, 1929.

22. Cheng, Z.L. *Insightful Medicine* (in Chinese). Beijing: People's Health Publishing House, 1955.

23. Zhang, X.C. *Records of Traditional Chinese Medicine in Combination with Western Medicine* (in Chinese). Hong Kong: Hong Kong Commercial Press, 1975.

24. Ou, M. et al. *Chinese Medical Prescriptions Handbook* (bilingual Chinese and English). Guangzhou: Wang Wen Press, 1988.

25. Wu, Qian. *The Golden Mirror of Medical Science* (in Chinese). Beijing: People's Health Publishing House, 1957.

26. Yeung, H.C. *Handbook of Chinese Herbs and Formulas, Volume II*. Los Angeles : Institute of Chinese Medicine, 1985.

27. Li, Z.Z. *Required Reading for Medical Professionals* (in Chinese). Shanghai: Shanghai Science and Technology Publishing House, 1958.

28. Hsu, H.Y. and Hsu, C.S. *Oriental Materia Medica: A Concise Guide*. Long Beach, Calif.: Oriental Healing Arts Institute, 1986.

Index of Conformations and Diseases

For the reader's convenience, we have alphabetized the conformations and diseases listed in the table of contents. The page numbers provided are those of the first pages of sections having the following names. For example, the section on abdominal pain begins on page 175.

English Index of Herbal Formulas

Page numbers on which formula charts appear are shown in boldface type. Though most formulas have charts, a few do not, either because they are patent medicines or because their ingredients are given in the text.

Index of Literal Translations of
Herbal Formula Names

This index provides literal translations of the names of herbal formulas which appear in this text. The majority of these translations are those of Dan Bensky and Randall Barolet, as found in their *Chinese Herbal Medicine: Formulas and Strategies*. The only page numbers are those pages on which formula charts appear.

Pinyin Index of Herbal Formulas

Page numbers on which formula charts appear are shown in boldface type. Though most formulas have charts, a few do not, either because they are patent medicines or because their ingredients are given in the text.

gan mai da zao tang **71**, 209, 301

ge gen huang lian huang qin tang **105**, 183

ge xia zhu yu tang **203**, 352

gu jing tang **425**

gua lou xie bai ban xia tang **73**, 156, 341

guan xin er hao **73**

gui pi tang **71**, 119, 158, 210, 214, 220, 225, 256, 302, 370, 375, 419, 420, 424

gui zhi fu ling wan 44, **45**

gui zhi long gu mu li tang **211**

gui zhi ren shen tang **341**

gui zhi shao yao zhi mu tang 319, **320**

gui zhi tang 51, **52**, 213, 319

hu qian wan **315**

huai hua san **260**

huang lian a jiao tang 119, **120**, 220

huang lian jie du tang **26**, 53, 84, 413

huang qi jian zhong tang 161, **162**, 177, 351, 355, 372, 411

huang tu tang 258, **259**

huo xiang zheng qi san **16**, 19, 171, 183, 195

ji jiao li huang wan **152**

jia jian shen fu you gui yin **157**

jia wei gui pi tang **302**

jia wei xiao yao san 135, **136**, 279

jiao tai wan **119**

jie geng tang **338**

jie yu dan **241**

jin ling zi san **354**

jin suo gu jing wan 110, **111**, 294, 382

jing fang bai du san **4**, 51, 52, 126, 227

juan bi tang 322, **323**

Cross–Reference Index of Formula Names

The following index allows the reader to access the English names and literal translations of formula names appearing in *pinyin*. Only pages on which formula charts appear are given.

zan mai da zao tang 71
Licorice and Jujube Combination
(Licorice, Wheat and Jujube Decoction)

ze gen huang lian huang qin tang 105
Pueraria, Coptis and Scute Combination
(Pueraria, Coptis and Scutellaria Decoction)

ze xia zhu yu tang 203
Persica and Carthamus Combination
(Drive Out Blood Stasis Below the Diaphragm Decoction)

zu jing tang 425
Tortoise Shell and Scute Combination
(Menorrhagia Decoction)

zua lou xie bai ban xia tang 73
Trichosanthes, Bakeri and Pinellia Combination
(Trichosanthes Fruit, Chinese Chive and Pinellia Decoction)

zuan xin er hao 73
Salvia and Carthamus Combination
(Coronary Heart Disease Formula No. II)

zui pi tang 71
Ginseng and Longan Combination
(Restore the Spleen Decoction)

zui zhi fu ling wan 45
Cinnamon and Hoelen Formula
(Cinnamon Twig and Poria Pill)

zui zhi long gu mu li tang 211
Cinnamon and Dragon Bone Combination
(Cinnamon Twig, Dragon Bone and Oyster Shell Decoction)

zui zhi ren shen tang 341
Cinnamon and Ginseng Combination
(Cinnamon Twig and Ginseng Decoction)

zui zhi shao yao zhi mu tang 320
Cinnamon and Anemarrhena Combination
(Cinnamon Twig, Peony and Anemarrhena Decoction)

qin jiao bie jia san 30
Chin-chiu and Turtle Shell Formula
(Gentian *Qinjiao* and Soft-shelled Turtle Shell Powder)

qing fei tang 39
Platycodon and Fritillaria Combination
(Clear Lung Heat Decoction)

qing shu yi qi tang 15
Lotus Stem and Ginseng Combination
(Clear Summer Heat and Augment the *Qi* Decoction)

qing wei san 31
Coptis and Rehmannia Formula
(Clear the Stomach Powder)

qing xin lian zi yin 32
Lotus Seed Combination
(Lotus Seed Decoction to Clear Heart Fire)

qing ying tang 132
Rhinoceros and Scrophularia Combination
(Clear Heat in *Ying Fen* Decoction)

qing zao jiu fei tang 23
Eriobotrya and Ophiopogon Combination
(Eliminate Dryness and Rescue the Lungs Decoction)

ren shen hu tao tang 111
Ginseng and Walnut Combination
(Ginseng and Walnut Decoction)

ren shen tang 12
Ginseng and Ginger Combination
(Regulate the Middle Pill)

ren shen yang rong tang 248
Ginseng Nutritive Combination
(Ginseng Decoction to Nourish the Nutritive *Qi*)

run chang tang 105
Linum and Rhubarb Combination
(Moisten the Intestines Pill)